Updates in the Management of Acute and Chronic Lesions of the Achilles Tendon

Editor

PHINIT PHISITKUL

FOOT AND ANKLE CLINICS

www.foot.theclinics.com

Consulting Editor

MARK S. MYERSON

September 2019 • Volume 24 • Number 3

ELSEVIER

1600 John F. Kennedy Boulevard • Suite 1800 • Philadelphia, Pennsylvania, 19103-2899

http://www.theclinics.com

FOOT AND ANKLE CLINICS Volume 24, Number 3
September 2019 ISSN 1083-7515, ISBN-978-0-323-68209-1

Editor: Lauren Boyle
Developmental Editor: Donald Mumford

Foot and Ankle Clinics (ISSN 1083-7515) is published quarterly by Elsevier, Inc., 360 Park Avenue South, New York, NY 10010-1710. Months of issue are March, June, September, and December. Periodicals postage paid at New York, NY, and additional mailing offices. Subscription price per year is $337.00 (US individuals), $552.00 (US institutions), $100.00 (US students), $371.00 (Canadian individuals), $663.00 (Canadian institutions), $215.00 (Canadian students), $465.00 (international individuals), $663.00 (international institutions), and $215.00 (international students). To receive student/resident rate, orders must be accompanied by name of affiliated institution, date of term, and the *signature* of program/residency coordinator on institution letterhead. Orders will be billed at individual rate until proof of status is received. Foreign air speed delivery is included in all *Clinics* subscription prices. All prices are subject to change without notice. **POSTMASTER:** Send address changes to *Foot and Ankle Clinics*, Elsevier Health Sciences Division, Subscription Customer Service, 3251 Riverport Lane, Maryland Heights, MO 63043. **Customer Service: 1-800-654-2452 (US and Canada). From outside of the United States and Canada, call 314-447-8871. Fax: 314-447-8029. E-mail: JournalsCustomerService-usa@elsevier.com (for print support); JournalsOnlineSupport-usa@elsevier.com (for online support).**

Reprints. For copies of 100 or more, of articles in this publication, please contact the Commercial Reprints Department, Elsevier Inc., 360 Park Avenue South, New York, NY 10010-1710. Tel.: 212-633-3874; Fax: 212-633-3820; E-mail: reprints@elsevier.com.

Contributors

CONSULTING EDITOR

MARK S. MYERSON, MD
Executive Director, Steps2Walk, Miami, Florida, USA

EDITOR

PHINIT PHISITKUL, MD
Chair, AOFAS Evidence-based Medicine Committee, Orthopaedic Surgeon, Tri-State Specialists, LLP, Sioux City, Iowa, USA

AUTHORS

SAMUEL B. ADAMS Jr, MD
Assistant Professor and Director of Foot and Ankle Surgery, Duke University Medical Center, Durham, North Carolina, USA

CRAIG C. AKOH, MD
Sports Medicine Fellow, Department of Orthopedics and Rehabilitation, University of Wisconsin-Madison School of Medicine and Public Health, Madison, Wisconsin, USA

ALEXEJ BARG, MD
Assistant Professor, Department of Orthopaedics, University of Utah, Salt Lake City, Utah, USA

JON-MICHAEL E. CALDWELL, MD
Resident, Department of Orthopedic Surgery, Columbia University Irving Medical Center/ NewYork-Presbyterian Hospital, New York, New York, USA

CHRISTOPHER CHEN, MD
Department of Orthopedic Surgery, University of Colorado School of Medicine, Aurora, Colorado, USA

RUTH L. CHIMENTI, DPT, PhD
Assistant Professor, Department of Physical Therapy and Rehabilitation Science, University of Iowa, Iowa City, Iowa, USA

RICCARDO D'AMBROSI, MD
IRCCS Istituto Ortopedico Galeazzi, Milan, Italy

KATHERINE M. DEDERER, MD
Resident Physician, Department of Orthopaedic Surgery, The University of North Carolina at Chapel Hill, Chapel Hill, North Carolina, USA

CONNOR P. DILGER, BS
Department of Physical Therapy and Rehabilitation Science, University of Iowa, Iowa City, Iowa, USA

MARK GLAZEBROOK, MD, MSc, PhD, FRCS(C)
Orthopedic Surgeon, Professor, Dalhousie University, Queen Elizabeth II Health Sciences Center, Halifax, Nova Scotia, Canada

KENNETH J. HUNT, MD
Director, Foot and Ankle Service, Department of Orthopedic Surgery, University of Colorado School of Medicine, Aurora, Colorado, USA

CRISTIAN INDINO, MD
IRCCS Istituto Ortopedico Galeazzi, Milan, Italy

ANISH R. KADAKIA, MD
Associate Professor, Department of Orthopaedic Surgery, Fellowship Director, Foot and Ankle Orthopedic Surgery, Northwestern Memorial Hospital, Northwestern University Feinberg School of Medicine, Chicago, Illinois, USA

JORDAN LILES, MD
Department of Orthopaedic Surgery, Duke University Medical Center, Durham, North Carolina, USA

CHO YAU LO, MBChB (CUHK), FRCSEd, FHKAM, FHKCOS
Resident Specialist, Department of Orthopaedics and Traumatology, North District Hospital, Hong Kong SAR, China

TODD LUDWIG, MD
Orthopaedic Resident, Department of Orthopaedics, University of Utah, Salt Lake City, Utah, USA

TUN HING LUI, MBBS (HK), FRCS (Edin), FHKAM, FHKCOS
Consultant, Department of Orthopaedics and Traumatology, North District Hospital, Hong Kong SAR, China

MILAP S. PATEL, DO
Clinical Instructor, Northwestern Memorial Hospital, Northwestern University Feinberg School of Medicine, Chicago, Illinois, USA

ANTHONY PERERA, MBChB, MRCS, MFSEM, PG Dip (Med Law), FRCS (Orth)
Consultant Orthopaedic Foot and Ankle Surgeon, University Hospital Llandough and University Hospital Wales, Cardiff, United Kingdom

PHINIT PHISITKUL, MD
Chair, AOFAS Evidence-based Medicine Committee, Orthopaedic Surgeon, Tri-State Specialists, LLP, Sioux City, Iowa, USA

DANIELA RUBINGER, BScPT
Physiotherapist, Citadel Physiotherapy, Halifax, Nova Scotia, Canada

YUK CHUEN SIU, MBChB (CUHK), FRCSEd, FHKAM, FHKCOS
Resident Specialist, Department of Orthopaedics and Traumatology, North District Hospital, Hong Kong SAR, China

TURAB ARSHAD SYED, MBChB, MRCS, MFSEM, DipSEM, DipSICOT, FRCS (Orth), MSc, MFST (Ed)
Consultant Trauma and Orthopaedic Surgeon, Royal Free London Hospital NHS Trust, London, United Kingdom

JOSHUA N. TENNANT, MD, MPH
Assistant Professor, Department of Orthopaedic Surgery, The University of North Carolina at Chapel Hill, Chapel Hill, North Carolina, USA

FEDERICO G. USUELLI, MD
Director, Foot and Ankle Department, Humanitas San Pio X, Milano, Italy

J. TURNER VOSSELLER, MD
Assistant Professor, Department of Orthopedic Surgery, Columbia University Irving Medical Center/NewYork-Presbyterian Hospital, New York, New York, USA

Editorial Advisory Board

Contents

Preface: Updates in the Management of Acute and Chronic Lesions of the Achilles Tendon **xv**

Phinit Phisitkul

Anatomical and Functional Considerations in Achilles Tendon Lesions **371**

Katherine M. Dederer and Joshua N. Tennant

The pathologic conditions of the Achilles tendon are best understood in the context of its unique anatomy and functional demands. Some of these unique considerations include its high physiologic load demands, microscopic tissue composition, muscular origin spanning the knee joint, intimate insertional relationship with the plantar fascia, sensory innervation, and vascular supply with watershed areas. Risks of both acute rupture and chronic tendinopathy are affected by the tendon's anatomy and its functional demands. The tendon's functional anatomy changes with advancing age, notably in its collagen composition and vascular supply.

Functional Rehabilitation for Nonsurgical Treatment of Acute Achilles Tendon Rupture **387**

Mark Glazebrook and Daniela Rubinger

The use of early functional rehabilitation in the treatment of nonoperative Achilles tendon ruptures has been shown to provide patients with outcomes similar to operative treatments. This article describes a high-quality accelerated functional rehabilitation program that begins with early diagnosis and appropriate patient selection to allow initiation of the nonoperative protocol. Complications with nonoperative treatment of Achilles ruptures are significantly lower than with operative treatment; however, re-rupture and elongation of the tendon resulting in decreased strength are problematic and more common if patients are non-compliant. These can be minimized with good patient education, close supervision, and good communication between physical therapist and physician.

Minimally Invasive Treatments of Acute Achilles Tendon Ruptures **399**

Milap S. Patel and Anish R. Kadakia

Achilles tendon rupture is a common injury to the lower extremity that requires appropriate treatment to minimize functional deficit. Available treatments of Achilles tendon ruptures include nonoperative, open surgical repair, percutaneous repair, and minimally invasive repair. Open surgical repair obtains favorable functional outcomes with significant potential for deep soft tissue complications, calling into question the value of open repair. Percutaneous repair is an alternative option with comparable functional results and minimal soft tissue complications; however, sural nerve injury is a complication. Minimally invasive Achilles repair offers optimal results with superior functional outcomes with minimal soft tissue complications and sural nerve injury.

Open Reconstructive Strategies for Chronic Achilles Tendon Ruptures 425

Christopher Chen and Kenneth J. Hunt

Chronic Achilles tendon ruptures typically are treated with surgical intervention except in low-demand patients or patients who are unable to tolerate surgery. Although several treatment strategies are described, most literature is case reports and case series. There is no widely accepted algorithm or gold standard for surgical treatment of chronic Achilles tendon ruptures. Treatment strategy depends on the size of the tendon gap after excision of nonviable tissue and scar tissue. Smaller gaps can be treated with direct end-to-end repair. Medium-sized gaps can be treated with tendon-lengthening procedures. Tendon transfers, autograft, allograft, xenograft, and synthetic grafting are described for the reconstruction of large defects.

Maximizing Return to Sports After Achilles Tendon Rupture in Athletes 439

Jon-Michael E. Caldwell and J. Turner Vosseller

Achilles tendon ruptures are devastating injuries to athletes, with return-to-sports rates around 70% and some risk for diminished performance post-injury. Surgical management in athletes is often favored for a number of reasons, although evidence guiding the optimal treatment is limited. Functional rehabilitation has been supported as a key component of operative and nonoperative treatment plans. Return-to-play protocols in the literature are sparse and varied due to often ambiguous definitions of what it means to return to sport and a lack of explicit criteria. Optimal sport-specific return-to-play milestones should be defined to guide the rehabilitation of injured athletes.

Management of Complications of Achilles Tendon Surgery 447

Jordan Liles and Samuel B. Adams Jr

There are multiple techniques to treat tendon defects in the event end-to-end repair cannot be achieved after débridement. In general, the choice of treatment technique is based on size of the resultant gap. Although each treatment technique has literature to support its use, there are no data to support the use of one technique over another. Treatment should be based on the experience and discretion of the treating surgeon. This article proposes an algorithm for wound breakdown, infection, and rerupture after Achilles tendon surgery. This algorithm should be used as a guide.

Endoscopic Management of Chronic Achilles Tendon Rupture 459

Turab Arshad Syed and Anthony Perera

Chronic ruptures of the Achilles tendon are often missed injuries, which is challenging for the surgeon. The complications from reconstruction are a considerable concern. Primary repair may be attempted, but the missed injury often presents later than 4 weeks with gaps greater than 4 cm, necessitating more complex reconstructions using local tissues such as turn-down flaps and VY plasty, requiring large incisions in an unfavorable area of the body. We describe a step-by-step technique of endoscopic flexor hallucis longus reconstruction for chronic Achilles rupture, which decreases local complications. This article reviews the available literature for endoscopic flexor hallucis longus reconstruction.

Biologics in the Treatment of Achilles Tendon Pathologies **471**

Cristian Indino, Riccardo D'Ambrosi, and Federico G. Usuelli

Regenerative medicine is gaining more and more space for the treatment of Achilles pathologic conditions. Biologics could play a role in the management of midportion Achilles tendinopathy as a step between conservative and surgical treatment or as an augmentation. Higher-level studies are needed before determining a level of treatment recommendation for biologic strategies for insertional Achilles tendinopathy. Combining imaging with patient's functional requests could be the way to reach a protocol for the use of biologics for the treatment of midportion Achilles tendinopathy and, for this perspective, the authors describe the Foot and Ankle Reconstruction Group algorithm of treatment.

Minimally Invasive and Endoscopic Approach for the Treatment of Noninsertional Achilles Tendinopathy **495**

Craig C. Akoh and Phinit Phisitkul

Minimally invasive treatment can offer an earlier recovery with less pain and scarring compared with traditional open surgeries. The goals of minimally invasive surgery are to debride degenerative tendon, stimulate healing, and, when appropriate, repair damaged tendon. Sclerotherapy and prolotherapy have been shown to reduce neovascularization and pain. Percutaneous stripping and endoscopic debridement are better options for diffuse tendinopathy. Plantaris release can be useful in diffuse disease in patients with primarily medial-sided Achilles pain. Overall, minimally invasive surgery provides similar benefits as open procedures with reduced complications and morbidity.

Nonsurgical Treatment Options for Insertional Achilles Tendinopathy **505**

Connor P. Dilger and Ruth L. Chimenti

Most nonoperative treatments for insertional Achilles tendinopathy (IAT) have insufficient evidence to support treatment recommendations. Exercise has the highest level of evidence supporting the ability of this treatment option to reduce IAT pain. The effects of exercise may be enhanced by a wide variety of other treatments, including soft tissue treatment, nutritional supplements, iontophoresis, education, stretching, and heel lifts. When exercise is unsuccessful, extracorporeal shock wave therapy seems to be the next best nonoperative treatment option to reduce IAT pain. After other nonoperative treatment options have been exhausted, injections may be considered, particularly to facilitate participation in an exercise program.

Minimally Invasive and Endoscopic Treatment of Haglund Syndrome **515**

Tun Hing Lui, Cho Yau Lo, and Yuk Chuen Siu

Haglund syndrome is a triad of posterosuperior calcaneal prominence (Haglund deformity), retrocalcaneal bursitis, and insertional Achilles tendinopathy. The sources of pain include the posterior calcaneal wall cartilage, retrocalcaneal and subcutaneous adventitial bursa, and the Achilles tendon. Resection of the posterosuperior calcaneal tubercle, bursectomy, excision of the Achilles tendon pathology, reattachment of the Achilles tendon, gastrocnemius aponeurotic recession, and flexor hallucis longus transfer have been proposed as surgical treatment options. All of them can be performed endoscopically or under minimally invasive approaches.

Surgical Strategies for the Treatment of Insertional Achilles Tendinopathy **533**

Alexej Barg and Todd Ludwig

Insertional Achilles tendinopathy is one of the most common Achilles tendon disorders and often results in substantial heel pain and functional disability. There is consensus that treatment of insertional Achilles tendinopathy should start with nonoperative modalities. Surgery should be reserved for patients who fail exhaustive conservative treatment for a period of 3 months to 6 months and include débridement of insertional calcifications. Intratendinous degenerative tissue should be débrided and any Haglund deformity resected. Different surgical techniques have been described for reattachment of the distal Achilles tendon. The authors' preferred surgical technique includes the knotless double-row footprint reconstruction. Postoperative complications are not rare.

FOOT AND ANKLE CLINICS

FORTHCOMING ISSUES

December 2019
Current Concepts of Treatment of Metatarsalgia
Gastón A. Slullitel, *Editor*

March 2020
Current Controversies in the Approach to Complex Hallux Valgus Deformity Correction
Sudheer Reddy, *Editor*

June 2020
Correction of Severe Foot and Ankle Deformities
Andy Molloy, *Editor*

RECENT ISSUES

June 2019
The Cavus Foot
Alexej Barg, *Editor*

March 2019
Avascular Necrosis of the Foot and Ankle
Kenneth J. Hunt, *Editor*

December 2018
Managing Instabilities of the Foot and Ankle
Andrea Veljkovic, *Editor*

RELATED SERIES

Clinics in Sports Medicine
Orthopedic Clinics
Physical Medicine and Rehabilitation Clinics

Preface

Updates in the Management of Acute and Chronic Lesions of the Achilles Tendon

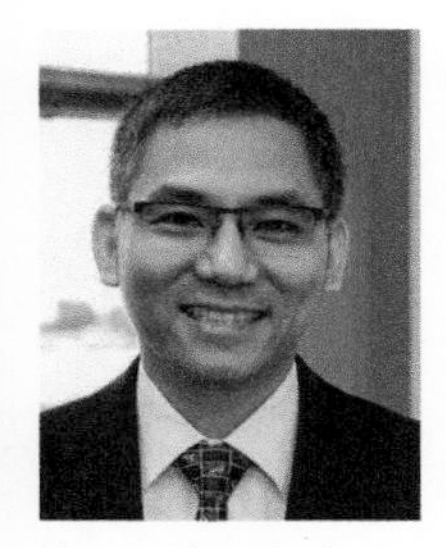

Phinit Phisitkul, MD
Editor

We are in a phase of evolution in that humans are demanding more service from the Achilles tendon than ever. With increases of diabetes and obesity, the widespread use of antibiotics, and poor lifestyles, children and adults are challenged by the popularity of sports and occasional high-impact activities. Insults to the Achilles tendon can manifest in various ways, ranging from an acute tendinitis to a complete rupture, to chronic conditions at various locations along the tendon or paratendinous tissue or bone.

Understanding of the pathophysiology of the Achilles tendon is evolving. We have surpassed the belief that inflammatory disease accounts for most Achilles tendon problems, as it was originally called "tendinitis." Various conditions are associated with Achilles tendon problems, including poor training techniques, underlying medical problems, inadequate healing response, antibiotic use, limb malalignment, contractures, and genetic predispositions. Emerging technologies are allowing the tendon to be treated by multitudes of options that could be geared to meet specific patient demands. High success rates were demonstrated from nonsurgical, biologic, minimally invasive, and open treatment for Achilles tendon conditions, provided the practice of proper patient selection and careful treatment implementation is followed.

Achilles, the strongest tendon in the human body, is named after a Greek hero, Achilleus, the central character and greatest warrior of Homer's *Iliad*, who fought in the Trojan War. This tendon bears great strength, but yet is still vulnerable, reminiscent of the death of Achilleus from a poison dart to the heel. This issue of *Foot and Ankle Clinics of North America* contains cutting-edge knowledge from thought leaders in the field of orthopedic foot and ankle surgery. We hope that you find the up-to-date

Foot Ankle Clin N Am 24 (2019) xv–xvi
https://doi.org/10.1016/j.fcl.2019.05.003
1083-7515/19/© 2019 Published by Elsevier Inc.

knowledge from this issue helpful in the treatment of patients suffering from Achilles tendon problems.

Phinit Phisitkul, MD
Tri-State Specialists, LLP
2730 Pierce Street, Suite 300
Sioux City, IA 51104, USA

E-mail address:
pphisitkul@gmail.com

Anatomical and Functional Considerations in Achilles Tendon Lesions

Katherine M. Dederer, MD, Joshua N. Tennant, MD, MPH*

KEYWORDS

• Achilles tendon • Anatomy • Rupture • Tendinitis • Blood supply

KEY POINTS

- Physiologic load is 10x body weight during highest levels of physical activity.
- Gastrocnemius and soleus origin, calcaneus and plantar fascia insertion.
- Collagen composition and crimp angle affect resiliency and flexibility of tendon.
- 90-degree twist from medial to posterior to lateral.
- Vascular watershed 2 to 5 cm proximal to calcaneal insertion predisposes to rupture.

INTRODUCTION

The Achilles tendon, named after the mythical hero of Homer's *The Iliad*, is the strongest tendon in the human body. At the same time, it is a frequent source of pain and dysfunction from tendinopathy or outright rupture due to the functional demands placed on it. The unique position of the Achilles musculotendinous unit spanning the knee, ankle, and subtalar joints necessitates flexibility and elasticity. Proper function is also closely tied to function of the gastrocnemius and soleus muscles, as well as the plantar fascia. The tendon's collagen composition changes with age as well as during its healing response to injury, changing its mechanical properties. Its dual blood supply, which produces a watershed region at the tendon's narrowest portion, also predisposes it to injury. Special considerations must be taken when undertaking surgical repair, particularly percutaneous repair, due to the close proximity of the sural nerve to the midsubstance of the tendon. Its anatomy and structure pose unique challenges to management, and a thorough understanding of these characteristics is crucial to successful treatment.

Neither of the authors have any relevant disclosures.
Department of Orthopaedic Surgery, University of North Carolina, 130 Mason Farm Rd, Chapel Hill, NC 27599, USA
* Corresponding author. UNC Orthopaedics, 3144 Bioinformatics Building, CB# 7055, Chapel Hill, NC 27599.
E-mail address: Josh_tennant@med.unc.edu

Foot Ankle Clin N Am 24 (2019) 371–385
https://doi.org/10.1016/j.fcl.2019.04.001
foot.theclinics.com
1083-7515/19/

ANATOMIC REGIONS OF THE ACHILLES TENDON

The Achilles tendon sees the highest loads in the body, experiencing up to 10 times body weight during running, skipping, and jumping.[1] Given such high demands for its function, Achilles tendon pathology is common in an environment of any level of physical activity, from ambulatory laborers to professional athletes. Achilles tendinopathy may exist in multiple areas and variable severity within the structure of the tendon. At the acute end of the spectrum, Achilles tendon rupture occurs 80% of the time between 2 and 6 cm proximal to the calcaneal insertion.[2,3] Chronic tendinopathies can be described by several frameworks, although there remains some ambiguity regarding descriptive terminology describing location within the tendon. Simply, the tendon can be divided into insertional (distal) and noninsertional (proximal) components. Additional classification systems have been proposed to stratify areas of the tendon into 3 regions: the insertional calcaneal region, the preinsertional region located 2 cm proximal to the calcaneal insertion, and the noninsertional, midportion of the tendon.[4]

TENDON STRUCTURE

Fibril Characteristics

The size of Achilles tendon fibrils has been shown to correlate with risk for tendon rupture (**Fig. 1**). Tendons containing shorter fibrils show an increased risk of rupture,[5] and decreased fibril width may also predispose a tendon to rupture.[6] Mechanical studies have been performed in animals, which correlate decreased fibril diameter with decreased strength, although these studies have not been replicated in humans.[7]

Collagen Composition

The normal Achilles tendon is composed of 95% type I collagen, accounting for about 70% of the dry weight of the tendon.[8] The parallel configuration of and covalent bonds between the collagen molecules within the fibrils gives the tendon its high tensile strength.[9] Ruptured and tendinopathic tendons show a decrease in type I collagen and an increased presence of type III collagen,[10] including when tenocytes are grown

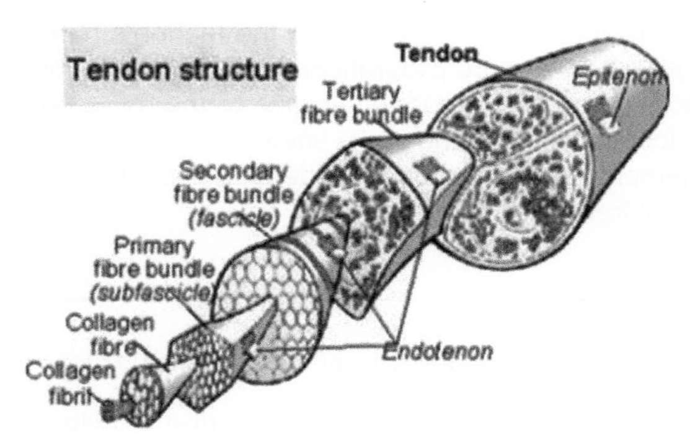

Fig. 1. Structure of the tendon. Fibrils are grouped together into fascicles, which are grouped together by epitenon and form the mass of the tendon. (*Adapted from* Doral, M. N., Alam, M., Bozkurt, M., Turhan, E., Atay, O. A., Donmez, G., & Maffulli, N. (2010). Functional anatomy of the Achilles tendon. Knee Surg Sports Traumatol Arthrosc 18(5):638–643; with permission.)

in vitro in monolayer cell culture.[11] Type III collagen yields lower tensile strength and therefore may predispose the healing tendon to rupture. Type II collagen is also produced by healing tendons.[12]

During the normal process of aging, the percentage of type I collagen in the tendon decreases. The fiber density and diameter also decrease, thus decreasing the elasticity of the tendon and increasing its predisposition to rupture.[12] Other studies have investigated the crimp angle, which is the angular measure of the sinusoidal pattern ("crimp") of the collagen network in the tendon. Crimps in tendon fibers act as a buffer within the tendon to avoid rupture from sudden stretch, allowing 1% to 3% stretching of the tendon tissue. A decrease in crimp angle in ruptured tendons compared with healthy controls has been demonstrated (**Figs. 2** and **3**).[6] Crimp angle also seems to decrease with age, leading to a loss of tendon elasticity.[13] This lends mechanistic support to the pathogenesis of Achilles tendon rupture and its increased frequency with age.

ACHILLES TENDON SIZE AND LENGTH

Based on cadaveric and radiologic studies, the average length of the Achilles tendon is 15 cm.[14] It is longer laterally than medially, due to the more distal extension of the medial gastrocnemius muscle compared with the lateral gastrocnemius.[15] The tendon's elasticity allows it to stretch about 4% of its length, with ruptures typically occurring after an 8% increase in length.[6,12]

The width of the Achilles tendon varies considerably throughout its length. It is widest proximally, measuring an average of 6.8 cm wide. The tendon reaches its narrowest diameter about 80% of the distance down the length of the tendon before widening again at its calcaneal insertion to 3.4 cm. At its narrowest point, the tendon averages only 1.8 cm in width.[2,14]

Tendon thickness averages 4.9 mm in healthy control subjects, although it has been shown that Achilles tendinopathy increases the tendon diameter, and ruptured tendons were substantially wider than controls (**Fig. 4**). Compared with this control population, one group found an average thickness of 11.7 mm in ruptured tendons and measured the contralateral, healthy tendons of the same patients to be 5.4 mm.[16] Population studies have found an increased rate of contralateral Achilles tendon

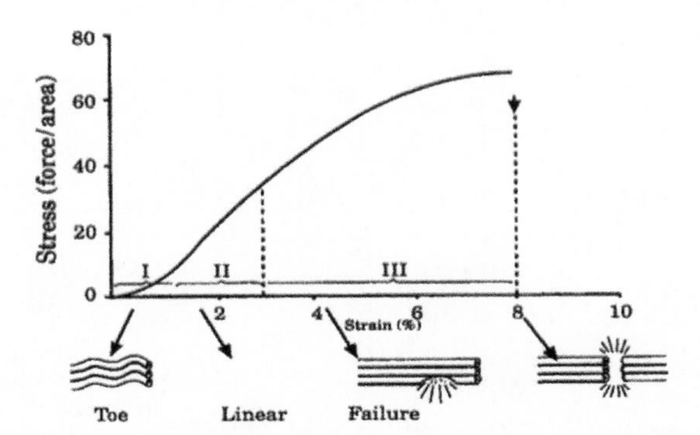

Fig. 2. Graph showing the role crimping plays in tendon elasticity. As lengthening increases, crimps are stretched and eventually macroscopic rupture occurs at greater than 8% increase in length. (*Adapted from* Doral, M. N., Alam, M., Bozkurt, M., Turhan, E., Atay, O. A., Donmez, G., & Maffulli, N. (2010). Functional anatomy of the Achilles tendon. Knee Surg Sports Traumatol Arthrosc 18(5):638–643; with permission.)

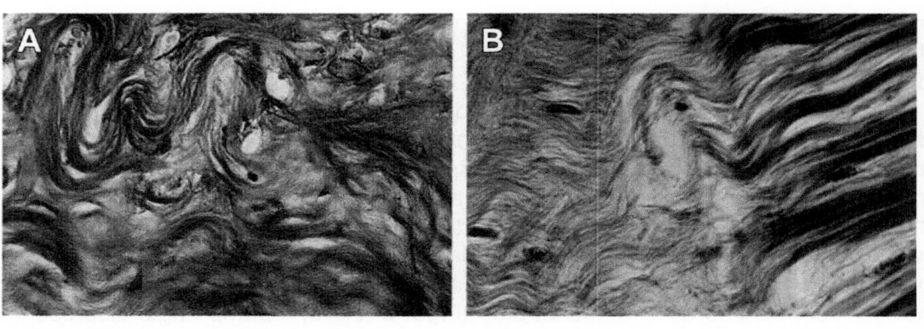

Fig. 3. Light micrograph revealing abnormal collagen patterning in a ruptured Achilles tendon (*A*) and an irregular crimping pattern in ruptured fibers (*B*). (*Adapted from* Järvinen, T. A. H. (2004). Collagen fibers of the spontaneously ruptured human tendons display decreased thickness and crimp angle. Journal of Orthopaedic Research 22(6):1303–1309; with permission.)

rupture in patients who have previously sustained a rupture compared with the uninjured population.[17] These findings together may support a correlation between tendon thickness and risk for Achilles rupture.

RELATIVE CONTRIBUTIONS OF THE GASTROCNEMIUS AND SOLEUS TO THE TENDON BODY

The Achilles tendon is the conjoint tendon of the medial and lateral gastrocnemius muscles as well as the soleus. A raphe forms where the two heads of the gastrocnemius join, which continues distally to join the soleus. The soleus arises from the posterior tibia and lies deep to the gastrocnemius (**Fig. 5**). It fuses with the gastrocnemius muscles to form the Achilles at the aforementioned average of 15 cm proximal to the calcaneus.[14] Variable contributions from the gastrocnemius and soleus exist in the Achilles tendon. A cadaveric study showed 52% of subjects had 52% contribution by the soleus, 48%

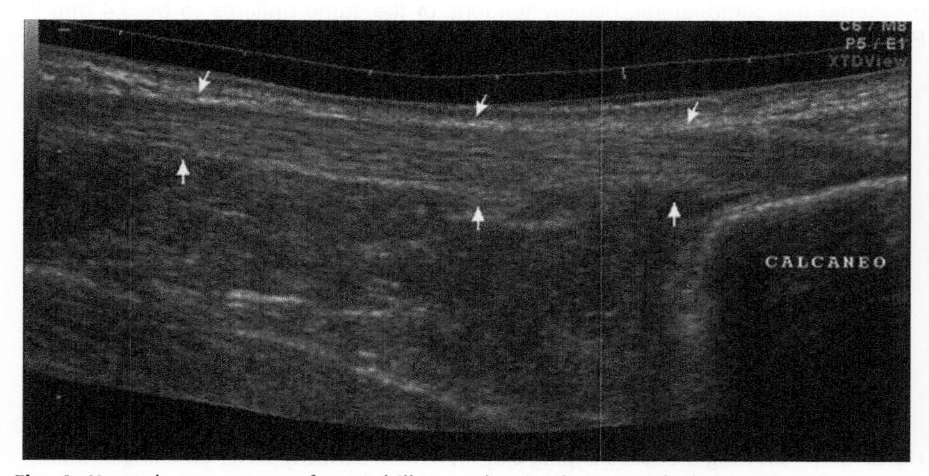

Fig. 4. Normal appearance of an Achilles tendon in the sagittal plane using ultrasound. (*Adapted from* Pierre-Jerome, C., Moncayo, V., & Terk, M. R. (2010). MRI of the Achilles tendon: a comprehensive review of the anatomy, biomechanics, and imaging of overuse tendinopathies. Acta Radiol 51(4):438–454; with permission.)

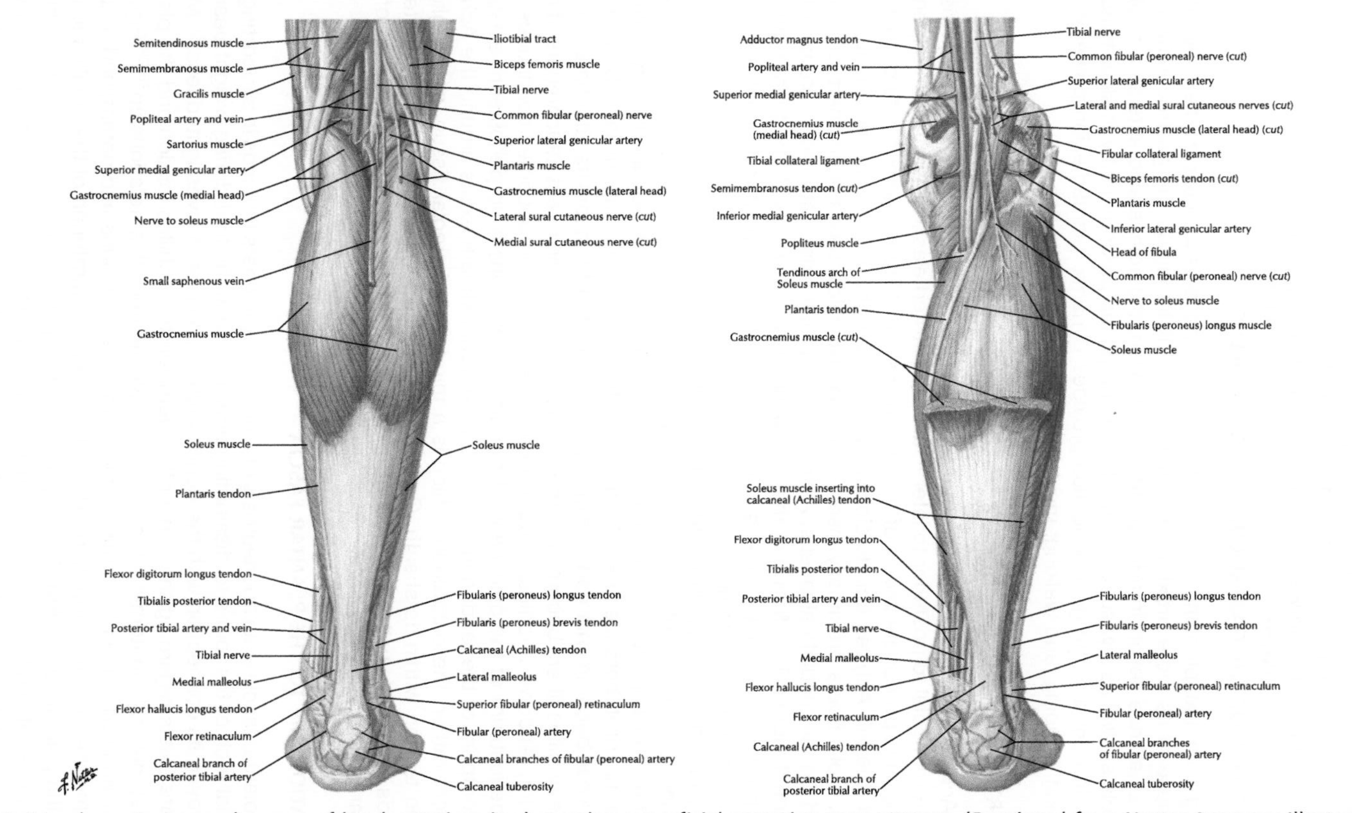

Fig. 5. Muscles, arteries, and nerves of leg (posterior view) muscles: superficial posterior compartment. (*Reprinted from* Netter Anatomy Illustration Collection © Elsevier Inc. All Rights Reserved.)

from the gastrocnemius. An equal contribution from the soleus and gastrocnemius was found in 35% of subjects. In 13% of subjects, the gastrocnemius contributed two-thirds of the tendon.[18] Variable lengths of tendon contributions exist, between 3 and 11 cm from the soleus and between 11 and 16 cm from the gastrocnemius.[19]

FUNCTIONS OF THE GASTROCNEMIUS AND SOLEUS

Along with the plantaris, the gastrocnemius and soleus muscles flex the ankle. Because of its more proximal insertion on the distal femur, the gastrocnemius also acts as a knee flexor. In addition to ankle flexion, the soleus also acts as a postural muscle as well as a vascular pump, being composed predominantly of slow-twitch fibers. In contrast, the gastrocnemius provides dynamic plantarflexion power during running, jumping, and walking; most of its fibers are fast-twitch.[13]

INSERTIONAL ANATOMY

The Achilles tendon spirals as it courses distally toward its calcaneal insertion, twisting 90° from medial to posterior to lateral, allowing stored elastic energy to be expended during the appropriate phase of gait or movement.[20] From a proximal to distal viewpoint, the left Achilles spirals clockwise and the right Achilles spirals counterclockwise. Tibial fibers proximally insert on the lateral calcaneus; fibular fibers proximally insert on the medial calcaneus. A double spiral may exist, with more rotation of the tendon if there is less fusion of the gastrocnemius and soleus.[21] The tendon twisting also produces an area of stress in the tendon, which is most significant between 2 and 5 cm from the insertion.[22,23]

The insertion of the Achilles tendon widens, varying from 1.2 to 2.5 cm wide at the calcaneus.[24] An area of fibrocartilage exists between the calcaneus and the attaching tendon. The superior and lateral aspect of the posterior calcaneus may have an abnormal protuberance, a Haglund deformity, over which a superficial subcutaneous bursa can become enlarged with irritation.[25] As the tendon nears its attachment, some of the Achilles fibers become Sharpey fibers, which are the direct attachments of periosteum, tendons, and ligaments to bone. The endotenon becomes continuous with the periosteum of the calcaneus at the attachment, where no periosteum exists on the footprint of the tendon insertion.[26] No synovial sheath exists around the Achilles tendon; rather, the paratenon, which is a thin layer of areolar tissue, allows gliding of the tendon within its sheath. Composed of mucopolysaccharides, the paratenon blends proximally with the fascia of muscle and distally with the periosteum of the calcaneus.

RELATIONSHIP TO THE PLANTAR FASCIA

The plantar fascia is an aponeurosis of type I collagen fibers that aids in supporting the medial arch of the foot and dissipating energy across the foot during weight bearing. However, its connection with the Achilles tendon has been investigated less.[27] Much debate exists regarding the connection between the Achilles tendon and the plantar fascia; several anatomic studies have investigated this relationship[28,29](**Fig. 6**). Snow and colleagues[30] examined cadavers of various ages and determined that a 1 to 2 mm periosteal connection existed between the paratenon of the Achilles tendon and the plantar fascia (**Fig. 7**). Others have shown that the robustness of the connection varies with age; the two are connected at birth, and the connection thins over time until only a thin connection remains by middle adulthood.[12] In a cadaveric study, only 5% of tendons inserted onto the distal one-third of the calcaneus.[31] The investigators

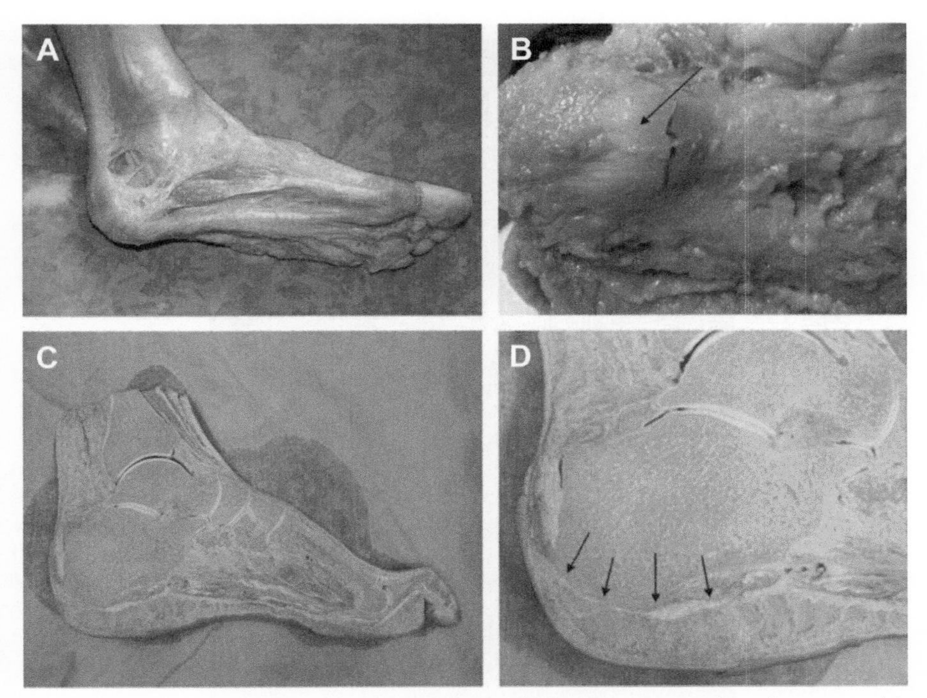

Fig. 6. Dissection of a fresh cadaver revealing the fibrous tissue over the calcaneus and its connection with the paratenon of the Achilles (*A, B*). Sagittal slice of foot again revealing this connection, from the anatomic collection of Padova University (*C, D*). Arrows show tissue of the plantar fascia origin (*B*) from the plantar view and (*D*) in sagittal cross section. (*Adapted from* Stecco, C., Corradin, M., Macchi, V., Morra, A., Porzionato, A., Biz, C., & De Caro, R. (2013). Plantar fascia anatomy and its relationship with Achilles tendon and paratenon. J Anat 223(6):665–676; with permission.)

recognized that the average age of their specimens was 67.8 years and subsequently performed an MRI investigation on younger patients. They found that younger patients on average had a more distal insertion of their tendon on the calcaneus and concluded that the average location of insertion in the living population is likely more distal than their cadaveric study reported.[32]

Further supporting the connection between the Achilles tendon and plantar fascia, MRI studies have shown a difference in thickness of the plantar fascia between healthy control patients and patients with evidence of Achilles tendonitis. The plantar fascia of healthy patients measured an average of 2.1 mm in thickness, whereas that of patients with Achilles tendonitis measured 3.4 mm.[27]

RELATIONSHIP OF THE PLANTARIS TO THE ACHILLES TENDON

The plantaris is a vestigial muscle that arises from the posterior aspect of the lateral femoral condyle proximal to the knee joint. It has a short muscle belly before becoming tendinous and traveling between the gastrocnemius and soleus muscles to insert in the medial aspect of the calcaneus (**Fig. 8**). In most patients, it has a distinct insertion

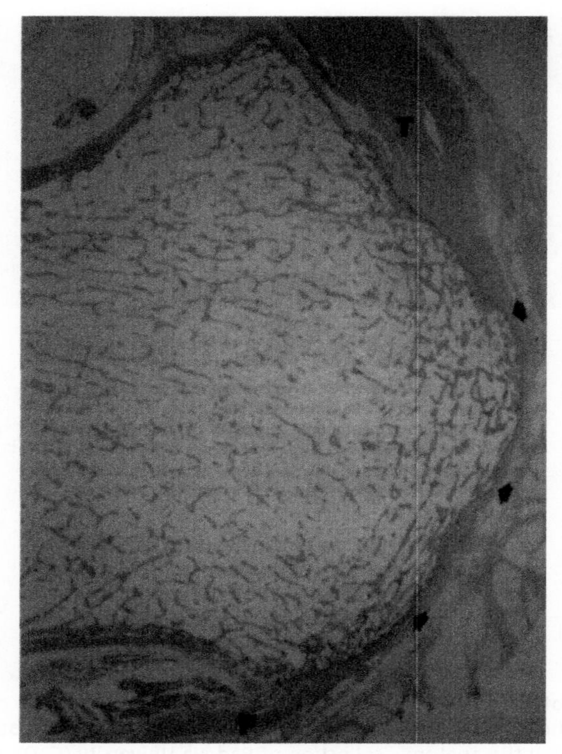

Fig. 7. Photomicrograph showing the insertions of both the Achilles tendon (T, *top arrow*), and the plantar fascia (F, *bottom arrows*) in a young adult. Note their common contribution to the calcaneal periosteum. (*Adapted from* Snow, S. W., Bohne, W. H., DiCarlo, E., & Chang, V. K. (1995). Anatomy of the Achilles tendon and plantar fascia in relation to the calcaneus in various age groups. Foot Ankle Int 16(7):418–421; with permission.)

separate from the Achilles but can share a common insertion in 6% to 8% of patients.[8] It is absent in nearly 10% of the population.[12] It contributes little to the function of the heel cord.

NERVES AND INNERVATION

Innervation to the muscles of the posterior compartment of the leg is provided predominantly by the tibial nerve, with contributions from the sural nerve to the Achilles tendon itself. The tibial nerve provides motor innervation to both the gastrocnemius and soleus muscles, as well as cutaneous sensation to the posterior leg.[13]

The sural nerve is a sensory nerve that receives contributions from both the tibial and peroneal nerves. It is frequently encountered during the approach to the Achilles tendon, particularly during minimally invasive repairs and may be injured. It frequently travels with the small saphenous vein. It crosses the posterior aspect of the Achilles tendon from medial to lateral on average 9 to 11 cm proximal to the calcaneal tubercle.[33,34] Others have reported it to cross the lateral border of the Achilles about 55% of the distance down the tendon from the musculotendinous junction[35] (**Fig. 9**). Most

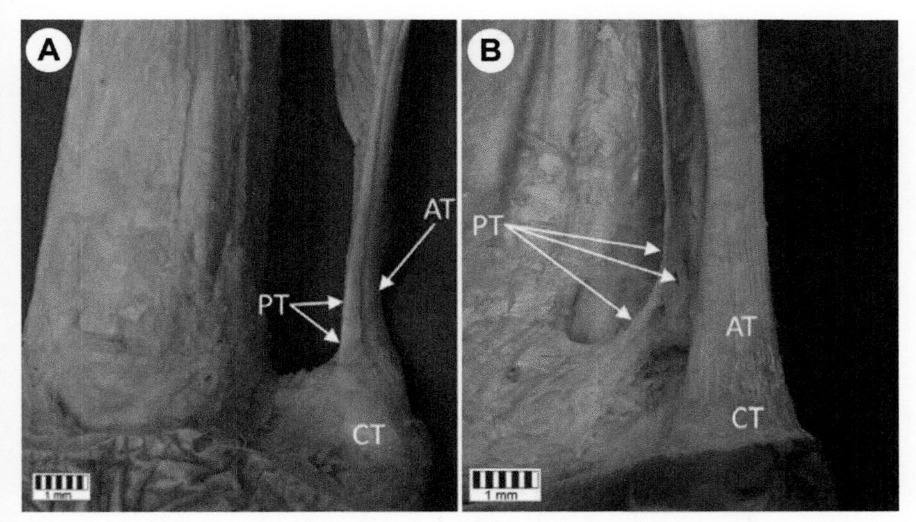

Fig. 8. Variances of plantaris anatomy in relation to the Achilles tendon. (*A*) Plantaris tendon inserting on the calcaneal tuberosity medial to the Achilles (most common), (*B*) Plantaris tendon inserting on deep medial fascia of the leg proximal to the calcaneal tuberosity (less common). (*Adapted from* Olewnick, L. et al. Anatomic study suggests that the morphology of the plantaris tendon may be related to Achilles tendonitis. Surg Radiol Anat 2017;39:69–75; with permission.)

investigators, however, agree that its course is variable and it is most at risk during surgery on the proximal half of the tendon. It is also intimately associated with the tendon for a longer course in shorter or older patients, placing these patients at increased risk for iatrogenic injury during surgery.[14]

VASCULAR SUPPLY

Most of the blood flow to the tendon is through a spidery network of small vessels in the paratenon. Most of the paratenon is supplied by the posterior tibial artery. This blood supply originates on the medial side of the lower leg and branches to supply the proximal and distal extents of the paratenon (**Fig. 10**). The peroneal artery originates laterally and branches to supply a small central section of tendon in the zone that is most frequently associated with ruptures (**Fig. 11**). The tendon is also at its narrowest in this middle section, and thus two watershed zones are created between capillaries from the tibial and peroneal arteries in the narrowest region of the tendon.[36] This may explain the high percentage of ruptures that occur in this zone.

Although the paratenon is highly vascular, this vascularity decreases with age. It does not have a true tendon sheath or synovium associated with it and thus can itself become enlarged and inflamed.[12]

TENDON DEGENERATION (TENDINOSIS)

Tendinosis is defined as diffuse thickening of the tendon in the absence of clinical signs of tendonitis and indicates intrasubstance degeneration. It occurs due to the repetitive microtrauma associated with weight-bearing activities and

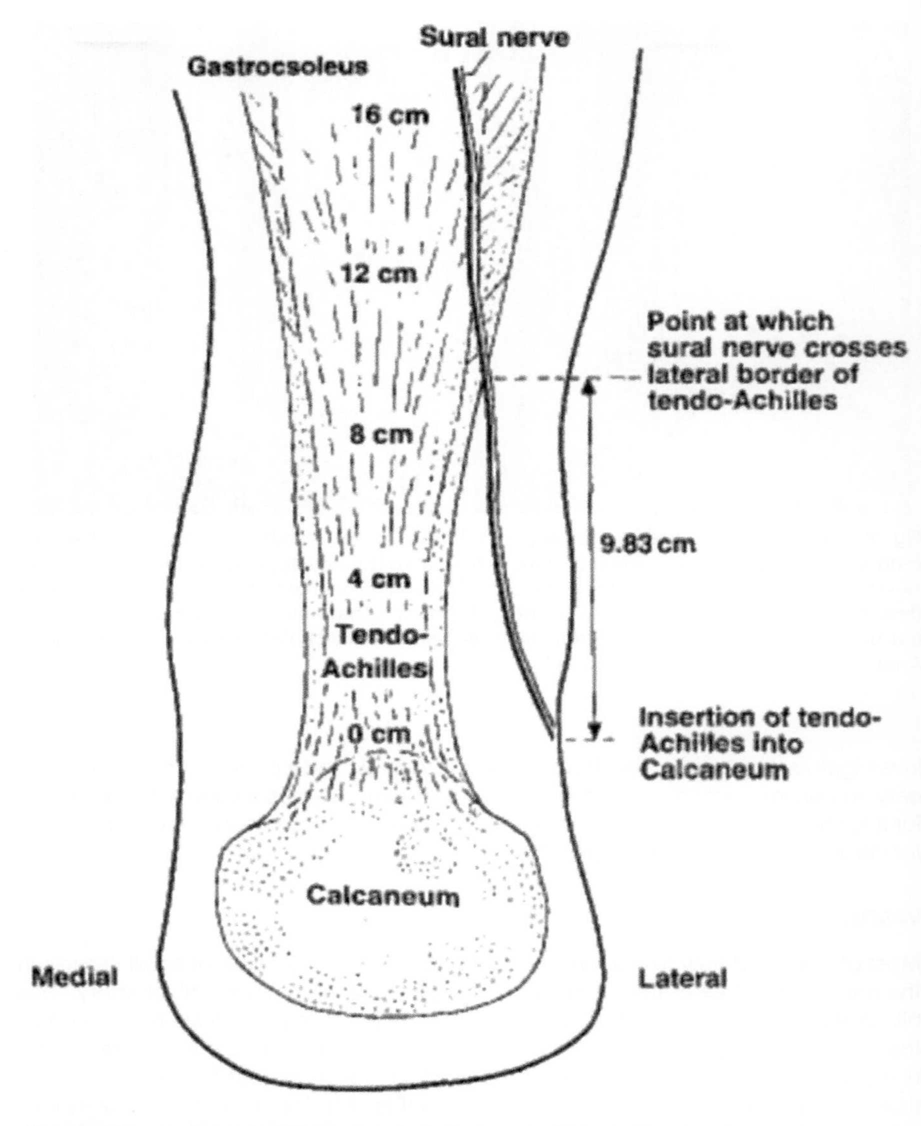

Fig. 9. The sural nerve's course in relation to the Achilles tendon. Note its average crossing distance of 9.8 cm proximal to the calcaneal insertion in this representation, although most investigators agree its course is variable. (*Adapted from* Webb, J., Moorjani, N., & Radford, M. (2000). Anatomy of the sural nerve and its relation to the Achilles tendon. Foot Ankle Int 21(6):475–477; with permission.)

exercises and is particularly common in runners. The limited vascular supply of the tendon impairs its ability to heal from these repetitive insults and instead thickens.

As the tendon thickens, its ability to glide smoothly within the paratenon becomes impaired. Degeneration can progress to palpable nodules or calcifications within the

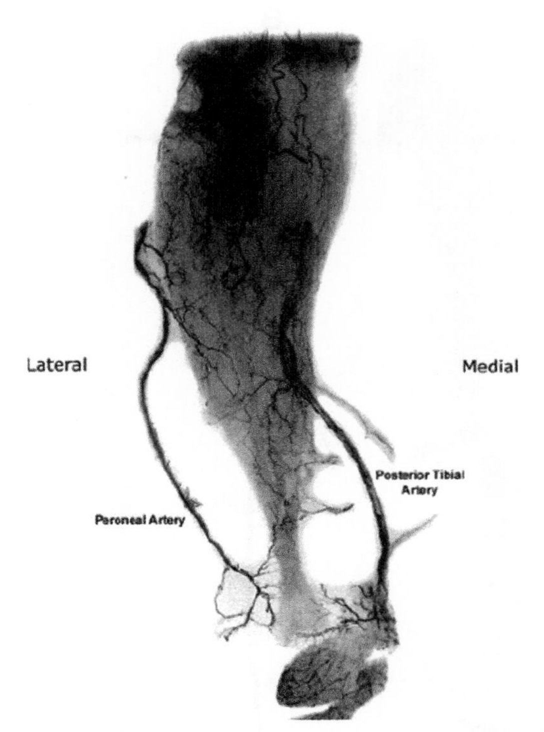

Fig. 10. Radiograph of the Achilles blood supply. The posterior tibial artery supplies the proximal and distal extent of the tendon while the peroneal artery supplies the central region. (*Adapted from* Chen, T. M., Rozen, W. M., Pan, W. R., Ashton, M. W., Richardson, M. D., & Taylor, G. I. The arterial anatomy of the Achilles tendon: anatomical study and clinical implications. Clin Anat 2009;22(3):377–385; with permission.)

tendon, both of which decrease the tensile strength of the tendon.[3] Tendinosis increases in frequency over the age of 35 years.

RISKS FOR RUPTURE

As previously mentioned, tendons typically require a stretch of greater than 8% of their length in order to rupture. This usually results from a sudden force placed on the tendon from strong plantarflexion or an eccentric load. Thus, injury often occurs during athletic participation.[13] Foot alignment when stress is placed on the tendon can also contribute to rupture risk. Excessively planovalgus foot alignment can generate eccentric stress across the tendon and predispose to tendonitis and rupture.[12]

Other risk factors for rupture include age greater than 60 years, male gender, higher body mass index, and history of prior oral corticosteroid or fluoroquinolone use. A history of diabetes mellitus, renal failure, and smoking has not been shown to significantly increase risk for tendon rupture.[2]

Fluoroquinolones are commonly used antibiotics that function by inhibiting DNA gyrase and have a strong affinity for connective tissues, with elevated concentrations

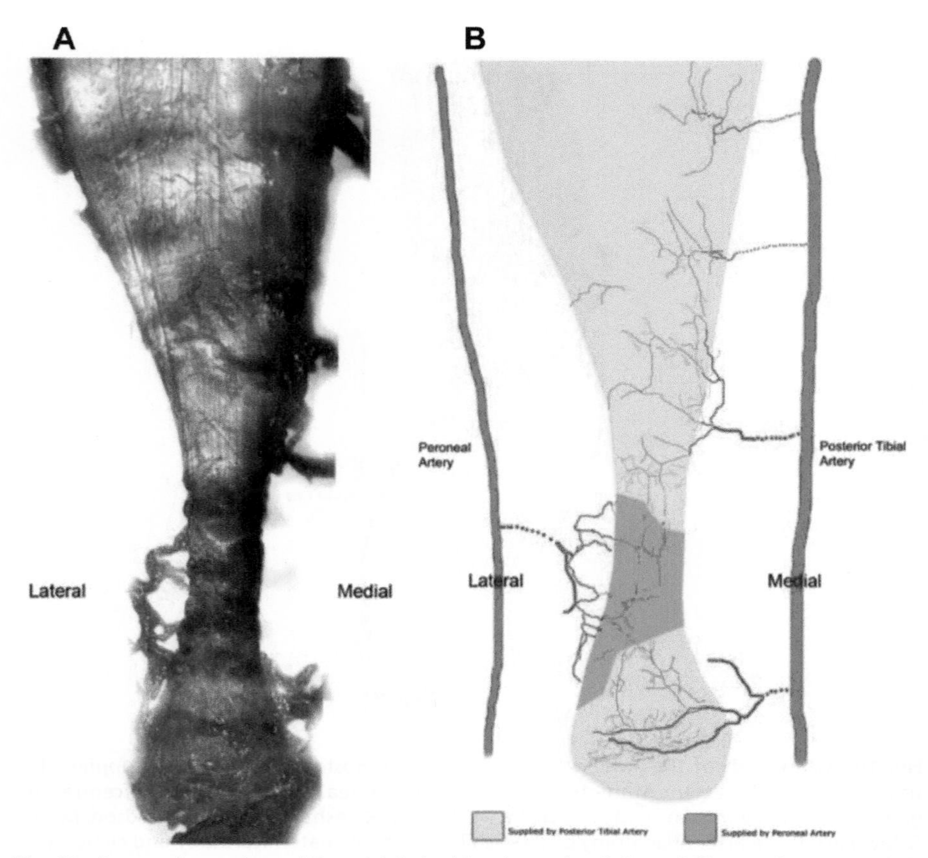

Fig. 11. Anatomic specimen (*A*) and (*B*) the blood supply of the Achilles tendon. Note that most of the tendon is supplied by the posterior tibial artery, whereas the narrowest preinsertional segment is supplied by the peroneal artery. (*Adapted from* Chen, T. M., Rozen, W. M., Pan, W. R., Ashton, M. W., Richardson, M. D., & Taylor, G. I. (2009). The arterial anatomy of the Achilles tendon: anatomical study and clinical implications. Clin Anat 22(3):377–385; with permission.)

in bone and cartilage relative to serum.[37] These medications have been shown to confer an odds ratio of 4.1 for Achilles tendon rupture for current exposure to fluoroquinolones, with a median onset from exposure to tendinopathy symptoms or rupture of 6 days.[38] Although the mechanism of the effect remains unclear, it is theorized that fluoroquinolones disproportionately affect human musculoskeletal tissue that is in a rapid-turnover state with impaired ability to heal, such as in older individuals with predisposition to tendinopathy.[39]

SUMMARY

- The strength of the Achilles tendon allows it to carry loads up to 10 times body weight.
- It acts as a connection between the gastrocnemius and soleus muscles and the calcaneus, spanning both the knee and ankle joints and providing explosive push-off.

- Crimped collagen provides elasticity to the tendon, and this crimping decreases over time and with injury. The collagen composition of the tendon also changes from predominantly type I collagen to type III collagen with age and injury.
- Eccentric contraction and abnormal foot alignment can cause rupture of the tendon.
- The tendon spirals 90° throughout its course to its insertion on the calcaneus.
- Relatively poor blood supply in the watershed region between the peroneal and posterior tibial arteries impairs healing from minor insults and results in tendinopathy.
- The plantar fascia connects the Achilles tendon to the plantar foot through a periosteal connection that thins over time. This may explain the success of treating plantar fasciitis with heel cord stretching.
- Surgical repair of the ruptured tendon is often undertaken, and special care must be taken to avoid injury to the sural nerve, given its close anatomic relationship to the tendon.

REFERENCES

1. Smart GT, Taunton JE, Clement DB. Achilles tendon disorders in runners–a review. Med Sci Sports Exerc 1980;12(4):231–43.
2. Claessen FMAP, de Vos R-J, Reijman M, et al. Predictors of primary achilles tendon ruptures. Sports Med 2014;44(9):1241–59.
3. Hess GW. Achilles tendon rupture: a review of etiology, population, anatomy, risk factors, and injury prevention. Foot Ankle Spec 2010;3(1):29–32.
4. Del Buono A, Chan O, Maffulli N. Achilles tendon: functional anatomy and novel emerging models of imaging classification. Int Orthop 2013;37(4):715–21.
5. Magnusson SP. Collagen fibril size and crimp morphology in ruptured and intact Achilles tendons. Matrix Biol 2002;21(4):369–77.
6. Järvinen TAH. Collagen fibres of the spontaneously ruptured human tendons display decreased thickness and crimp angle. J Orthop Res 2004;22(6): 1303–9.
7. Parry DA, Barnes GR, Craig AS. A comparison of the size distribution of collagen fibrils in connective tissues as a function of age and a possible relation between fibril size distribution and mechanical properties. Proc R Soc Lond B Biol Sci 1978;203(1152):305–21.
8. O'Brien M. Functional anatomy and physiology of tendons. Clin Sports Med 1992; 11(3):505–20.
9. Bailey AJ, Lapiere CM. Effect of an additional peptide extension of the N-terminus of collagen from dermatosparactic calves on the cross-linking of the collagen fibres. Eur J Biochem 1973;34(1):91–6.
10. Jozsa L, Balint BJ, Reffy A, et al. Fine structural alterations of collagen fibers in degenerative tendinopathy. Arch Orthop Trauma Surg 1984;103(1):47–51.
11. Maffulli N. Tenocytes from ruptured and tendinopathic achilles tendons produce greater quantities of type III collagen than tenocytes from normal achilles tendons. An in vitro model of human tendon healing. Am J Sports Med 2000; 28(4):499–505.
12. Pierre-Jerome C, Moncayo V, Terk MR. MRI of the Achilles tendon: a comprehensive review of the anatomy, biomechanics, and imaging of overuse tendinopathies. Acta Radiol 2010;51(4):438–54.
13. Wong M, Kiel J. Anatomy, lower limb, calf, tendons, Achilles. Treasure Island (FL): StatPearls; 2018.

14. Apaydin N. Relationships of the sural nerve with the calcaneal tendon: an anatomical study with surgical and clinical implications. Surg Radiol Anat 2009; 31(10):775–80.
15. O'Brien M. The anatomy of the Achilles tendon. Foot Ankle Clin 2005;10(2): 225–38.
16. Bleakney RR. Long-term ultrasonographic features of the Achilles tendon after rupture. Clin J Sport Med 2002;12(5):273–8.
17. Arøen A. Contralateral tendon rupture risk is increased in individuals with a previous Achilles tendon rupture. Scand J Med Sci Sports 2004;14(1):30–3.
18. Cummins EJ, Anson BJ. The structure of the calcaneal tendon (of Achilles) in relation to orthopedic surgery, with additional observations on the plantaris muscle. Surg Gynecol Obstet 1946;83:107–16.
19. Curwin S SW. Tendonitis: its etiology and treatment. Lexington (MA): Collamore Press; 1984.
20. Alexander RM, Bennet-Clark HC. Storage of elastic strain energy in muscle and other tissues. Nature 1977;265(5590):114–7.
21. Jones FW. Structure and function as seen in the foot. Baltimore: Baillière, Tindall and Cox; 1944.
22. Barfred T. Experimental rupture of the Achilles tendon. Comparison of various types of experimental rupture in rats. Acta Orthop Scand 1971;42(6):528–43.
23. Benjamin M, Evans EJ, Copp L. The histology of tendon attachments to bone in man. J Anat 1986;149:89–100.
24. Schepsis AA, Jones H, Haas AL. Achilles tendon disorders in athletes. Am J Sports Med 2002;30(2):287–305.
25. Kang S, Thordarson DB, Charlton TP. Insertional Achilles tendinitis and Haglund's deformity. Foot Ankle Int 2012;33(6):487–91.
26. Kvist M. Achilles tendon injuries in athletes. Sports Med 1994;18(3):173–201.
27. Stecco C, Corradin M, Macchi V, et al. Plantar fascia anatomy and its relationship with Achilles tendon and paratenon. J Anat 2013;223(6):665–76.
28. Bolívar YA, Munuera PV, Padillo JP. Relationship between tightness of the posterior muscles of the lower limb and plantar fasciitis. Foot Ankle Int 2013; 34(1):42–8.
29. Garrett TR. The effectiveness of a gastrocnemius-soleus stretching program as a therapeutic treatment of plantar fasciitis. J Sport Rehabil 2013;22(4): 308–12.
30. Snow SW, Bohne WH, DiCarlo E, et al. Anatomy of the Achilles tendon and plantar fascia in relation to the calcaneus in various age groups. Foot Ankle Int 1995; 16(7):418–21.
31. Kim PJ. The variability of the Achilles tendon insertion: a cadaveric examination. J foot Ankle Surg 2010;49(5):417–20.
32. Kim PJ. Variability of insertion of the Achilles tendon on the calcaneus: an MRI study of younger subjects. J foot Ankle Surg 2011;50(1):41–3.
33. Doral MN, Alam M, Bozkurt M, et al. Functional anatomy of the Achilles tendon. Knee Surg Sports Traumatol Arthrosc 2010;18(5):638–43.
34. Webb J, Moorjani N, Radford M. Anatomy of the sural nerve and its relation to the Achilles tendon. Foot Ankle Int 2000;21(6):475–7.
35. Kammar H, Carmont MR, Kots E, et al. Anatomy of the sural nerve and its relation to the achilles tendon by ultrasound examination. Orthopedics 2014;37(3): e298–301.
36. Chen TM, Rozen WM, Pan WR, et al. The arterial anatomy of the Achilles tendon: anatomical study and clinical implications. Clin Anat 2009;22(3):377–85.

37. Melhus A, Apelqvist J, Larsson J, et al. Levofloxacin-associated Achilles tendon rupture and tendinopathy. Scand J Infect Dis 2003;35(10):768–70.
38. Corrao G, Zambon A, Bertu L, et al. Evidence of tendinitis provoked by fluoroquinolone treatment: a case-control study. Drug Saf 2006;29(10):889–96.
39. Williams RJ 3rd, Attia E, Wickiewicz TL, et al. The effect of ciprofloxacin on tendon, paratenon, and capsular fibroblast metabolism. Am J Sports Med 2000;28(3):364–9.

Functional Rehabilitation for Nonsurgical Treatment of Acute Achilles Tendon Rupture

Mark Glazebrook, MD, MSc, PhD, FRCS(C)[a,*], Daniela Rubinger, BScPT[b]

KEYWORDS

• Achilles • Tendon • Rupture • Functional rehabilitation • Nonoperative
• Physical therapy

KEY POINTS

- Current available literature suggests that when treating an acute Achilles tendon midsubstance rupture with accelerated functional rehabilitation, the clinical outcomes for nonoperative and operative treatments are similar.
- If an appropriate accelerated functional rehabilitation program cannot be utilized properly, then consideration should be given to operative treatment.
- The initial diagnosis and initiation of nonoperative treatment with functional rehabilitation must be started within 48 hours with the foot immobilized in plantar flexion and non-weight bearing.
- Patient education and supervision with a physical therapist experienced in functional rehabilitation are essential for success. Patient compliance also is essential for success.
- A problematic complication of nonoperative treatment of Achilles tendon ruptures is weakness secondary to overstretching of the Achilles. This can be mitigated or prevented with close supervision of the rehabilitation protocol and communication between physical therapist and physician, with adjustments in the protocol when necessary.

INTRODUCTION

Rupture of the Achilles tendon is one of the most common sports-related injuries in the adult population[1]. Despite the increased incidence, there is no consensus on the best method of treatment, because both operative and nonoperative treatments present unique benefits and disadvantages. It is essential to present patients with the risks and benefits of both operative and nonoperative treatments to allow patients to make an informed choice on the course of their treatment.

[a] Queen Elizabeth II Health Sciences Center, Halifax Infirmary (Room 4867), 1796 Summer Street, Halifax, Nova Scotia B3H 3A7, Canada; [b] Citadel Physiotherapy, 1554 Dresdon Row, Suite 3070, Halifax, Nova Scotia B3J 2X2, Canada
* Corresponding author.
E-mail address: markglazebr@hotmail.com

Foot Ankle Clin N Am 24 (2019) 387–398
https://doi.org/10.1016/j.fcl.2019.05.001 foot.theclinics.com
1083-7515/19/

The operative treatment of an Achilles tendon rupture includes open repairs and minimally invasive and percutaneous techniques, all involving the placement of sutures, which provide extra protection during the healing process at the cost of disruption of blood supply. The obvious benefits include additional protection from rerupturing from minor forces and elongation of tendon from careless aggressive rehabilitation. Surgical repair, however, can place patients at increased risk for wound infection, deep infection, scarring, sural nerve sensory disturbances, and deep vein thrombosis (**Table 1**).[2]

The nonoperative treatment of Achilles tendon ruptures offers the benefit of no further disruption of blood supply at healing site and decreased rates of surgical complications but requires appropriate monitoring by the medical team and patient compliance with functional rehabilitation. Compliance with the accelerated rehabilitation protocol by patient and physiotherapist is of utmost importance because deviation can lead to tendon elongation, leading to residual weakness. It has been found that clinical outcomes correlate with the degree of tendon lengthening and that early, well-supervised mobilization can reduce the degree of tendon elongation.[3]

Most importantly, the current available evidence in the literature shows that when the accelerated rehabilitation protocol is administered correctly, there is no significant difference in the clinically important outcomes for patients who receive operative or nonoperative treatments. If the nonoperative treatment functional rehabilitation protocol cannot be supervised and administered correctly, however, then strong consideration should be given to operative treatment.[3]

Nonoperative treatment methods include several different techniques. A functional rehabilitation protocol can include early weight bearing, early controlled range of motion (ROM), or both.[4] The degree to which a patient is weight bearing and the amount

Table 1
Risks and benefits of operative treatment and nonoperative treatments

Benefits	Risks
Operative treatment	
• Low rate of rerupture similar to nonoperative treatment • Good functional outcome similar to nonoperative treatment • Possible slightly earlier return to high demanding activity by weeks not months • More robust with sutures able to resist poor compliance with rehabilitation program in in early healing phase and possible prevention of rerupture with low force earlier in recovery • Improved high torque strength[2]	• General risks of operative treatment • Risk of wound infection • Risk of nerve injury • Risk of wound healing problems • Scar • Blood clot
Nonoperative treatment	
• Low rate of rerupture similar to operative treatment • Avoid operation and associated risks • Similar rate of rerupture to operative treatment • Similar functional outcome to operative treatment	• Blood clot • Weakness as a result of tendon over stretching if poor compliance with GAPNOT • Rerupture with minor force less than that of the additional strength provided by sutures • Possibly slower return to high demanding activity by weeks not months

of time before controlled ROM exercises begin are variable between protocols, but there is evidence in the literature that suggests they are important components in the success of nonoperatively treated Achilles tendon ruptures. Nilsson-Helander and colleagues[4] found that using functional braces results in more favorable outcomes than casting, as demonstrated by a lower rerupture rate. Suchak and colleagues[5] investigated early weight bearing and its consequence on health-related quality of life and found it increased the quality of life in the early stages of rehabilitation. Lastly, a study conducted by Olsson and colleagues[6,7] demonstrated early controlled ROM and early loading of the tendon resulted in favorable clinical outcomes. The best studied accelerated rehabilitation protocol for nonoperative treatment of a midsubstance Achilles rupture was described by Willits and colleagues[2] in a high-quality level 1 randomized controlled trial. This article describes the Glazebrook/Rubinger Achilles protocol for nonoperative treatment (GAPNOT), which is standardized accelerated rehabilitation protocol (see **Table 3**) modified from the previous study of Willits and colleagues.[2]

The intent of this article is to provide a comprehensive description of the GAPNOT protocol with key points of the treatment emphasized to provide guidance to rehabilitation team in order to achieve optimal clinical outcomes for patients.

METHODS

Diagnosis

Diagnosis of an acute Achilles tendon rupture is made with careful history, physical examination, and review of diagnostic imaging if necessary. The key history features include complaints of sudden snap, acute severe pain localized to rupture site, and often difficulty with weight-bearing activities.

The physical examination is best done with the patient in the prone position and the feet hanging over the end of the bed (**Fig. 1**A). The key physical examination features that confirm an acute Achilles tendon rupture include a midsubstance palpable gap (**Fig. 2**), a lack of plantar-flexion response with calf squeeze (Thompson test), and localized pain, swelling, and ecchymosis (see **Fig. 2**). Tests are repeated with the knee in flexion and extension (**Fig. 1**B). Although not essential, ultrasound or magnetic resonance imaging (MRI) can assist in confirming Achilles tendon rupture if clinical history and physical examination are not definitive. Furthermore, a lateral plain radiograph projection excludes a bony avulsion, which may be important in choosing treatment.

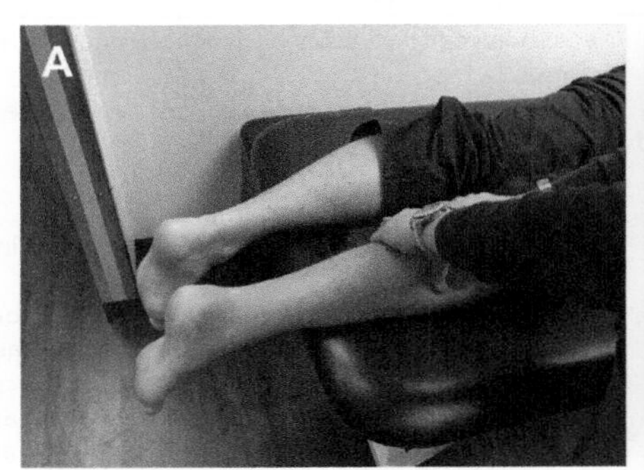

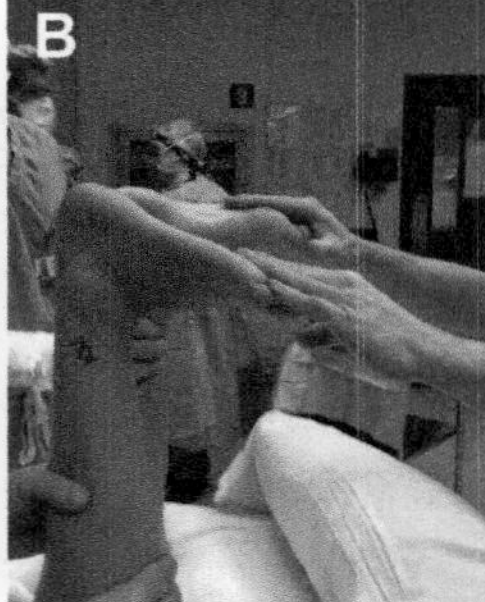

Fig. 1. (*A*) Patient positioning for examination of suspected acute Achilles rupture. (*B*) Patient positioned with knee flexed for examination.

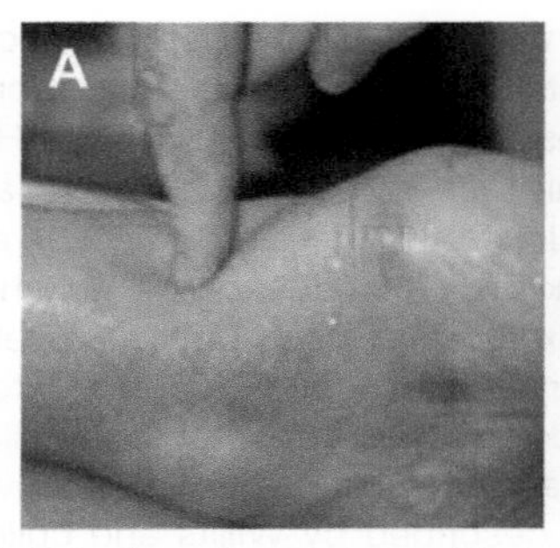

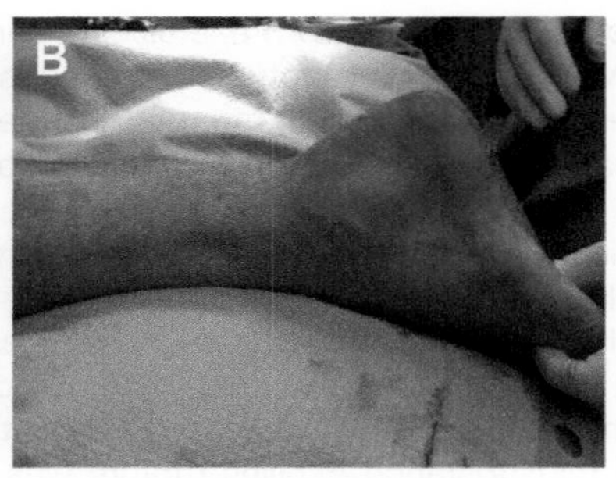

Fig. 2. (*A, B*) Defect of complete midsubstance Achilles tendon rupture.

An MRI has a high sensitivity for identifying a complete versus rupture partial rupture. Caution should be exercised, however, with interpretation of the MRI signal. Radiologists tend to use this to report a gap size. It is more likely that the gap reported is a zone of trauma where the frayed ends of the ruptured Achilles tendon produce an MRI signal different from that of a normal tendon. Furthermore, the current best available evidence in a randomized controlled study[2] ignored the presence or absence of the gap, when using nonoperative treatment, and showed similar results to operative treatment.

Criteria for Nonoperative Treatment

Patients with confirmed diagnosis of acute Achilles tendon rupture are appropriate for nonoperative treatment if they are diagnosed within 2 days of injury and had minimal weight-bearing activities during that period. It is important that they meet the criteria listed in **Table 2**. If not, they should proceed with surgical repair.

Glazebrook/Rubinger Achilles Protocol for Nonoperative Treatment

Once patients are deemed appropriate for nonoperative treatment, they should be educated on the benefits, risks, and limitations of both operative and nonoperative

Table 2
Inclusion and exclusion criteria for nonoperative versus operative treatment of Achilles tendon ruptures

Inclusion Criteria	Exclusion Criteria
• Complete, midsubstance Achilles tendon rupture (diagnosed by Thompson squeeze test, palpable gap on the tendon, and confirmed by MRI) • Willingness and ability to comply with the functional rehabilitation protocol • Treatment began within the first 7 d of injury • Informed consent was completed	• Achilles tendon avulsion from calcaneus or calf muscle tear • Not placed in plantar-flexed cast within the first 48 h of injury • Open Achilles tendon • Any additional injury to injured leg • Prior rerupture or significant injury to the injured Achilles tendon • Any physical or mental impairment that would affect a patient's ability to closely follow the protocol • Any factors known to increase the risk for an Achilles tendon rupture (diabetes mellitus and immunosuppressive therapy, including local and systemic steroids and fluoroquinolones)

treatments. Patients who choose to undergo nonoperative treatment of Achilles tendon ruptures should be immobilized (preferably in plaster cast) in maximum passive plantar-flexion position (**Fig. 3**) and instructed to remain non–weight bearing for 2 weeks.

At the 2-week follow-up visit, the patients are placed in the Achilles-specific walking boot with 40° heel lifts (**Fig. 4**) or a similar boot, and the GAPNOT protocol should be initiated under the supervision of a physiotherapist. The detailed physiotherapy protocol is outlined in **Table 3**. Key features are outlined later but it is important to establish a weight-bearing schedule and guidelines with patient on the initial physiotherapy visit. Determining a weight-bearing schedule, as well as dates for the heel lifts to be removed and weaning from the boot walker, may help create compliance in the patient, which is key for successful outcome.

The physician follow-up, supervision, and care should continue at 6 weeks, 12 weeks, 26 weeks, and 52 weeks after the rupture. During these visits, the healing is assessed with history and physical examination, looking for and assessing resolving pain, swelling, ecchymosis, gradual return to activity specified by the GAPNOT protocol, and filling of the palpable defect. The physician also should examination patient length of the Achilles tendon ROM using careful passive dorsiflexion with the knee in extended position compared with the contralateral side. Patients should be counseled on avoiding a fall or stumble and avoiding activities that may force the ankle beyond the 90° dorsiflexion position.

The GAPNOT protocol involves progressive weight bearing, increasing by 25% body weight per week during weeks 3 to 6. During this time, patients commenced

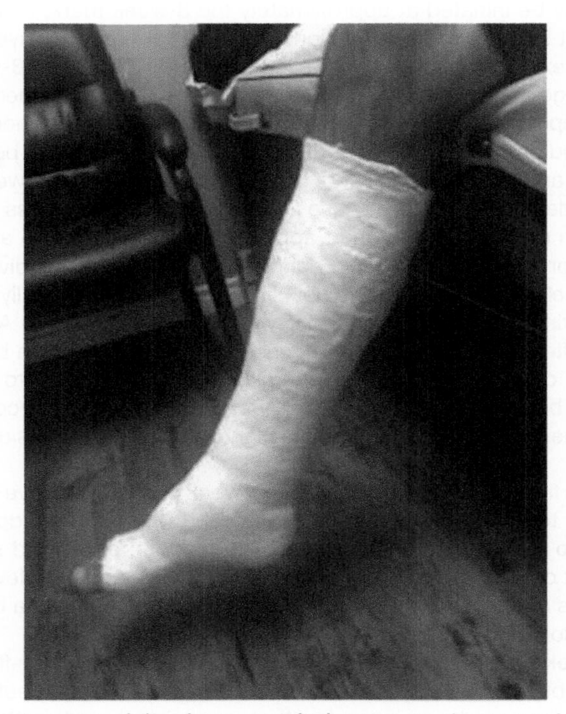

Fig. 3. Achilles rupture immobilized non–weight bearing maximum passive plantar-flexion cast.

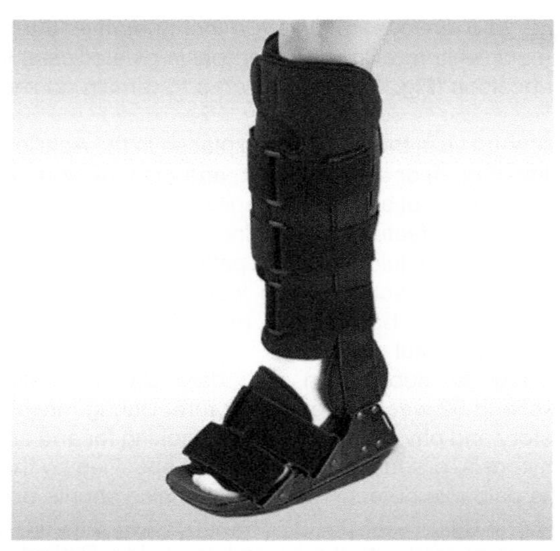

Fig. 4. Achilles-specific boot walker with heel wedges. (Achilles Boot image courtesy of Breg, Inc.)

pain-free, gradual active plantar and dorsiflexion exercises below 90° of ankle dorsiflexion, and conventional physiotherapy modalities are used for control of pain and swelling as needed. Electrical muscle stimulation with active heel raises in the sitting position also may be initiated at approximately the 3-week mark, ensuring the ankle does not go past 90° of ankle dorsiflexion. It is important that passive ranging of the ankle into dorsiflexion beyond 90° is avoided during the 2-week to 8-week stage.

During this stage, communication between physician and physiotherapist is optimal to deal with complications, such as reruptures, tendon elongation, noncompliance of patient, and blood clots. It is important that all exercises and weight bearing are pain-free and patients are decreasing activity if they are noticing any pain, swelling, or tension on the injured side. Patients typically use 2 crutches as they progress through weight bearing but often reduce to 1 crutch at approximately weeks 4 to 5 and no crutches by week 6. This progression of weight bearing status, however, is individualized.

Between 6 weeks and 8 weeks, the heel lifts are reduced gradually in height while fully weight bearing, followed by a further week to wean from the Achilles-specific boot. Patients often use assistance of a cane while weaning from a boot walker. An Achilles-specific compression garment (**Fig. 5**) is recommended to patients when weaning from a boot walker but is not mandatory. Physiotherapy continues during this stage with the addition of resisted ankle plantar-flexion exercises using resistance tubing.

While weaning from the boot walker at end of week 8, it is imperative to do this gradually with a step to gait initially, so as not lengthen the Achilles tendon. Patients are recommended to wear shoes at all times, even indoors, and avoid shoes with low heel rise. Patient cans lengthen their stride gradually over the next few weeks as the tendon lengthens naturally. They are still instructed to do stairs 1 at a time, protecting the Achilles tendon.

Between 8 weeks and 12 weeks, patients can initiate active plantar-flexion strengthening exercises but avoid activities that dorsiflex the ankle past neutral. Thereafter, strength, power, and endurance are worked on. It is imperative that patients are educated to avoid activities that place the foot beyond 90° of ankle dorsiflexion and

Table 3
Glazebrook/Rubinger Achilles protocol for nonoperative treatment

Time Period	Protocol
0–2 wk	• Plaster cast with ankle in maximum passive plantar flexion; non–weight bearing with crutches
2–4 wk	• Achilles-specific (or other) walking boot with maximum passive plantar-flexed heel lifts • Protected weight bearing with crutches: ○ Weeks 2–3—25% ○ Weeks 3–4—50% ○ Weeks 4–5—75% ○ Weeks 5–6—100% • Active plantar and dorsiflexion ROM exercises to neutral, inversion/eversion below neutral • Modalities to control swelling (ultrasound, interferential current with ice, acupuncture, light/laser therapy) • Electrical muscle stimulation to calf musculature with seated heel raises when tolerated. • Patients being seen 2–3 times/wk depending on availability and degree of pain and swelling in the foot and ankle • Knee/hip exercises with no ankle involvement, for example, leg lifts from sitting, prone, or side-lying • Non–weight-bearing fitness/cardio work, for example, biking with 1 leg (with boot walker on), deep water running (usually not started until 3–4 wk point) • Hydrotherapy if available (within motion and weight-bearing limitations) • Emphasize need of patient to use pain as guideline. If in pain, back off activities and weight bearing.
4–6 wk	• Continue weight bearing as tolerated • Continue 2–4 wk protocol • Progress electrical muscle stimulation to calf with lying calf raises on shuttle with no resistance as tolerated approximately weeks 5–6. Please ensure that ankle does not go past neutral while doing exercises. • Continue with physiotherapy 2–3 times/wk. • Emphasize patient doing non–weight-bearing cardio activities as tolerated with boot walker on.
6–8 wk	• Continue physiotherapy 2 times/wk • Continue with modalities for swelling as needed. • Continue with electrical muscle stimulation on calf with strengthening exercises. Do not go past neutral ankle position. • Remove heel lifts in stages dependent on Achilles length. Remove 1 lift daily as tolerated. Always leave 1–2 lifts in to represent regular shoe lift, depending on boot design. • Weight bearing as tolerated, usually 100% weight bearing in boot walker now. • Graduated resistance exercises (open and closed kinetic chain as well as functional activities)—start with resisted tubing exercises • With weighted-resisted exercises, do not go past neutral ankle position. • Gait retraining now that 100% weight bearing • Fitness/cardio to include weight bearing as tolerated, for example, biking • Hydrotherapy
8–12 wk	**Ensure patient understands that tendon is still very vulnerable, and patients need to be diligent with activities of daily living and exercises. Any sudden loading of the Achilles (trip, step up stairs, etc.) may result in a rerupture.** • Wean off boot (usually over 2–5 d process—varies per patient), at night as well

(*continued on next page*)

Table 3
(*continued*)

Time Period	Protocol
	• Wear Achilles compression ankle brace to provide extra stability and swelling control once boot walker is removed. • Return to crutches/cane as necessary and gradually wean off. Have patient always wear shoes, limiting time in bare/sock feet. • Continue to progress to ROM, strength, and proprioception exercises. • Add exercises, such as stationary bicycle, elliptical, and walking on treadmill, as patient tolerates. • Add balance board activities—standing with block to prevent dorsiflexion past neutral position. • Add calf stretches in standing (gently). Do not allow ankle to go past neutral position. • Add double-heel raises and progress to single-heel raises when tolerated. Do not allow ankle to go past neutral position. • Continue physiotherapy 1–2 times/wk depending on how independent patient is at doing exercises and access to exercise equipment.
12–16 wk	• Continue to progress ROM, strength, and proprioception exercises. • Retrain strength, power, endurance. Ensure patient understands that tendon is still very vulnerable and patients need to be diligent with activities of daily living and exercises. Avoid lunges, squats, etc., because these places excessive stretch on tendon.
16+ weeks	• Increase dynamic weight-bearing exercise, including sport-specific retaining (ie, skipping, jogging, and weight training).
6–9 mo	• Return to normal sporting activities that do not involve contact or sprinting, cutting jumping, etc., if patient has regained 80% strength
12 mo	• Return to sports that involve running/jumping as directed by medical team and tolerated if patient has regained 100% strength.

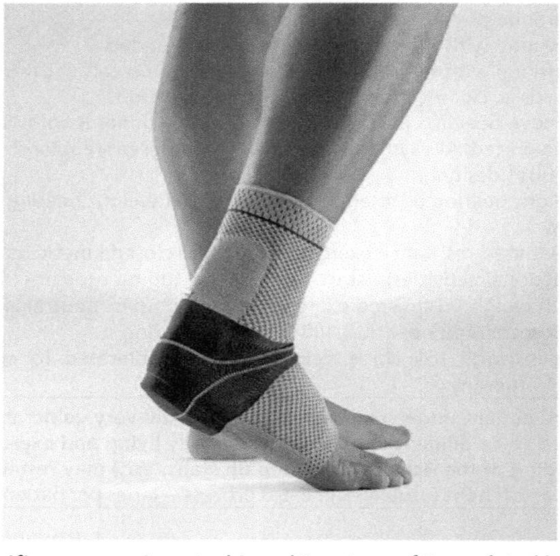

Fig. 5. Achilles-specific compression stocking. (*Courtesy of* Bauerfeind.)

allow normal activities of daily activities set the appropriate length of Achilles tendon. Physical therapy should still avoid stretching to achieve normal ROM at this stage.

During this stage, patients initiate using a stationary bicycle with little resistance, being careful to point their toes on the affected side while pedaling. They also can initiate closed kinetic chain strengthening exercises on resistance machines with care placed on not going past neutral (**Fig. 6**). They also are able to start double-heel raises multiple times daily. Initially, most of the weight and strength are coming from the nonaffected side; however, as they get stronger, they are encouraged to balance weight between both sides and slowly start to put more weight on the affected side, increasing its strength. Balance and proprioceptive retraining exercises can be initiated using a balance board device, which is blocked to prevent dorsiflexion (**Fig. 7**).

From 12 weeks to 16 weeks, they continue to attend physiotherapy, working on strengthening exercises and progressing the double-heel raises to modified double-heel raises with the nonaffected leg placed behind the affected side to isolate the calf raise on the affected side. Clinically, patients often are not able to do a single-heel raise until the 4-month mark postinjury. Patients also can continue with stationary bicycle, elliptical machine, and strengthening exercises at the gym, that is, seated and standing calf raises with weights if not going past neutral. Patients are cautioned to avoid lunges and squats till 6 months.

During the stage of 10 weeks to 16 weeks, the complication of rerupture and elongation of the tendon may be more common due to patients regaining a more normal activity pattern. Education and careful monitoring of activities that a patient is doing are essential to help prevent rerupture elongation. Patients often stop attending physical therapy during this period because they feel they are better when they can walk normal again. Patient compliance to program is essential for best outcomes.

From 4 months to 6 months, patients usually are doing strengthening exercises on their own at home or in a gym, with periodic rechecks with physiotherapists to ensure that they are not elongating the tendon and that strength in Achilles tendon is returning. Patients may initiate light skipping activities during this stage and light jogging can be initiated if they are able to do 25 consecutive single-heel raises.

From 6 months, gradual return to sporting activities is encouraged but patients are advised to avoid contact sports and high-intensity activities, such as sprinting, cutting, and jumping. From 9 months to 12 months, full return to sporting activity is allowed.

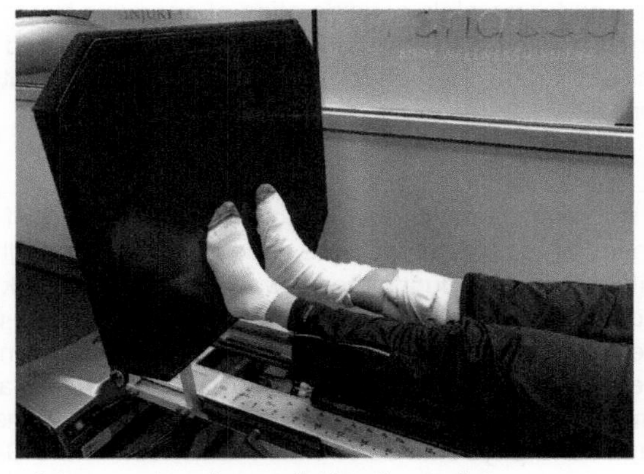

Fig. 6. Resistance training—active plantar flexion in week 8.

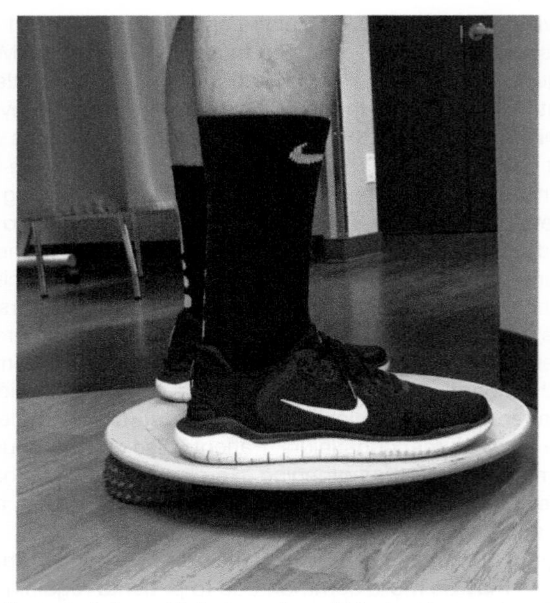

Fig. 7. Proprioceptive retraining with balance board blocked in rear to prevent dorsiflexion.

COMPLICATIONS

Complete Rerupture

Complete rerupture is an uncommon but devastating complication of both operative and nonoperative treatment, with rates reported in the literature between 3% and 4%.[2] Patients who are identified with complete reruptures should be assessed by a surgeon for consideration of operative treatment. Although repeat nonoperative treatment is an option, it has not been studied. Patients should be educated on this.

Partial Rerupture

Partial rerupture is an uncommon complication of both operative and nonoperative treatments. When patients are identified with partial reruptures, they should be immediately immobilized in plantar-flexed position and made non–weight bearing and assessed by a surgeon for possible consideration of operative treatment. If operative treatment is deemed unnecessary, the protocol should be adjusted with consensus between the physical therapist and physician as to which time point in the GAPNOT protocol the patient needs to revert to.

Elongation

Elongation likely is more common with nonoperative treatment if protocol is not administered properly or in patients who are noncompliant. Although this may occur at any time point, it is more likely during the 10-week to 16-week mark as patients start walking and gain confidence. Elongation can be identified on follow-up visits by poor progression of strengthening and careful examination of patient extent of passive dorsiflexion with knee in extended position compared with contralateral side (**Fig. 8**). If elongation is identified, the protocol should be adjusted with consensus between the physical therapist and physician as to which time point in the GAPNOT protocol the patient may need to revert to. If elongation is extreme, patients should be advised

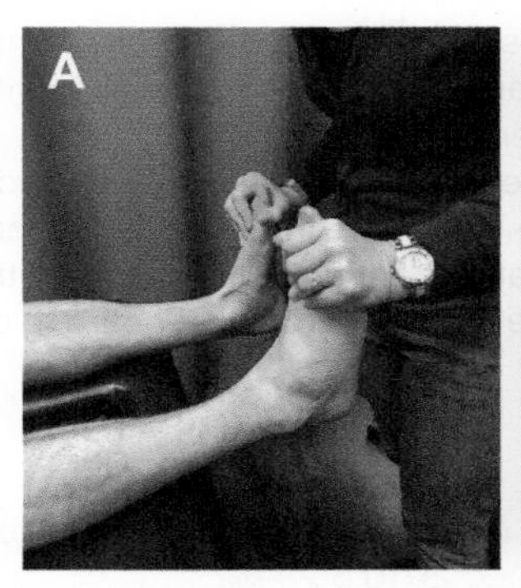

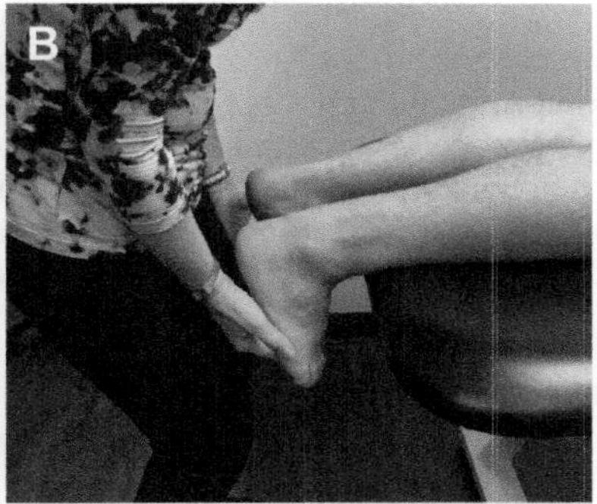

Fig. 8. (*A, B*) Examination of the patient's Achilles tendon length with knee in extended position.

of risks and benefits of surgical shortening of the tendon and continued nonoperative treatment with shortening surgery as necessary.

Deep Vein Thrombosis and Pulmonary Embolism

Deep vein thrombosis and pulmonary embolism are rare occurrences but serious potential complications with immobilization and casting. They should be considered with calf pain, swelling, and shortness of breath, and emergency treatment should be sought immediately.

Calf Atrophy and Poor Strength

With proper Achilles tendon length, calf atrophy and poor strength are minor complications in the long term when patients do not complete the physical therapy protocol. They often result because patients can resume all normal activities of daily living and sporting events and do not understand the need for doing isolated and specific calf-strengthening exercises. When calf weakness is identified, patients are educated on the importance of isolated Achilles strengthening exercises on the affected side.

SUMMARY

Historically, when functional rehabilitation was not used for the nonoperative treatment of an acute midsubstance rupture of the Achilles tendon, the benefits of surgical treatment have been cited as increased strength, decreased rerupture, and a faster return to high-level activity. However, two high-quality level 1 studies[2,3] have demonstrated that nonoperative treatment with functional rehabilitation provides equivalent outcomes to surgical treatment. As a result, there has been an increased incidence of patients avoiding the risks of surgery and choosing nonoperative treatment.

It is essential that patients and surgeons alike understand that nonoperative treatment does not mean no treatment. Nonoperative treatment protocols, such as the GAPNOT protocol described in this article, must be closely supervised by an experienced physiotherapist and physician, with open communication to allow optimal results and avoid complications. If this cannot be done, patients should be educated on the historical benefits of surgery in the absence of functional rehabilitation.

Treatment failure and resultant complications with nonoperative treatment almost always are due to noncompliance, overzealous activity, or neglect by physiotherapist or physician. As such, patient selection and education are important and following the

GAPNOT protocol is essential. Furthermore, close supervision and good communication by both physical therapist and physician are mandatory to avoid, identify, and treat the complications of nonoperative treatment.

In summary, nonoperative treatment of acute midsubstance Achilles tendon ruptures with functional rehabilitation, such as the GAPNOT protocol, described in this article, provides clinical outcome similar to operative treatment. It is essential that physicians and physiotherapist work closely to supervise and administer care to optimize outcomes and avoid complications.

REFERENCES

1. Hess GW. Achilles tendon rupture: a review of etiology, population, anatomy, risk factors, and injury prevention. Foot Ankle Spec 2010;3:29–32.
2. Willits K, Amendola A, Bryant D, et al. Operative versus nonoperative treatment of acute Achilles tendon ruptures: a multicenter randomized trial using accelerated functional rehabilitation. J Bone Joint Surg Am 2010;92:2767–75.
3. Soroceanu A, Sidhwa F, Aarabi S, et al. Surgical versus nonsurgical treatment of acute achilles tendon rupture. J Bone Joint Surg Am 2012;94:2136–43.
4. Nilsson-Helander K, Silbernagel KG, Thomeé R, et al. Acute achilles tendon rupture: a randomized, controlled study comparing surgical and nonsurgical treatments using validated outcome measures. Am J Sports Med 2010;38:2186–93.
5. Suchak AA, Bostick GP, Beaupré LA, et al. The influence of early weight-bearing compared with non-weight-bearing after surgical repair of the Achilles tendon. J Bone Joint Surg Am 2008;90:1876–83.
6. Olsson N, Silbernagel KG, Eriksson BI, et al. Stable surgical repair with accelerated rehabilitation versus nonsurgical treatment for acute Achilles tendon ruptures: a randomized controlled study. Am J Sports Med 2013;41:2867–76.
7. Stathakis A, Wadden C, Glazebrook M. Asymmetric Z-Tendon shortening to maximize excision of abnormal tendon tissue: a technique tip to treat elongated tendons with pathology. Techniques in Foot & Ankle Surgery 2019;18(1):43–7.

Minimally Invasive Treatments of Acute Achilles Tendon Ruptures

Milap S. Patel, DO[a], Anish R. Kadakia, MD[b,*]

KEYWORDS

- Achilles rupture • Achilles repair • Minimally invasive Achilles repair
- Percutaneous Achilles repair

KEY POINTS

- Achilles tendon rupture is a common injury to the lower extremity that requires appropriate treatment to minimize functional deficit.
- Current available treatments of Achilles tendon ruptures include nonoperative, open surgical repair, percutaneous repair, and minimally invasive repair.
- Open surgical repair obtains favorable functional outcomes with a significant potential for deep soft tissue complications, calling into question the value of open repair.
- Percutaneous repair is an alternative option with comparable functional results and minimal soft tissue complications; however, the risk of sural nerve injury is a known complication.
- Minimally invasive Achilles repair offers optimal results with superior functional outcomes with minimal soft tissue complications and sural nerve injury.

INTRODUCTION

Should minimally invasive Achilles tendon repair be the new standard of treatment of acute Achilles tendon ruptures?

Incidence of Achilles tendon rupture is highest in men between 30 years and 39 years of age.[1,2] This incidence has been steadily increasing due to patients living an increasingly active lifestyle.[2–7] The Achilles tendon is one of the strongest tendons in the body, yet it is most commonly affected by spontaneous ruptures. Ruptures occur primarily in patients who participate in activities involving explosive acceleration and maximal effort. Untreated Achilles tendon ruptures hinder an active lifestyle and

[a] Northwestern Memorial Hospital, Northwestern University Feinberg School of Medicine, 259 East Erie, 13th Floor, Chicago, IL 60611, USA; [b] Department of Orthopaedic Surgery, Northwestern Memorial Hospital, Northwestern University Feinberg School of Medicine, 259 East Erie, 13th Floor, Chicago, IL 60611, USA
* Corresponding author.
E-mail address: kadak259@gmail.com

Foot Ankle Clin N Am 24 (2019) 399–424
https://doi.org/10.1016/j.fcl.2019.05.002 foot.theclinics.com
1083-7515/19/

additionally have a detrimental effect on activities of daily living. Increased functional length of the tendon in untreated patients results in significant weakness and altered gait and is the underlying reason why operative fixation is considered for this pathology.

Optimal treatment options for acute Achilles ruptures have been debated in the orthopedic literature for decades. In the past, the debate was concentrated on whether conservative treatment was a superior option to open surgical management. Currently, as technology and techniques have advanced, the debate has evolved to include minimally invasive options that offer a similar advantage of tendon apposition with limited surgical risk.

Modern treatment options for an acute Achilles tendon rupture include conservative care (functional rehabilitation) and open, percutaneous, and minimally invasive or limited open Achilles repair for acute midsubstance Achilles tendon ruptures. The optimal treatment continues to be highly debated even though there have been rapid advances in understanding of Achilles tendon injuries, surgical strategies, and surgical techniques. Each option plays an important role in a carefully selected patient population while providing unique risks and benefits. Current literature grazes over these unique characteristics and seems to demonstrate many similar outcomes with small differences. These small differences are important to understand and need to be scrutinized in great detail in order to provide patients with optimal care. The goal of treatment is to return patients to full activity and try to achieve preinjury strength by restoring physiologic tendon length and tension while subjecting patients to the fewest complications.

Individual patients have different functional needs of their lower extremity depending on age, occupation, and/or activity level. Choice of treatment regimen ultimately is up to the patient; the job of surgeons is to educate patients with current evidence-based results. Outcomes also differ depending on patient compliance with treatment regimen. The debate is not as simplistic as whether surgery or conservative treatment is the best for an Achilles rupture; the real question is which treatment is best for a patient's physiology and athletic demands.

ANATOMIC IMPLICATIONS

Because percutaneous and minimally invasive repair techniques are becoming more prevalent, it is important to understand several important and relevant anatomic implications. With a thorough understanding of the anatomy, the safety of a minimally invasive approach can be maximized.

The sural nerve has a variable course in the lower extremity, making it difficult to utilize anatomic landmarks to trace out the nerve. Webb and colleagues[8] performed dissection of sural nerve in 30 cadavers. Proximally, the sural nerve crossed over to the lateral border of the Achilles tendon at an average of 9.8 cm proximal to the Achilles insertion. At the Achilles insertion at the calcaneus, the sural nerve is 1.88 cm anterior and lateral. Its pathway is crucial to understand because the sural nerve invariably is in close proximity to the repair site on the lateral border of the Achilles tendon. The sural nerve is located between fascia cruris and paratenon[9,10]; therefore, any repair techniques that utilize sutures outside of the paratenon theoretically are at risk of incarcerating sural nerve.

The Achilles tendon derives its vascular supply from posterior tibial artery and the peroneal artery. The posterior tibial artery vascularizes the proximal and distal aspects of the tendon and the peroneal artery vascularizes the central aspect of the tendon.[11] The midsection of the tendon, approximately 4 cm to 7 cm from insertion, is considered a hypovascular area with the poorest blood supply and has the highest propensity to rupture.[11]

The skin over the Achilles tendon has a fragile vascular supply, which has resulted in known complications, such as delayed wound healing and infection. Yepes and colleagues[12] performed a digital vascular mapping of skin and subcutaneous tissue over the Achilles tendon with arteriography to provide vascular safe zones for skin incision. A pattern of vascularity was noted in 10 fresh human cadaver legs over posteromedial, posterolateral, and posterior skin borders of tendon. More consistently, the greatest amount of vascularization was noted between the axis of the medial malleolus and the medial border of Achilles tendon. Additionally, the least vascularization of skin and subcutaneous tissue was directly posterior. This vascular anatomy may contribute to the wound complication risk in extensile open approaches.

Ankle position in a splint/cast after repair also can play an important role in providing oxygenation to the skin over surgical repair site. Poynton and O'Rourke[13] determined skin perfusion by measuring transcutaneous skin oxygen pressure over the Achilles tendon. It was determined that skin perfusion is maximal at 20° of ankle plantar flexion and perfusion diminished by 49% at 40° of plantar flexion. Casting the ankle in 20° of plantar flexion maximizes wound healing potential while taking tension off the repair site. The authors have taken this concept to all posterior incisions, given the universal nature of improving blood flow to the skin after surgery.

The Achilles tendon is unique in that it does not have a true synovial sheath but rather a highly vascular paratenon. Paratenon serves several essential functions, including providing a passageway for vascular supply in addition to allow for smooth tendon gliding. Carr and Norris[14] investigated vascularity of Achilles tendons in 16 fresh cadavers by injecting barium sulfate and India ink. They were able to demonstrate numerous vessels evenly distributed throughout the length of paratenon even over the watershed area of the tendon. During repair, it is imperative to minimize violation to paratenon and preserve its integrity to limit vascular insult to tendon as well as prevent formation of future adhesion. The importance of paratenon repair has been emphasized in recent literature as well.[15]

Carr and Norris[14] also demonstrated several other vessels that ran into the mesotenon toward the anterior aspect of the tendon providing additional blood supply. Therefore, it is crucial to minimize any dissection at the anterior aspect of the tendon during attempts at mobilizing a scarred down tendon. Although repair of the paratenon is important, avoiding injury to the tendon via a minimally invasive approach is superior.

RATIONALE FOR NONSURGICAL MANAGEMENT

Proponents of nonsurgical management have always cited surgical complications as the main disadvantage for surgical management.

Nonsurgical management options include cast immobilization or early functional rehabilitation with functional bracing. Historically, cast immobilization has been the preferred method of nonsurgical management. This consisted of immobilization in a non–weight-bearing cast for 4 weeks followed by weight-bearing cast for another 4 weeks with restoration of ankle motion for a total of approximately 8 weeks in cast immobilization.[16–20] Several disadvantages with this management included significant muscle atrophy, ankle stiffness, and loss of coordination and proprioception.

As more evidence-based data are presented, cast immobilization no longer is justified and nonsurgical management has evolved toward use of early functional rehabilitation with functional bracing. The term, *functional rehabilitation*, implies early range of motion, protected weight bearing, or a combination of both.

Nilsson-Helander and colleagues[21] performed a randomized controlled study, which indicated that early functional rehabilitation is beneficial regardless of nonsurgical or surgical management. Additionally, they were not able to demonstrate any statistically significant difference between the 2 groups. Willits and colleagues[22] also performed a randomized controlled study demonstrating support for nonsurgical treatment with accelerated functional rehabilitation compared with surgical treatment. Soroceanu and colleagues[23] performed a meta-analysis of randomized trials that demonstrated nonsurgical treatment with early functional rehabilitation resulted in similar functional outcomes as surgical treatment. Twaddle and Poon[24] and Olsson and colleagues[25] presented similar outcomes in their randomized study. Wallace and colleagues[26] achieved 2.8% rerupture rate with early functional rehabilitation in nonsurgically treated patients. Surgical complications can be avoided with nonsurgical management with comparable outcomes, according to the previously discussed studies.

Furthermore, functional rehabilitation has the added benefit of improved strength characteristics of healed tendon,[27–34] greater patient satisfaction,[35–39] and improved cartilage nutrition to hindfoot joints with preservation of range of motion.[40] These studies have convinced some surgeons to modify their practice into treating ruptures predominantly nonsurgically.[3,41]

Failure of nonsurgical management is due primarily to improper apposition of tendon stumps. Normal tendon healing response takes place regardless of tendon stump proximity. With elongated Achilles tendon, end-range plantar flexion power is decreased significantly through gastrocnemius-soleus complex.[42] The musculotendinous junction is relatively lengthened and cannot shorten effectively to generate normal plantar flexion power. Weakness with toe-off and fatigue is a common complaint in these patients.

Surgical management relies on complete apposition of tendon stumps to restore tendon length and tension. Effective nonsurgical management relies on similar principals, which is why there are several objective measurements that ensure successful outcome. These measurements utilize magnetic resonance imaging or dynamic ultrasound during initial evaluation. Nonsurgical management is effective if there is less than 5 mm of gap with maximum plantar flexion, less than 10 mm of gap with foot in neutral position, or with greater than 75% tendon apposition with foot in 20° of plantar flexion.[43,44]

Ideal timing for initiation of successful nonsurgical treatment also has been questioned.

Delayed presentation may hinder appropriate apposition of tendon stumps by a well-organized hematoma. Young and colleagues[45] were able to obtain rerupture rates as low as 3% to 5% with casting by excluding patients from nonsurgical management who presented after 72 hours. Another study[46] reported ideal timing for nonsurgical management initiation to be less than 48 hours with inferior outcome with plantar flexion strength after 1 week. The investigators did not comment on ideal treatment between 3 days and to days from injury. Wallace and colleagues[26] reported clinically insignificant rerupture rate with nonsurgical management even with delayed presentation at 2 weeks. Additionally, delayed presentation may lead to more retraction of the tendon ends with interposed hematoma and predispose to rerupture.

Ideal candidates for nonsurgical management include patients with significant medical comorbidities that preclude anesthesia or those who cannot tolerate appropriate positioning required for surgical repair. Patients who have sedentary lifestyle with low-functional demand also may benefit from nonsurgical management.

RATIONALE FOR SURGICAL MANAGEMENT WITH MINIMALLY INVASIVE TECHNIQUE

Historically, nonsurgical management have had significantly higher rerupture rates compared with surgical management; however, surgical management is associated with inherent risks to any surgery as well as increased risk of wound-related complications.[16,20,47–53] Outcomes, in regard to rerupture rates, are not as well defined with integration of functional rehabilitation.[21–26] Even with advent of functional rehabilitation, there are numerous benefits to surgical management that need to be discussed further.

Willits and colleagues[22] randomized 144 patients to either nonsurgical or open surgical repair along with accelerated functional rehabilitation; 72 patients were randomized to nonsurgical treatment group and the other 72 to surgical treatment group. Rerupture occurred in 2 of the surgical treatment group and in 3 of the nonsurgical treatment group. There were 4 superficial infections, 1 deep infection, 2 wound complications, 1 skin puckering, and 1 with hypertrophic scar in the surgical group. None of these complications was found in the nonsurgical treatment group. Deep venous thrombosis (DVT) was present in 1 in surgical and nonsurgical group whereas pulmonary embolism was present in 1 surgical group. Overall, the surgical group had a total of 13 complications compared with 6 in the nonsurgical group. A majority of surgical complications were soft tissue related. Overall, this study demonstrated clinically similar outcomes between 2 managements. At 1-year and 2-year velocity testing, the surgical group demonstrated higher plantar flexion strength ratio at 240°/s compared with the nonsurgical group. The difference was small but statistically significant. Although clinical relevance of this increase in plantar flexion strength may be unclear, it can provide increased power to an athlete. Cetti and colleagues[16] demonstrated a higher rate of resuming sports activities after surgical repair.

Soroceanu and colleagues[23] recently performed a meta-analysis of randomized trials comparing surgical to nonsurgical management demonstrating similar rerupture rates between managements if functional rehabilitation is used. Surgical management did have lower rerupture rate, however, if functional rehabilitation was not used in nonsurgical patients. Additionally, surgical patients returned to work 19.16 days sooner. Earlier return to work with less sick leave absences in surgical compared with nonsurgical patients is a clear benefit in returning patients to routine daily function and has been demonstrated by multiple studies.[16,18,20,39,54]

Olsson and colleagues[25] performed a randomized controlled study involving 100 patients randomized to nonsurgical management and surgical management with open repair followed by an accelerated rehabilitation protocol. No significant difference between groups in terms of symptoms, physical activity level, or quality of life was observed. The surgical group had 0 reruptures compared with the nonsurgical group, with 5; however, this difference was not statistically significant. There were 6 superficial infections in the surgical group all managed with antibiotics without any long-term deficit. In functional testing, the surgical group demonstrated a trend toward superior results; however, significantly superior results in drop countermovement jump and hopping were noted.

Nilsson-Helander and colleagues[21] performed a randomized controlled trial with 49 patients in surgical group and 48 in nonsurgical group. Open surgical repair was used followed by accelerated functional rehabilitation. There were 6 (12%) reruptures in nonsurgical group, as opposed to 2 (4%) in surgical group. This was not statistically significant; however, this may be a function of the relatively small number of patients. The surgical group achieved greater improvement in muscle function test in heel-rise work, heel-rise height, concentric power, and hopping tests at the 6-month evaluation than did the nonsurgical group. There were no differences, however, between groups at the 12-month evaluation, except on the heel-rise work test in which the surgical group performed significantly better than the nonsurgical group. It is possible that surgically managed patients were more confident in their surgical repair and were more aggressive during rehabilitation, resulting in faster improvement in function.

Existing randomized controlled trials comparing surgical and nonsurgical management may not be adequately powered to detect differences in function and overall outcomes. After reviewing the literature and analyzing small important differences, however, surgical management clearly demonstrates increased plantar flexion strength,[22] higher rate of resuming sporting activities,[16] earlier return to work,[16,18,20,23,39,54] superior functional outcome especially in drop countermovement jump and hopping,[25] and faster rehabilitation.[21] Although a majority of these studies do not demonstrate statistically significant difference in rerupture rates, all studies have less number of reruptures in surgical groups compared with nonsurgical groups, and this may be clinically relevant to some surgeons.

A major advantage of surgical management is the ability to approximate the ruptured tendon stumps to re-establish tendon length. With restoration of tendon length, gastrocnemius–soleus–Achilles tendon complex tension and muscle integrity are restored, resulting in improved functional outcome. Surgical management generally is divided into open, percutaneous, and minimally invasive or limited open repair.

Potential complications include superficial and/or deep infection, delayed wound healing, wound necrosis, adhesion formation, sural nerve injury, rerupture, and DVT.

Injury to the sural nerve results in symptoms that can range from simple annoyance to severe pain, resulting in significant debilitation by making routine tasks, such as dressing, finding comfortable shoes, and foot/ankle position, difficult. If a painful neuroma does not respond to conservative management, including medication, desensitization therapy, or nerve blocks, proximal sural nerve excision and burial are recommended. Open repair is associated with as high as 6% sural nerve injury[51]; meanwhile, with percutaneous repair, it has been reported as high as 60%.[55] Minimally invasive techniques with a subparatenon placement of the suture, however, have significantly lower rates of injury compared with both open and percutaneous, as discussed later.

Delayed wound healing can be managed with wet to dry dressing or silver sulfadiazine cream. A larger wound dehiscence occasionally needs a negative-pressure wound therapy to assist with wound closure. Persistently large soft tissue defect after appropriate management warrants plastic surgery involvement for definitive wound coverage.

Superficial wound infection is managed with oral antibiotics if evaluated early. Deep infection is a major complication that has to be managed surgically. In some cases, irrigation and débridement along with intravenous antibiotic are sufficient. In most cases, all infected tissue and foreign material used for repair should be excised. If primary repair is compromised, revision should be performed after infection has been eradicated at a delayed setting. Depending on quality of tendon at time of revision, allograft, fascial augmentation, or flexor hallucis longus tendon transfer may be necessary to augment the repair. Deep infection requiring reconstruction can provide acceptable function; however, it carries morbidity to the patient and high cost to the health care system and does not compare to a successful open repair with regard to function.

Because open surgical repair is associated with high complication rates and potentially devastating outcomes, percutaneous repair techniques were developed. This technique indirectly approximates ruptured tendon stumps without exposure at the rupture site, thereby sparing any violation to paratenon and surrounding soft tissue.

Ma and Griffith[56] initially developed a method of percutaneously repairing Achilles tendon ruptures to create a compromise between nonsurgical and surgical open repair pitfalls. Repair was performed within 3 days of injury under local anesthesia without tourniquet. This technique involves 3 small stab incisions through subcutaneous tissue on medial and lateral aspect of the Achilles tendon followed by passage of nonabsorbable suture through the tendon. The sutures were tied on the medial aspect of the rupture site outside of the paratenon; 18 patients underwent this repair and ankle power was restored to 89% of contralateral lower extremity at 2 years. There were 2 minor complications reported. Both were related to symptomatic suture knot, which resolved after excision of these suture knots. Complications, including superficial and/or deep infection, wound necrosis, and sural nerve injury, were not reported. This was not a randomized study, but it was able to effectively restore tendon function without a formal open approach while avoiding associated complications.

Hockenbury and Johns[55] performed an in vitro study comparing 5 specimens repaired with percutaneous repair using the Ma and Griffith technique and 5 specimens repaired with an open technique in fresh-frozen below-the-knee specimens. Postrepair dissection demonstrated 3 of 5 cadaver specimens having sural nerve entrapment in percutaneous group.

Other percutaneous techniques[57,58] have surfaced in literature since the introduction of the Ma and Griffith technique but are not popularized due to associated complications. Delponte and colleagues[58] developed a modified percutaneous technique by using 2 harpoon-like devices, called Tenolig, FH Orthopedics (Chicago, IL), which are preloaded with sutures, to be inserted approximately 6 cm proximal to rupture site and exit 4 cm to 5 cm distal to the rupture site. The sutures have a metallic barblike structure that adheres to the proximal tendon stump and pulls the tendon distally when the sutures are pulled. When appropriate tension is obtained, the sutures are locked to a metallic disc by a crimper that sits superficial to skin for 6 weeks at exit site. This technique had promising results initially; however, Maes and colleagues[59] demonstrated unusually high complication rates in 124 cases, including unbending of harpoon in 5 cases, wire rupture in 1 case, skin necrosis at entrance wound in 10 cases, tendon rerupture in 12 cases, and sural nerve injury in 8 cases.

There is not abundant literature that compares outcomes between nonoperative and percutaneous repair. Rowley and Scotland[60] compared outcomes in 14 patients who underwent immobilization in equinus position casting and 10 patients who underwent percutaneous repair. No complications were noted in equinus casted patients. One of 10 patients who underwent percutaneous repair suffered from sural nerve entrapment. Patients who were managed with percutaneous repair were more likely to regain nearly normal plantar flexion strength and returned to activity sooner than the group managed with equinus casting. This study does demonstrate percutaneous repair group did functionally better against immobilization group; however, accelerated functional rehabilitation has showed to be a superior nonsurgical management and should ideally be compared to this. There are several studies that compare outcomes of conventional open repair techniques with that of percutaneous.

Haji and colleagues[61] conducted a retrospective analysis comparing 70 open Achilles repairs to 38 modified Ma and Griffith percutaneous repairs. Subjective analysis of functional outcomes demonstrated higher percentage of patients with normal range of motion and higher plantar flexion power in the percutaneously repaired group. There were 4 (5.7%) ruptures in open repair compared with 1 (2.6%) in percutaneous.

Increased deep infections were noted in open repair at 4 (5.7%) compared with 0 (0%) in percutaneous. Decreased sural nerve injury were noted in open repair at 1 (1.4%) compared with 4 (10.5%) in percutaneous. The sural nerve lesions in percutaneous repairs were transient in nature and resolved during the follow-up period.

Recently, Rozis and colleagues[62] performed a prospective study with 82 patients who were randomized into open repair group or percutaneous repair group using the Ma and Griffith technique. The open repair group had 3 (7%) infections whereas percutaneous repair had 0 (0%). There were 2 patients with superficial infection, which were eradicated with oral antibiotics, and 1 patient developed skin necrosis, which necessitated plastic surgery coverage with rotational skin flap. The percutaneous repair group had 3 (7.3%) patients with sural nerve injury and 0 (0%) in open repair group. There were no reruptures in either group.

Compared with open repair, percutaneous techniques did bring the wound-related complication to a negligible amount; however, they do increase iatrogenic injury to the sural nerve. Incidence of sural nerve injury rates after percutaneous repair vary according to literature. Ma and Griffith[56] reported 0 cases of iatrogenic sural nerve injury. Meanwhile, Klein and colleagues[63] used the Ma and Griffith technique in 38 patients and reported 5 (13%) sural nerve entrapment as well as 3 (7.8%) reruptures. Other investigators have noted sural nerve injury rate as low as 7.3%[62] and as high as 60%.[55] Majewski and colleagues[64] published a retrospective case-control study demonstrating how to avoid sural nerve injury during percutaneous repair. A total of 84 patients were retrospectively analyzed at 2 different hospitals undergoing the same percutaneous repair technique, except that the sural nerve was exposed in 1 hospital and sural nerve was not exposed in the other. The overall incidence of sural nerve injury was 18% in the nonexposed group and 0% in the exposed group. Percutaneous repair strength was called into question by Hockenbury and Johns[55] who performed an in vitro biomechanical testing in 5 cadavers after repair demonstrated that tendons that underwent open repair were able to resist almost twice the amount of ankle dorsiflexion (27.6°) before appearance of a 10-mm gap compared with percutaneous repair (14.4°). These results are not clinically relevant because during the early postoperative period, accelerated rehabilitation does not allow for forced dorsiflexion. Cretnik and colleagues[65] performed a biomechanical testing on 36 cadavers demonstrating the modified Ma and Griffith technique having greater tensile strength and gapping resistance compared with the standard Ma and Griffith technique. This does not compare directly open to percutaneous repair strength, but it does demonstrate the modified techniques to have greater mechanical strength immediately after surgery. More recently, Goren and colleagues[66] compared 10 patients with the Ma and Griffith percutaneous repair to 10 patients with open repair. Dynamometer strength evaluation revealed 16% loss of strength in percutaneous group and 18.2% in open group compared with the contralateral side. Even if the rate of sural nerve injury can be minimized by exposing sural nerve and comparable repair strength can be obtained by integrating a different technique, another major drawback of percutaneous technique is its inability to visualize direct apposition of ruptured stumps, which can potentially result in malalignment of tendon stumps.

Both open and percutaneous repair techniques provide similar functional outcome. The major difference lies in that open repair is much more destructive to soft tissue that may account for the significant thickening associated with the repair and the deep wound complication rate. Percutaneous techniques provide soft tissue friendly repair, but it has its own unique complications with sural nerve injury and inability to visualize tendon apposition. Minimally invasive repair techniques take the benefit of both the open and percutaneous techniques while minimizing their associated complications.

Amlang and colleagues[57] developed a technique where a Dresden instrument was inserted 2 cm to 3 cm proximal to rupture site through a small incision. The instrument was advanced distal to rupture site between fascia cruris and paratenon. Sutures were inserted percutaneously through this instrument and pulled out through proximal incision. After appropriate tension was obtained, the sutures were tied in the proximal portion of the rupture. The investigators claimed 2 of 62 cases having reruptures and 0 cases of sural nerve injury with 62% with very good outcomes. Keller and colleagues[67] also demonstrated favorable outcomes with 100 percutaneous repairs with Dresden technique. This technique has garnered a significant following in Europe and South America.

Kakiuchi[68] took advantage of best aspects from open and percutaneous repair techniques and applied them to a newer technique, where looped Kirschner wires were inserted deep to paratenon from the tendon rupture site using a limited open incision. This allowed sutures to be placed deep to paratenon and retrieved from the ruptured site. With this technique, there was decreased chance of injury to the sural nerve and direct visualization of end-to-end tendon apposition at repair site. With increased functional outcomes[69] along with minimal wound and sural nerve complication rates compared with open and percutaneous repair, this technique laid the foundation for current minimally invasive repair techniques.

Assal and colleagues[70] developed the Achillon (Integra LifeSciences, Plainsboro, New Jersey) device based on Kakiuchi's technique. This device is a guiding instrument with inner and outer corresponding arms. This instrument is inserted deep to paratenon around the Achilles tendon from the rupture site using a 2-cm longitudinal incision. When the instrument is around proximal ruptured stump, 3 sutures are passed and instrument is removed, leaving 6 suture strands exiting from the incision. The same is done for distal tendon stump using same incision. After appropriate tension is achieved, the sutures are tied to each other in a proximal to distal fashion creating 3 box suture configurations. In 82 patients, there were 0 cases of wound complications, 0 cases of infection, 0 sural nerve disturbances, and 3 reruptures. Two patients were noncompliant with postoperative protocol and a third patient fell at 12 weeks. Mean AOFAS score at 26-month follow-up was 96 points and all patients returned to previous work/sporting activities. There was no significant difference in the mean number of single-limb hops and plantar flexion strength between injured and uninjured sides.

Calder and Saxby[71] published outcome in 46 repairs with Achillon. There was 1 superficial wound infection, which subsided after oral antibiotics; 2 cases of temporary sural nerve paresthesias, which resolved spontaneously at 3 months; and 0 reruptures. An average American Orthopaedic Foot & Ankle Society score of 98.4 was obtained and all patients returned to previous levels of sporting activities by 6 months. They suggested Achilles repair allowed active mobilization and earlier return to sporting activities.

Several studies were published comparing outcomes between Achillon and open repairs.[72–76] Atkas and Kocaoglu[72] prospectively analyzed outcomes in 40 patients. There was no significant difference in AOFAS score at 22.4-month follow-up. Local tenderness, skin adhesions, and scar and tendon thickness were better in the Achillon group. In the Achillon group, there was 0 reruptures, 0 sural nerve injuries, 0 superficial or deep infections, and 0 adhesions. Bhattacharyya and Gerber[74] prospectively compared 59 patients and showed decreased operating time, less bed usage, less consumption of postoperative analgesics, fewer associated indirect costs to the health care provider, and no postoperative morbidity. In the Achillon group, there were 0 reruptures, 0 sural nerve injuries, 0 superficial or deep infections, and 0 adhesions. Kolodziej and colleagues[75] randomized 47 patients and were able to demonstrate 0 reruptures, 0 sural nerve injuries, 0 deep infections, 1 superficial infection, and 0 adhesions. Valencia and Alcalá[76] demonstrated 0 reruptures, 0 sural nerve injuries, 0 superficial or deep infections, and 1 adhesion in the Achillon group. More recently, a meta-analysis by Alcelik and colleagues[73] demonstrated similar outcomes.

To assess strength, Ismail and colleagues[77] compared pull-out strength of Achillon and Kessler repairs in ovine (sheep) tendons. Mean load to failure with 3-strand Achillon repair was 153 N ± 60 N and in Kessler repair was 123 N ± 24 N. This demonstrates that the Achillon system is capable of producing a biomechanically sound repair. Huffard and colleagues[78] demonstrated similar results in 10 cadavers when compared Krackow suture configuration to Achillon. Mean load to failure in Krackow suture configuration was 276 N; meanwhile, it was 342 N in Achillon. Similar results were demonstrated by Heitman and colleagues.[79]

Achillon was able to effectively provide benefits of percutaneous repair without the complications of open repair, but there were some deficiencies. The jig is not very stout and has a risk of missing needle passes through bending moment because it was made out of polycarbonate. It is a single-use device that resulted in increased cost to health care system. The jig is straight and nonanatomic by design. As a result of the design, occasionally, it is difficult to pass around the torn tendon stump while pulling counterpressure. All 3 sutures pass through the tendon in the same transverse plane predisposing it to early failure through suture cut-out. Lastly, all sutures were sliding suture and there was no option of locking suture construct. In 2010, a newer instrumentation, called Percutaneous Achilles Repair System (PARS) (Arthrex, Naples, Florida), was developed by making improvements on these shortcomings. The PARS jig is metallic and nondisposable to save costs to health care. The metallic characteristic makes it stout and less prone to bending during passage, decreasing the risk of the needles missing the inner arms of the jig. Its design is more anatomic with anterior contour, which easily glides around the tendon stumps while applying counterpressure. Lastly, there is possibility of inserting up to 7 different sutures at once in multiple planes with an option of making all sutures transverse or up to 2 locked suture configurations.

To date, there has only been 1 study published comparing outcomes between PARS to open repair. Hsu and colleagues[80] retrospectively reviewed 101 PARS to 169 open repair patients. It demonstrated a greater number of patients returning to baseline physical activities by 5 months in PARS (98%) compared with the open group (82%). In the open group, there were 0 reruptures, 0 DVT, 5 cases (3%) of sural neuritis, 7 cases (4%) of superficial wound dehiscence, 3 cases (2%) of superficial infection, and 3 reoperations (2%) for deep infection. In the PARS group, there were 0 reruptures, 0 cases of sural neuritis, 0 cases of DVT, 3 cases (3%) of superficial wound dehiscence, and 2 operations (2%) for superficial foreign-body reaction to FiberWire, Arthrex (Naples, FL) without concurrent infection. Overall, the complication rates in the open group were 10.6% (18 cases) and 5.0% (5 cases) in PARS group.

Several biomechanical tests have been published demonstrating superior construct strength of PARS. Demetracopoulos and colleagues[81] compared strength of minimally invasive repair using nonlocking sutures (Achillon) to a combination of locking and nonlocking sutures (PARS) in 31 cadavers. It was clearly demonstrated that locking suture construct was able to without more cyclical loading prior to detection of 2-mm and 9.5-mm tendon gaps as well as withstanding significantly greater load to failure compared with a nonlocking suture construct (299.6 N vs 385 N). Recently, Dekker and colleagues[82] biomechanically compared Krackow suture construct to limited open repair using PARS in 18 cadavers. Average load to failure was 353.6 N in the open group compared with 313.3 N in the PARS group, which was not statistically significant. Mean initial linear clinical findings since testing is done representing the immediate intraoperative repair; meanwhile, it is a known that early motion along with progressive loading increased tendon strength.

Another advantage of minimally invasive repair is cosmesis. Although this may not directly improve functional outcome, patient satisfaction is increased if similar outcomes are provided with smaller incision. Del Buono and colleagues[83] performed a systematic review of 12 studies comparing open and minimally invasive repairs in 781 patients. They reported 3.4-cm average length of incision for the minimally invasive group compared with 12 cm for the open repair group (**Fig. 1**).

Appropriate selection and meticulous surgical techniques maximize functional outcomes while minimizing complications. Repair is advocated in all active patients if optimum performance is desired. It should be used in athletes and in patients who have high activity level. Nonsurgical management is reserved for older (over 60), sedentary, or debilitated patients. Minimally invasive surgery provides benefits of functional outcome that is obtained with open surgical approach without the soft tissue complications. With advances in surgical instrumentations and techniques, minimally invasive Achilles tendon repair has provided sufficient data to justify its use for repairs. Minimally invasive repair has definitively demonstrated superior overall outcomes with decreased surgical complications compared with open repair. Because there is no agreed-on treatment regimen, the choice of treatment is based largely on preference of surgeon and the patient; however, the authors believe, based on their experience and the evidence provided by the literature, that minimally invasive repair techniques should be the new gold standard treatment of acute midsubstance Achilles tendon ruptures. Regardless of surgical technique that is chosen, a functional rehabilitation protocol is advocated to maximize the functional outcome (**Table 1**).

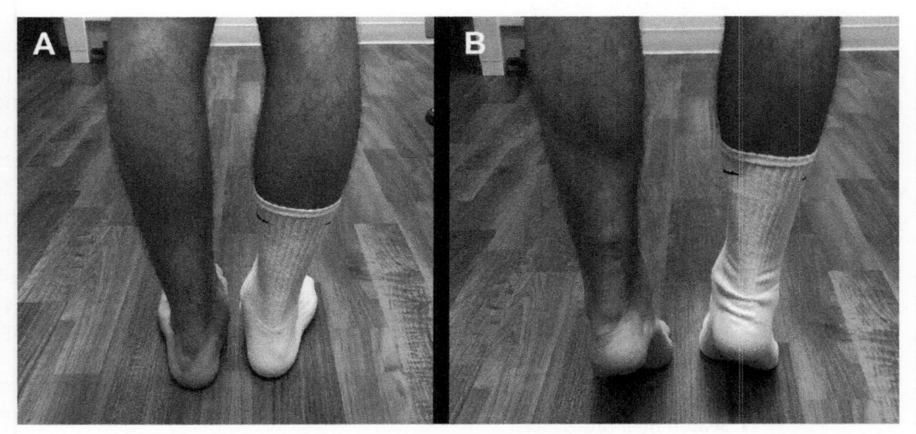

Fig. 1. A 3-month postoperative photograph after PARS repair of an acute Achilles tendon rupture (*A* - at neutral, *B* - plantarflexion). Note the minimal thickening and the ability to perform a double limb heel rise with minimal calf atrophy seen.

Table 1
Postoperative functional rehabilitation protocol

Week 0–2	• Non–weight-bearing splint in place
Week 2	• Postoperative splint is removed and removable boot is applied with heel lifts to maintain 20° plantar flexion. • Weight bearing is initiated and progressed as tolerated • Soft tissue/scar mobilization • ROM exercise: plantar flexion/dorsiflexion from 20° to full plantar flexion, 2 sets of 20 repetitions; circumduction (both directions), 2 sets of 10 repetitions • Strengthening exercise: isometric inversion/eversion, 2 sets of 10 repetitions with ankle at 20° of plantar flexion; toe curls with towel and weight; hamstring curls in prone with boot on for resistance, 2 sets of 10 repetitions • Cryotherapy
Week 3	• Progress weight bearing to full weight as tolerated in boot with 2 heel lifts. • Soft tissue/scar mobilization • Begin stationary bike in boot with low resistance. • Aqua therapy may begin without any weight bearing by using a flotation device. ROM, walking, or running in the water is done to preserve fitness level. Aqua therapy is not necessary but, if available, may be used. • ROM exercise: continue as before; may progress to gentle stretch to neutral ankle position with use of strap or towel • Strengthening: isometric inversion/eversion, dorsiflexion/plantar flexion 2 sets of 10 repetitions to progress to 2 sets of 20 repetitions over the course of week 3; begin light band–resisted inversion, eversion, dorsiflexion, and plantar flexion, 2 sets of 10 repetitions. Prone knee flexion, 2 sets of 20 repetitions • Cryotherapy
Weeks 4–6	• Weight bearing to full in boot brace with heel lift • Take 1 lift out at week 5. • Take the other lift out at week 6; therefore, at 6 weeks should be in the boot with no lifts. • Gentle cross-fiber massage to Achilles tendon • Ultrasound, phonophoresis, electrical stimulation used to decrease inflammation and scar formation. • Stationary bike up to 20 minutes, with minimal resistance and aqua therapy as outlined in week 3 • Gentle stretching of Achilles tendon with towel or in standing (if limited to less than neutral position only). Stretch with knee extended and flexed to 40°. • Strengthening: isometric exercise as on week 3; increase resistive band exercise for plantar flexion, dorsiflexion, inversion, and eversion; 3 sets of 20 repetitions. • Hamstring curls to facilitate gastrocnemius muscle without flexing the ankle. May be done in prone or standing with light resistance; 3 sets of 20 repetitions
Weeks 6–7	• Patient progresses from boot to shoe with heel lift. • Stationary bike without boot and with progressive resistance • Gentle stretching exercise to neutral ankle position • BTE passive ROM, isometric, and isotonic exercise • Weight shifting and unilateral balance exercise seated on therapeutic ball • Closed chain, partial weight-bearing strengthening of plantar flexors (neutral through full plantar flexion) • Seated heel raises • Total gym heel raises (low angle)

(*continued on next page*)

Table 1 (*continued*)	
	• Hamstring curls with light resistance • Open chain strengthening of foot and ankle musculature band (light to medium resistance) • Gait training with concentration on weight shifting heel to toe over involved foot and side to side weight shifting • Begin stair stepper with involved limb only. • Aqua therapy (especially good for obese patients to initiate weight bearing activity and athletes to maintain conditioning): walking in water (waist deep or greater), standing heel raises (water at least waist deep or greater), flutter kick with kick board (with or without fins as tolerated), conditioning exercise • Soft tissue mobilization • Modalities to control edema and pain
Weeks 8–9	• Patient is wearing shoe full time with heel lift • Stationary bike—increased resistance and time • Gentle stretching up to neutral ankle dorsiflexion if needed • Gait training—step over progressively higher steps as able • BTE isotonic and isometric exercise for plantar flexion strengthening (eccentric bias) • Band-resisted inversion and eversion in seated position with foot flat on the floor and band around ankle • Band-resisted dorsiflexion (open chain) • Total gym with increased angle for heel raises and short arc squats. Begin unilateral eccentric plantar flexion exercise. • Short arc squats in standing • Hamstring curls (progressive resisted exercise) • Progress to standing heel raises using uninvolved LE to assist involved LE • Progress to standing balance exercise in tandem and then single-leg support • Aqua therapy (obese patients may progress more slowly and refine ambulation quality in pool): walking in water, standing heel raises (water at least waist deep), flutter kick with kick board (with or without fins), plyometrics, conditioning exercise

Weeks 10–12	• Patient wearing shoe without lift
	• Stationary bike (warm up and/or aerobic conditioning)
	• Gentle stretching in standing past neutral
	• BTE strengthening
	• Standing balance exercise with/without eyes closed
	• Perturbation
	  ○ BOSU ball
	  ○ Airex pad
	  ○ Band resist
	  ○ Ball toss
	• Squats with moderated resistance (limit ankle dorsiflexion)
	• Hamstring curls with resistance
	• Standing heel raises (2 feet with progression to single limb for eccentric strengthening, then eccentric/concentric strengthening as able)
	• Total gym single-heel raise
	• Resisted walking: free motion machine, pulleys, bands
	• Elliptical trainer
	• Aqua therapy (for obese patients to progress walking tolerance and endurance, heel raises and aerobic conditioning; for athletes to progress plyometrics and aerobic conditioning)

(*continued on next page*)

Table 1 (*continued*)	
Weeks 12–14	• Stationary bike (warm up and/or aerobic conditioning) • Gentle stretching • Balance exercise with perturbation in single limb support unless within normal limits and equal bilaterally • Resisted bilateral heel rises with free motion, calf machine • Unilateral heel rises if able or eccentric unilateral heel rises • Elliptical trainer
Week 14 and beyond	• If patient is able to perform a single leg heel rise 10 times and has low pain rating may progress to ○ Stair stepper ○ Plyometrics training (begin with 1 feet and progress to single-limb jumps) ○ Jogging—slow speed and limited distance, with progression as symptoms permit

Abbreviations: LE, lower extremity; ROM, range of motion.

AUTHORS' PREFERRED TECHNIQUES FOR MINIMALLY INVASIVE ACHILLES REPAIR

Percutaneous Achilles Repair System

Indications

- Primary repair of Achilles tendon rupture occurring approximately 2 cm to 7 cm proximal to calcaneal insertion
- Acute Achilles tendon ruptures (<3 weeks) are ideal with this technique. Tears that are older than 3 weeks are amenable with this technique as long as scar tissue adhesions between tendon and paratenon are freed up and tendon is mobilized adequately.

Contraindications

- Insertional Achilles tendon ruptures are not amenable to be repaired with this technique and the use the Midsubstance SpeedBridge (Arthrex) technique is preferred.
- Chronic Achilles tendon ruptures of greater than 6 weeks occasionally require additional procedures to augment repair, which is routinely performed through an open approach.

Equipment

- PARS jig and PARS suture system

Patient positioning

- General or regional anesthesia can be used, although regional is preferred when feasible. The authors do not use a tourniquet; however, if desired, the tourniquet should be placed on the thigh, not the calf, to avoid limiting the excursion of the gastrocnemius-soleus complex.
- This technique is performed with patient in prone position. The affected extremity is at the edge of the table and propped up with blankets so it is sitting higher than contralateral extremity. Passing of needles through the PARS jig is easier with affected extremity positioned higher.

Surgical technique

- A 2-cm longitudinal incision is made paramedially, beginning 1 cm proximal to distal stump extending superiorly. This can be extended proximally or distally as required. A transverse incision is another alternative; however, a Z-shaped extension of incision is required if more visualization is needed proximally or distally. Given the ability to plantar flex the foot that allows the distal stump to be delivered into the wound, the incision is ideally based at the level of the proximal stump (**Fig. 2**).

- Skin hooks are used for retraction to minimize damage to skin with pickups. Paratenon is sharply incised followed by blunt dissection.
- A finger or freer elevator is used for blunt dissection to free up any adhesions at the proximal and distal stumps.
- An Allis clamp is used to grasp proximal stump within the paratenon and pulled longitudinally through the incision (**Fig. 3**). Occasionally, a second Allis clamp can be used to grasp the tendon more proximally while pulling on the first Allis clamp to grasp better quality tendon. If questioning whether the proximal stump is grasped adequately, a hand can be placed over the calf while tugging on an Allis clamp and the gastrocnemius-soleus complex should be palpated and distal translation should be noted.
- The PARS jig is now inserted into the proximal paratenon sheath with the inner arms around the proximal stump. Once the arms are within the paratenon sheath, the arms are opened up progressively and advanced proximally while keeping counterpressure on the Allis clamp.
- If the inner arms are correctly positioned next to the tendon, the outer aiming arms should be positioned in the posterior one-fourth of the leg longitudinally

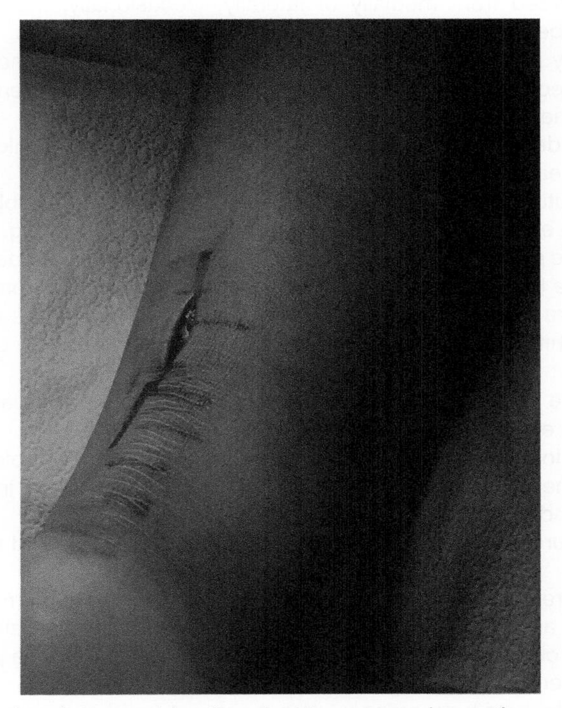

Fig. 2. Patient is placed prone with a 2-cm incision centered over the proximal stump. On first utilizing this technique, a larger incision can be used; however, with repeated use, the incision can be routinely made less than 2 cm.

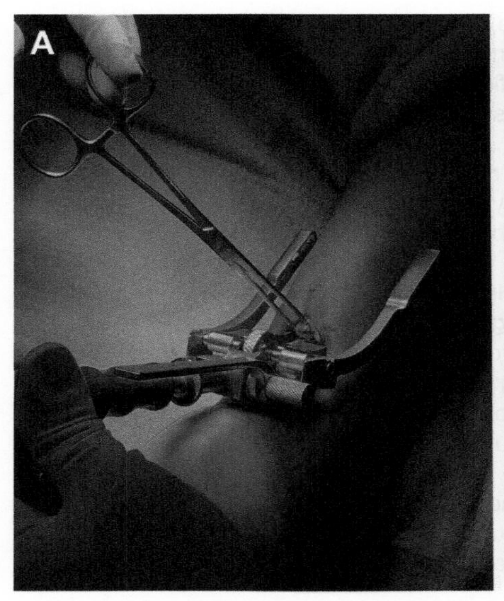

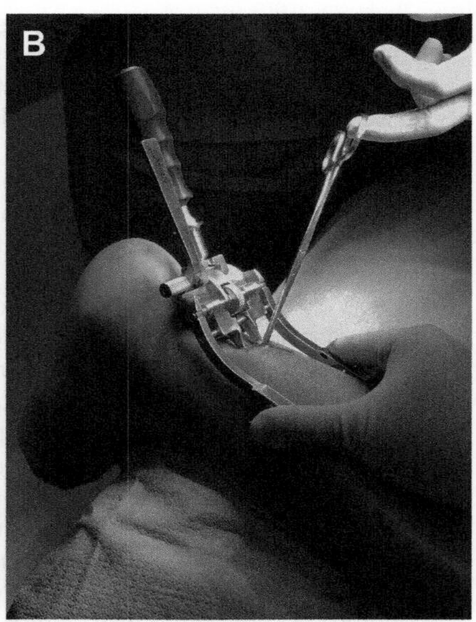

Fig. 3. An Allis clamp is utilized to hold tension while the PARS jig is inserted (*A* - inferior view, *B* - superior view).

when visualized from medially or laterally. Occasionally, the Achilles tendon stump can be easily palpated sitting between the 2 inner arms.

- While gently pulling on the Allis clamp and the jig in neutral position, a suture passing needle is inserted through hole 1. This needle essentially locks the tendon to the jig and is left in this position.
- A bump made out of stacked towel can be placed under the ankle to make needle passes easier.
- A second suture passing needle is passed through hole 2. Pass blue/white suture through the eyelet and the needle is pulled out from hole 2 (**Fig. 4**).
- Same suture passing needle is passed through hole 3. Pass looped end of green/white suture through the eyelet and the needle is pulled out from hole 3.
- Same suture passing needle is passed through hole 4. Pass nonlooped end of green/white suture through the eyelet and the needle is pulled out from hole 4.
- Same suture passing needle is passed through hole 5. Pass black/white suture through the eyelet and the needle is pulled out from hole 5.
- If a second locked suture is desired, black/white suture from hole 5 can be used in this manner by passing looped sutures through hole 6 and 7 in similar fashion as hole 3 and 4.
- A white suture is passed through eyelet of needle in hole 1 and needle is pulled out (**Fig. 5**).
- PARS jig is retracted out of the wound while closing the inner arms. This ensures the sutures are through the tendon and within the paratenon sheath. Once the sutures are out of the wound, carefully pull out sutures from the jig and organize them in order they were inserted.
- On each side, hold both green/white sutures in 1 hand and pass the blue suture around the 2 green/white sutures twice and pass end of blue suture through the loop.

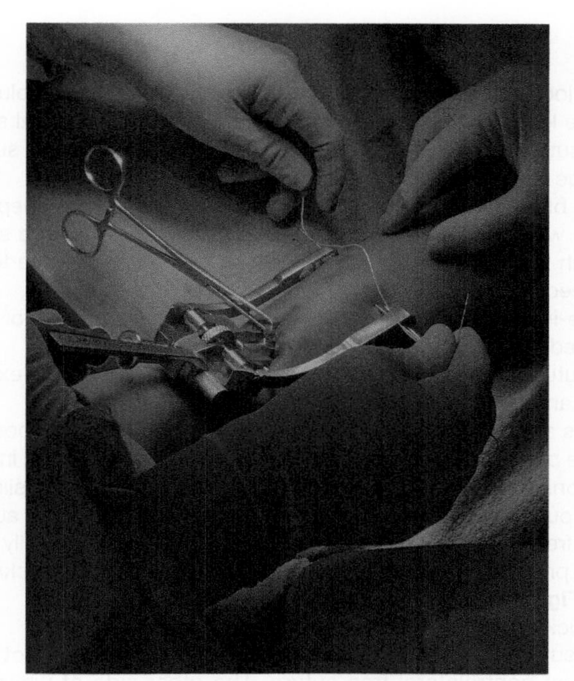

Fig. 4. The first needle is left in place allowing the PARS jig to hold the position of the proximal stump. The second suture is passed with ease, followed by the remaining 4 sutures in sequential order.

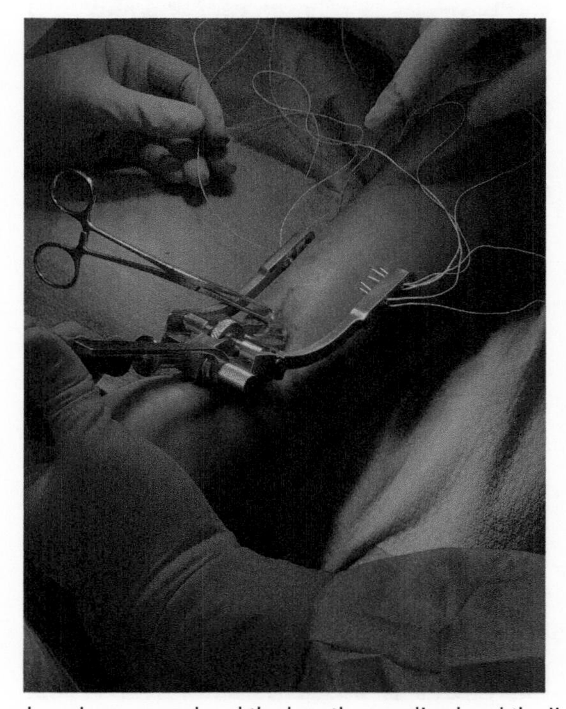

Fig. 5. All 5 sutures have been passed and the lengths equalized and the jig is then removed followed by locking of the central suture.

- Pull the unlooped green/white suture on each side while the blue suture is still through the loop. This pulls the blue suture to the contralateral side and create a locking suture construct. Make sure not to dispose looped sutures because these will be used for distal stump.
- Pull on the blue sutures to remove any slack and minimize creep.
- Pull on the white and black/white suture individually to ensure suture does not pull through tendon. If either suture pulls out, the jig is reinserted and suture-passing needle is passed with its designated suture.
- The jig is re-inserted into the distal stump and the same order for suture passing is conducted as detailed for the proximal stump.
- Once all sutures are passed, there should be 3 sutures with excellent tension proximally and distally on each side (**Fig. 6**).
- The sutures are tied down with the foot held in plantar flexed position by an assistant. The black/white sutures are tied on 1 side of the tendon initially. Because this is a nonlocked suture, the knot on the tied side can be slid proximally or distally by pulling on the free suture on contralateral side. The authors prefer to pull on the free suture to pull knot on contralateral side proximally into the wound so it is not prominent under the incision. The other side of black/white suture is tied next (**Fig. 7**).
- The blue locking sutures are tied on both sides.
- The white suture is tied on 1 side followed by shuttling the knot more proximal by pulling on contralateral free suture. The other side of white suture is tied next.

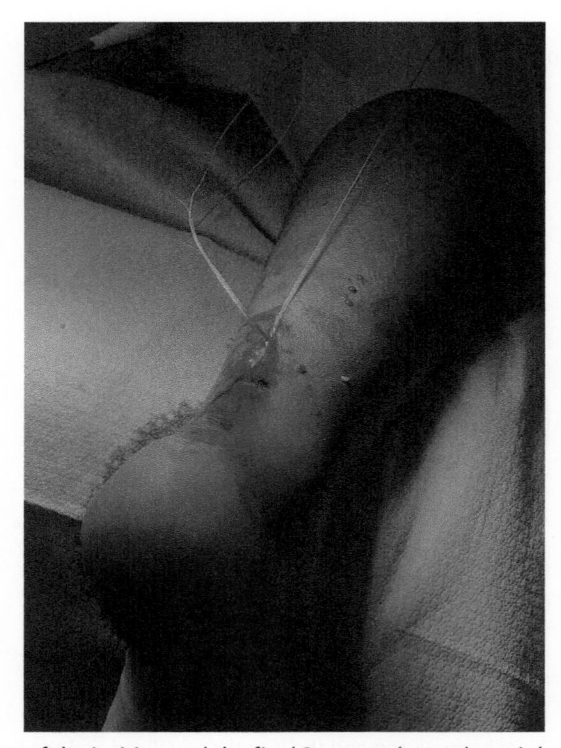

Fig. 6. Appearance of the incision and the final 3 sutures (central one is locked) securing the proximal stump.

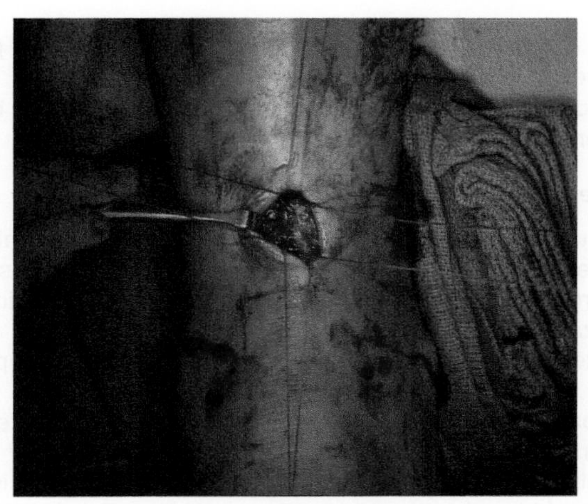

Fig. 7. Visualization of tendon apposition during placement of the knots to complete the repair. The ability to visualize the apposition of the tendon without requiring a large soft tissue exposure is a key advantage of this technique compared with an open or percutaneous approach.

- The repair is tested by restoration of Thompson test and with moderate dorsiflexion pressure on the foot. If the repair fails with gentle pressure or there is no plantar flexion with calf squeeze, the quality of the repair should be reevaluated and revised if needed.
- Paratenon is approximated with 2-0 Vicryl suture.
- Subcutaneous tissue is approximated with 3-0 Monocryl suture.
- Skin is approximated with 3-0 nylon suture.

Midsubstance Speed Bridge Repair

Indications

- Primary repair of Achilles tendon rupture occurring approximately 1 cm to 7 cm proximal to calcaneal insertion.
- Acute Achilles tendon ruptures (<3 weeks) are ideal with this technique. Tears that are older than 3 weeks are amenable with this technique as long as scar tissue adhesions between tendon and paratenon are freed up and tendon is mobilized adequately.

Contraindications

- Chronic Achilles tendon ruptures of greater than 6 weeks occasionally require additional procedures to augment repair, which is routinely performed through an open approach.

Equipment

- PARS jig and PARS suture system
- Achilles Midsubstance SpeedBridge system

Patient positioning

- General or regional anesthesia can be used.
- This technique is performed with patient in prone position. The affected extremity is at the edge of the table and propped up with blankets so it is sitting higher than

contralateral extremity. Passing of needles through the PARS jig is easier with affected extremity positioned higher.
- The authors do not use a tourniquet, but a thigh tourniquet can be used per surgeon preference.

Surgical technique

- A 3-cm longitudinal incision is made paramedially 1 cm proximal to distal stump. This can be extended proximally or distally as required. A transverse incision is another alternative; however, a Z-shaped extension of incision is required if more visualization is needed proximally or distally.
- The PARS technique is used in the proximal tendon stump, as described previously.
- A stab incision is made over the calcaneus on the medial and lateral aspect of the Achilles insertion site.
- A 3.4-mm drill bit is used to create anchor point at these stab incisions. Trajectory of the drill should be distally and toward the midline. Bony debride in these anchor points is irrigated with fluid.
- These holes are then tapped with 4.75-mm Bio-SwiveLock (Arthrex) anchors.
- A Banana SutureLasso (Arthrex) tip is passed retrograde via these stab incisions passing through medial and lateral aspect of the distal tendon stump (**Fig. 8**).
- The nitinol wire loop is advanced within the Banana SutureLasso to allow passage of proximal sutures.
- The Banana SutureLasso and the nitinol wire are pulled simultaneously out from the distal stab incisions. This delivers proximal suture through the stab incisions. The same is done for opposite side.
- While applying maximal tension across the sutures, the ankle is cycled through dorsiflexion and plantar flexion approximately 10 times to minimize any creep from suture. Tendon apposition should be noted (**Fig. 9**).
- All 3 sutures are passed through Bio-SwiveLock eyelet on each side. While the assistant holds the ankle in a plantar-flexed position, so that 2 tendon stumps

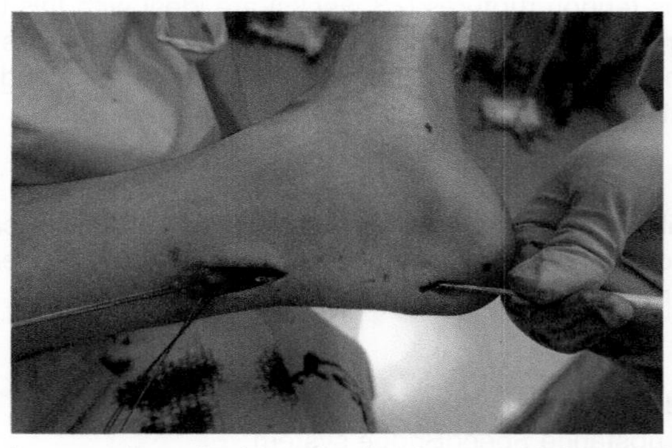

Fig. 8. Passage of the curved needle from the distal aspect of the Achilles tendon. Ideally, the needle should pass through the stump of the tendon, one passage is medial and the other lateral. By passing the needle through the distal stump, this may decrease the risk of over-tightening the tendon because the tendons edges engage each other as opposed to sliding on top of each other if the suture was placed either anterior or posterior to the tendon.

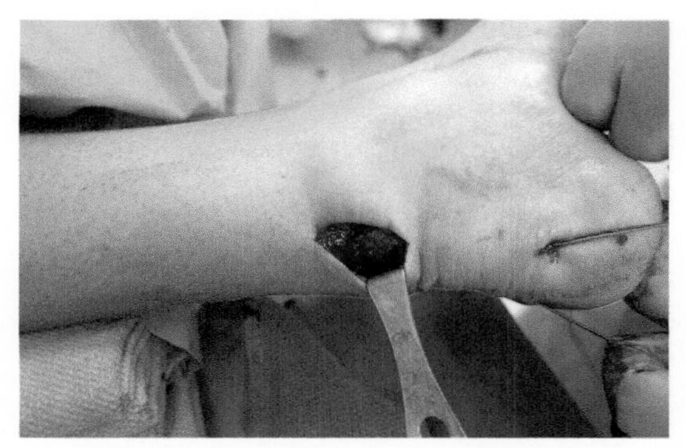

Fig. 9. With tension placed on the distal ends of the suture and slight plantar flexion of the limb, direct tendon apposition can be seen.

are opposed, and applies tension on opposite side sutures, the Bio-SwiveLock anchor is inserted into the anchor hole. Opposite side anchor is inserted in the same manner (**Fig. 10**).

- The repair is tested by restoration of the Thompson test.
- Paratenon is approximated with 2-0 Vicryl suture.
- Subcutaneous tissue is approximated with 3-0 Monocryl suture.
- Skin is approximated with 3-0 nylon suture (**Fig. 11**).

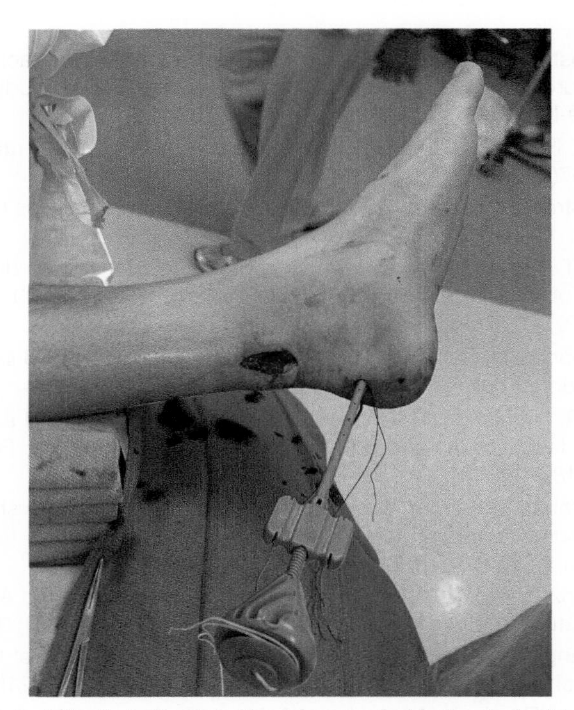

Fig. 10. Placement of the SwivelLock in the calcaneus holds the desired tension and maintains tendon apposition without the need knots at the level of the rupture.

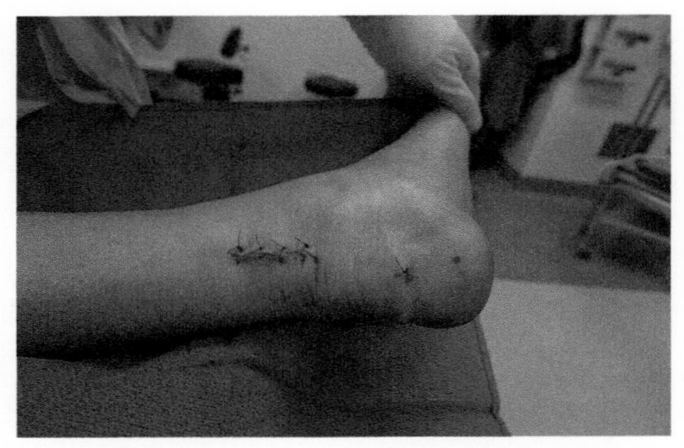

Fig. 11. Final appearance of the repair with dorsiflexion pressure placed on the foot, noting excellent final tension and stability of the construct.

REFERENCES

1. Gwynne-Jones DP, Sims M. Epidemiology and outcomes of acute achilles tendon rupture with operative or nonoperative treatment using an identical functional bracing protocol. Foot Ankle Int 2011;32(4):337–43.
2. Maffulli N, Waterston SW, Squair J, et al. Changing incidence of Achilles tendon rupture in Scotland: a 15-year study. Clin J Sport Med 1999;9(3):157–60.
3. Huttunen TT, Kannus P, Rolf C, et al. Acute Achilles tendon ruptures: incidence of injury and surgery in Sweden between 2001 and 2012. Am J Sports Med 2014;42(10):2419–23.
4. Jozsa L, Kvist M, Balint BJ, et al. The role of recreational sport activity in Achilles tendon rupture: a clinical, pathoanatomical, and sociological study of 292 cases. Am J Sports Med 1989;17(3):338–43.
5. Leppilahti J, Puranen J, Orava S. Incidence of Achilles tendon rupture. Acta Orthop 1996;67(3):277–9.
6. Möller A, Åström M, Westlin NE. Increasing incidence of Achilles tendon rupture. Acta Orthop 1996;67(5):479–81.
7. Nyyssönen T, Lüthje P, Kröger H. The increasing incidence and difference in sex distribution of Achilles tendon rupture in Finland in 1987–1999. Scand J Surg 2008;97(3):272–5.
8. Webb J, Moorjani N, Radford M. Anatomy of the sural nerve and its relation to the Achilles tendon. Foot Ankle Int 2000;21(6):475–7.
9. Carmont MR, Highland AM, Rochester JR, et al. An anatomical and radiological study of the fascia cruris and paratenon of the Achilles tendon. Foot Ankle Surg 2011;17(3):186–92.
10. Porter KJ, Robati S, Karia P, et al. An anatomical and cadaveric study examining the risk of sural nerve injury in percutaneous Achilles tendon repair using the Achillon device. Foot Ankle Surg 2014;20(2):90–3.
11. Chen TM, Rozen WM, Pan WR, et al. The arterial anatomy of the Achilles tendon: anatomical study and clinical implications. Clin Anat 2009;22(3):377–85.
12. Yepes H, Tang M, Geddes C, et al. Digital vascular mapping of the integument about the Achilles tendon. J Bone Joint Surg Am 2010;92(5):1215–20.
13. Poynton AR, O'Rourke K. An analysis of skin perfusion over the Achilles tendon in varying degrees of plantarflexion. Foot Ankle Int 2001;22(7):572–4.

14. Carr AJ, Norris SH. The blood supply of the calcaneal tendon. J Bone Joint Surg Br 1989;71(1):100–1.
15. Müller SA, Evans CH, Heisterbach PE, et al. The role of the paratenon in Achilles tendon healing: a study in rats. Am J Sports Med 2018;46(5):1214–9.
16. Cetti R, Christensen SE, Ejsted R, et al. Operative versus nonoperative treatment of Achilles tendon rupture: a prospective randomized study and review of the literature. Am J Sports Med 1993;21(6):791–9.
17. Coombs RH. Prospective trial of conservative and surgical treatment of Achilles tendon rupture. J Bone Joint Surg Br 1981;63:288.
18. Majewski M, Rickert M, Steinbrück K. Achilles tendon rupture. A prospective trial assessing various treatment possibilities. Orthopade 2000;29(7):670–6.
19. Nistor LA. Surgical and non-surgical treatment of Achilles Tendon rupture. A prospective randomized study. J Bone Joint Surg Am 1981;63(3):394–9.
20. Möller M, Movin T, Granhed H, et al. Acute rupture of tendo Achillis: a prospective, randomised study of comparison between surgical and non-surgical treatment. J Bone Joint Surg Br 2001;83(6):843–8.
21. Nilsson-Helander K, Grävare Silbernagel K, Thomee R, et al. Acute Achilles tendon rupture: a randomized, controlled study comparing surgical and nonsurgical treatments using validated outcome measures. Am J Sports Med 2010; 38(11):2186–93.
22. Willits K, Amendola A, Bryant D, et al. Operative versus nonoperative treatment of acute Achilles tendon ruptures: a multicenter randomized trial using accelerated functional rehabilitation. J Bone Joint Surg Am 2010;92(17):2767–75.
23. Soroceanu A, Sidhwa F, Aarabi S, et al. Surgical versus nonsurgical treatment of acute Achilles tendon rupture: a meta-analysis of randomized trials. J Bone Joint Surg Am 2012;94:2136–43.
24. Twaddle BC, Poon P. Early motion for Achilles tendon ruptures: is surgery important? A randomized, prospective study. Am J Sports Med 2007;35(12):2033–8.
25. Olsson N, Silbernagel KG, Eriksson BI, et al. Stable surgical repair with accelerated rehabilitation versus nonsurgical treatment for acute Achilles tendon ruptures: a randomized controlled study. Am J Sports Med 2013;41(12):2867–76.
26. Wallace RG, Heyes GJ, Michael AL. The non-operative functional management of patients with a rupture of the tendo Achillis leads to low rates of re-rupture. J Bone Joint Surg Br 2011;93(10):1362–6.
27. Eliasson P, Andersson T, Aspenberg P. Achilles tendon healing in rats is improved by intermittent mechanical loading during the inflammatory phase. J Orthop Res 2012;30(2):274–9.
28. Enwemeka CS, Spielholz NI, Nelson AJ. The effect of early functional activities on experimentally tenotomized Achilles tendons in rats. Am J Phys Med Rehabil 1988;67(6):264–9.
29. Gelberman RH, Woo SL, Lothringer K, et al. Effects of early intermittent passive mobilization on healing canine flexor tendons. J Hand Surg Am 1982;7(2):170–5.
30. Hammerman M, Aspenberg P, Eliasson P. Microtrauma stimulates rat Achilles tendon healing via an early gene expression pattern similar to mechanical loading. J Appl Physiol 2013;116(1):54–60.
31. Michna H, Hartmann G. Adaptation of tendon collagen to exercise. Int Orthop 1989;13(3):161–5.
32. Mosler E, Folkhard W, Knörzer E, et al. Stress-induced molecular rearrangement in tendon collagen. J Mol Biol 1985;182(4):589–96.

33. Schepull T, Aspenberg P. Early controlled tension improves the material properties of healing human achilles tendons after ruptures: a randomized trial. Am J Sports Med 2013;41(11):2550–7.
34. Woo SL, Gelberman RH, Cobb NG, et al. The importance of controlled passive mobilization on flexor tendon healing: a biomechanical study. Acta Orthop Scand 1981;52(6):615–22.
35. Barfod KW, Bencke J, Lauridsen HB, et al. Nonoperative, dynamic treatment of acute achilles tendon rupture: influence of early weightbearing on biomechanical properties of the plantar flexor muscle–tendon complex—a blinded, randomized, controlled trial. J Foot Ankle Surg 2015;54(2):220–6.
36. Costa ML, MacMillan K, Halliday D, et al. Randomised controlled trials of immediate weight-bearing mobilisation for rupture of the tendo Achillis. J Bone Joint Surg Br 2006;88(1):69–77.
37. McComis GP, Nawoczenski DA, DeHaven KE. Functional bracing for rupture of the Achilles tendon. Clinical results and analysis of ground-reaction forces and temporal data. J Bone Joint Surg Am 1997;79(12):1799–808.
38. Mortensen NH, Skov O, Jensen PE. Early motion of the ankle after operative treatment of a rupture of the Achilles tendon: a prospective, randomized clinical and radiographic study. J Bone Joint Surg Am 1999;81(7):983–90.
39. Saleh M, Marshall PD, Senior R, et al. The Sheffield splint for controlled early mobilisation after rupture of the calcaneal tendon. A prospective, randomised comparison with plaster treatment. J Bone Joint Surg Br 1992;74(2):206–9.
40. Salter RB, Simmonds DF, Malcolm BW, et al. The biological effect of continuous passive motion on the healing of full-thickness defects in articular cartilage. An experimental investigation in the rabbit. J Bone Joint Surg Am 1980;62(8):1232–51.
41. Mattila VM, Huttunen TT, Haapasalo H, et al. Declining incidence of surgery for Achilles tendon rupture follows publication of major RCTs: evidence-influenced change evident using the Finnish registry study. Br J Sports Med 2015;49(16):1084–6.
42. Mullaney MJ, McHugh MP, Tyler TF, et al. Weakness in end-range plantar flexion after Achilles tendon repair. Am J Sports Med 2006;34(7):1120–5.
43. Hufner TM, Brandes DB, Thermann H, et al. Long-term results after functional nonoperative treatment of achilles tendon rupture. Foot Ankle Int 2006;27(3):167–71.
44. Kotnis R, David S, Handley R, et al. Dynamic ultrasound as a selection tool for reducing Achilles tendon reruptures. Am J Sports Med 2006;34(9):1395–400.
45. Young SW, Patel A, Zhu M, et al. Weight-bearing in the nonoperative treatment of acute Achilles tendon ruptures: a randomized controlled trial. J Bone Joint Surg Am 2014;96(13):1073–9.
46. Carden DG, Noble JO, Chalmers JO, et al. Rupture of the calcaneal tendon. The early and late management. J Bone Joint Surg Br 1987;69(3):416–20.
47. Bhandari M, Guyatt GH, Siddiqui F, et al. Treatment of acute Achilles tendon ruptures a systematic overview and meta analysis. Clin Orthop Relat Res 2002;400:190–200.
48. Jiang N, Wang B, Chen A, et al. Operative versus nonoperative treatment for acute Achilles tendon rupture: a meta-analysis based on current evidence. Int Orthop 2012;36(4):765–73.
49. Jones MP, Khan RJ, Smith RL. Surgical interventions for treating acute Achilles tendon rupture: key findings from a recent Cochrane review. Achilles tendon

ruptures: a meta-analysis of randomized, controlled trials. J Bone Joint Surg Am 2012;94(12):e88.
50. Khan RJ, Fick D, Keogh A, et al. Treatment of acute Achilles tendon ruptures: a meta-analysis of randomized, controlled trials. J Bone Joint Surg Am 2005; 87(10):2202–10.
51. Lo IK, Kirkley A, Nonweiler B, et al. Operative versus nonoperative treatment of acute Achilles tendon ruptures: a quantitative review. Clin J Sport Med 1997; 7(3):207–11.
52. Wilkins R, Bisson LJ. Operative versus nonoperative management of acute Achilles tendon ruptures: a quantitative systematic review of randomized controlled trials. Am J Sports Med 2012;40(9):2154–60.
53. Zhao HM, Yu GR, Yang YF, et al. Outcomes and complications of operative versus non-operative treatment of acute Achilles tendon rupture: a meta-analysis. Chin Med J (Engl) 2011;124:4050–5.
54. Metz R, Verleisdonk EJ, van der Heijden GJ, et al. Acute Achilles tendon rupture: minimally invasive surgery versus nonoperative treatment with immediate full weightbearing—a randomized controlled trial. Am J Sports Med 2008;36(9): 1688–94.
55. Hockenbury RT, Johns JC. A biomechanical in vitro comparison of open versus percutaneous repair of tendon Achilles. Foot Ankle 1990;11(2):67–72.
56. Ma GW, Griffith TG. Percutaneous repair of acute closed ruptured achilles tendon: a new technique. Clin Orthop Relat Res 1977;(128):247–55.
57. Amlang M, Christiani P, Heinz P, et al. The percutaneous suture of the Achilles tendon with the Dresden instrument. Oper Orthop Traumatol 2006;18(4):287–99.
58. Delponte P, Potier L, Buisson P. Treatment of subcutaneous ruptures of the Achilles tendon by percutaneous ténorraphie. Rev Chir Orthop Reparatrice Appar Mot 1992;78(6):404–7.
59. Maes R, Copin G, Averous C. Is percutaneous repair of the Achilles tendon a safe technique? A study of 124 cases. Acta Orthop Belg 2006;72(2):179–83.
60. Rowley DI, Scotland TR. Rupture of the Achilles tendon treated by a simple operative procedure. Injury 1982;14(3):252–4.
61. Haji A, Sahai A, Symes A, et al. Percutaneous versus open tendo achillis repair. Foot Ankle Int 2004;25(4):215–8.
62. Rozis M, Benetos IS, Karampinas P, et al. Outcome of percutaneous fixation of acute Achilles tendon ruptures. Foot Ankle Int 2018;39(6):689–93.
63. Klein W, Lang DM, Saleh M. The use of the Ma-Griffith technique for percutaneous repair of fresh ruptured tendo Achillis. Chir Organi Mov 1991;76(3):223–8.
64. Majewski M, Rohrbach M, Czaja S, et al. Avoiding sural nerve injuries during percutaneous Achilles tendon repair. Am J Sports Med 2006;34(5):793–8.
65. Cretnik A, Zlajpah L, Smrkolj V, et al. The strength of percutaneous methods of repair of the Achilles tendon: a biomechanical study. Med Sci Sports Exerc 2000;32(1):16–20.
66. Goren D, Ayalon M, Nyska M. Isokinetic strength and endurance after percutaneous and open surgical repair of Achilles tendon ruptures. Foot Ankle Int 2005;26(4):286–90.
67. Keller A, Ortiz C, Wagner E, et al. Mini-open tenorrhaphy of acute Achilles tendon ruptures: medium-term follow-up of 100 cases. Am J Sports Med 2014;42(3): 731–6.
68. Kakiuchi M. A combined open and percutaneous technique for repair of tendo Achillis: comparison with open repair. J Bone Joint Surg Br 1995;77(1):60–3.

69. Rebeccato A, Santini S, Salmaso G, et al. Repair of the Achilles tendon rupture: a functional comparison of three surgical techniques. J Foot Ankle Surg 2001;40(4): 188–94.
70. Assal M, Jung M, Stern R, et al. Limited open repair of Achilles tendon ruptures: a technique with a new instrument and findings of a prospective multicenter study. J Bone Joint Surg Am 2002;84(2):161–70.
71. Calder JD, Saxby TS. Early, active rehabilitation following mini-open repair of Achilles tendon rupture: a prospective study. Br J Sports Med 2005;39(11): 857–9.
72. Aktas S, Kocaoglu B. Open versus minimal invasive repair with Achillon device. Foot Ankle Int 2009;30(5):391–7.
73. Alcelik I, Saeed ZM, Haughton BA, et al. Achillon versus open surgery in acute Achilles tendon repair. Foot Ankle Surg 2018;24(5):427–34.
74. Bhattacharyya M, Gerber B. Mini-invasive surgical repair of the Achilles tendon—does it reduce post-operative morbidity? Int Orthop 2009;33(1):151–6.
75. Kołodziej L, Bohatyrewicz A, Kromuszczyńska J, et al. Efficacy and complications of open and minimally invasive surgery in acute Achilles tendon rupture: a prospective randomised clinical study—preliminary report. Int Orthop 2013; 37(4):625–9.
76. Valencia JA, Alcalá MÁ. Reparación de la ruptura aguda del tendón calcaneo. Estudio comparativo entre dos tecnicas quirúrgicas. Acta Ortopedica Mexicana 2009;23(3):125–9.
77. Ismail M, Karim A, Shulman R, et al. The Achillon Achilles tendon repair: is it strong enough? Foot Ankle Int 2008;29(8):808–13.
78. Huffard B, O'loughlin PF, Wright T, et al. Achilles tendon repair: Achillon system vs. Krackow suture: an anatomic in vitro biomechanical study. Clin Biomech 2008;23(9):1158–64.
79. Heitman DE, Ng K, Crivello KM, et al. Biomechanical comparison of the Achillon tendon repair system and the Krackow locking loop technique. Foot Ankle Int 2011;32(9):879–87.
80. Hsu AR, Jones CP, Cohen BE, et al. Clinical outcomes and complications of percutaneous Achilles repair system versus open technique for acute Achilles tendon ruptures. Foot Ankle Int 2015;36(11):1279–86.
81. Demetracopoulos CA, Gilbert SL, Young E, et al. Limited-open Achilles tendon repair using locking sutures versus nonlocking sutures: an in vitro model. Foot Ankle Int 2014;35(6):612–8.
82. Dekker RG, Qin C, Lawton C, et al. A biomechanical comparison of limited open versus krackow repair for achilles tendon rupture. Foot Ankle Orthop 2017; 2(4):1–7.
83. Del Buono A, Volpin A, Maffulli N. Minimally invasive versus open surgery for acute Achilles tendon rupture: a systematic. Br Med Bull 2013;1:14.

Open Reconstructive Strategies for Chronic Achilles Tendon Ruptures

Christopher Chen, MD, Kenneth J. Hunt, MD*

KEYWORDS

- Primary Achilles repair • Achilles reconstruction • V-Y advancement
- FHL tendon transfer • Autograft • Allograft • Xenograft

KEY POINTS

- Multiple reconstructive strategies exist for the treatment of chronic Achilles tendon rupture.
- Choosing a treatment strategy typically depends on the quality of the existing tissue, gap size, and surgeon comfort with each technique.
- Patients should be counseled on the likelihood of generalized calf atrophy, and ankle plantar flexion strength deficits compared with the uninjured side.
- Most patients return to leisure and athletic activities without functional deficits.
- Patients should be counseled on the risk of thromboembolic events, and pharmaceutical anticoagulation should be considered and discussed.

INTRODUCTION

Although the management of acute Achilles tendon ruptures is not without advances and controversy, surgical treatment is the mainstay of treatment of symptomatic chronic Achilles tendon ruptures. Improved awareness and education among musculoskeletal providers have reduced the rate of chronic ruptures because most are identified and addressed acutely. Nonoperative treatment may be considered for low-demand patients or patients who cannot safely tolerate surgical intervention. In such cases, a low-profile brace, such as a carbon-fiber ground reaction force ankle-foot orthosis, can be used. In patients with compromised function related to a chronic rupture, surgical repair methods have demonstrated satisfactory results in most cases. The primary goal of surgery is to

---

Disclosure Statement: No authors have financial relationships or conflicts related to this work.
Department of Orthopedic Surgery, University of Colorado School of Medicine, 12631 East 17th Avenue, B202, Aurora, CO 80045, USA
* Corresponding author.
E-mail address: kenneth.j.hunt@ucdenver.edu

Foot Ankle Clin N Am 24 (2019) 425–437
https://doi.org/10.1016/j.fcl.2019.04.002
foot.theclinics.com
1083-7515/19/

restore appropriate length and tension for the triceps surae with adequate and healthy tendon tissue.

Several reconstructive strategies exist for chronic Achilles tendon ruptures. The Myerson classification (**Table 1**), which classifies Achilles tendon ruptures by defect size, is useful when determining reconstructive strategy.[1] In this classification, type 1 lesions measure no more than 1 cm to 2 cm long. Defects of this size often can be managed with direct end-to-end repair. Type 2 defects range from 2 cm to 5 cm. These injuries can be managed with tendon-lengthening procedures, with or without tendon transfer. Type 3 lesions are greater than 5 cm and may require a tendon transfer, with or without a tendon-lengthening procedure. Other novel techniques, including the use of allograft for reconstruction, may be useful for the reconstruction of large defects. Because the reported outcomes for reconstructive strategies for chronic Achilles tendon ruptures largely are limited to case reports and case series, there is no clear gold standard surgical treatment option. Factors, such as patient age, activity level, defect size, body habitus, medical comorbidities, and quality of soft tissue envelope, should be considered when choosing a reconstructive strategy.

PRIMARY REPAIR

For chronic Achilles tendon ruptures with less than 2 cm of retraction after débridement of scar tissue, primary repair without augmentation can be performed. Primary repair can be performed with either imbrication or excision of the scar tissue.

Prior histologic and clinical studies have demonstrated that scar tissue within the paratenon contains prominent granulation tissue response as well as dense and thick collagen fibers with vessels.[2–4] Degenerative changes, including tendolipomatosis, mucoid degeneration, and vascular changes, typically are not present in scar tissue.[3]

To perform a primary repair, the patient is positioned in the prone position with the feet hanging from the edge of a padded operating table. Bilateral legs, ankle, and feet are prepped and draped to allow for comparison of appropriate tension to be used in the repair. A longitudinal incision is made along the posteromedial aspect of the Achilles tendon (**Fig. 1**). Care should be taken to avoid damaging the sural nerve and the small saphenous vein, which commonly are entrapped in scar tissue above the level of the paratenon. Both the paratenon and interposed scar tissue can be incised longitudinally. The underlying scar tissue then is inspected and the healthy tendon ends can be palpated and identified. In most cases, the gap between the tendon stumps is filled with scar tissue. In cases of tendon healed in an elongated position, it may be

Table 1
Size-based classification for surgical treatment of chronic Achilles tendon ruptures, originally described by Myerson

Defect Size	Surgical Procedure
1–2 cm	End-to-end anastomosis and posterior compartment fasciotomy
2–5 cm	V-Y lengthening and augmented with a tendon transfer if needed
>5 cm	Tendon transfer alone or in combination with V-Y advancement or turndown[a].

[a] Due to the bulk of the tendon at the point at which it is passed inferiorly, some surgeons prefer not to use a turndown flap.

Data from Myerson MS. Achilles tendon ruptures. Instr Course Lect.1999; 48:219-230.

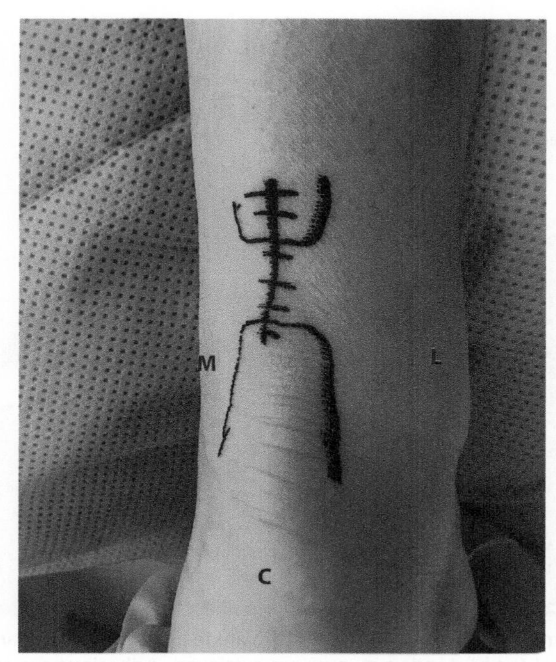

Fig. 1. A longitudinal incision is made along the posteromedial aspect of the Achilles tendon.

necessary to resect an adequate amount of scar tissue to address the laxity, which may cause decreased plantarflexion power and gait mechanics.[3] The ends of the tendon stumps should be approximated with the ankle in approximately 20° to 30° of plantarflexion. To ensure that the triceps surae moves freely after the repair, it is important to release the adhesions between the tendon and sheath as well as the gastrocnemius and soleus (**Fig. 2**).

Once scar tissue has been removed and healthy collagen tissue is available for repair, heavy nonabsorbable suture, such as no. 2 or no. 5 nonabsorbable polyfilament suture, can be used to primarily repair the tendon ends with a modified Krackow suture technique (**Fig. 3**). The paratenon should be repaired as a separate layer to avoid excessive scar tissue formation, followed by subcutaneous tissue and skin.

With the technique outlined previously, Yasuda and colleagues[3] reported excellent outcomes in 30 consecutive patients, with postoperative mean American Orthopaedic Foot and Ankle Society (AOFAS) score of 98.1 and Achilles Tendon Total Rupture Score (ATRS) of 92.0. At 2-year follow-up, there were no reruptures, and no patients reported difficulty with walking and climbing stairs; 14 athletes in the group returned to play at preinjury level of participation. Similarly, Porter and colleagues[2] also reported excellent outcomes in the treatment of 41 chronic Achilles tendon ruptures treated with proximal release of the gastrocsoleus complex, imbrication of early fibrous scar without excision of local tissue, and primary repair of the tendinous ends with heavy nonabsorbable polyfilament suture. All patients returned to preinjury level of activity at 5.8 months (range 2.5–9 months) and no patients sustained reruptures at 18-month follow-up.

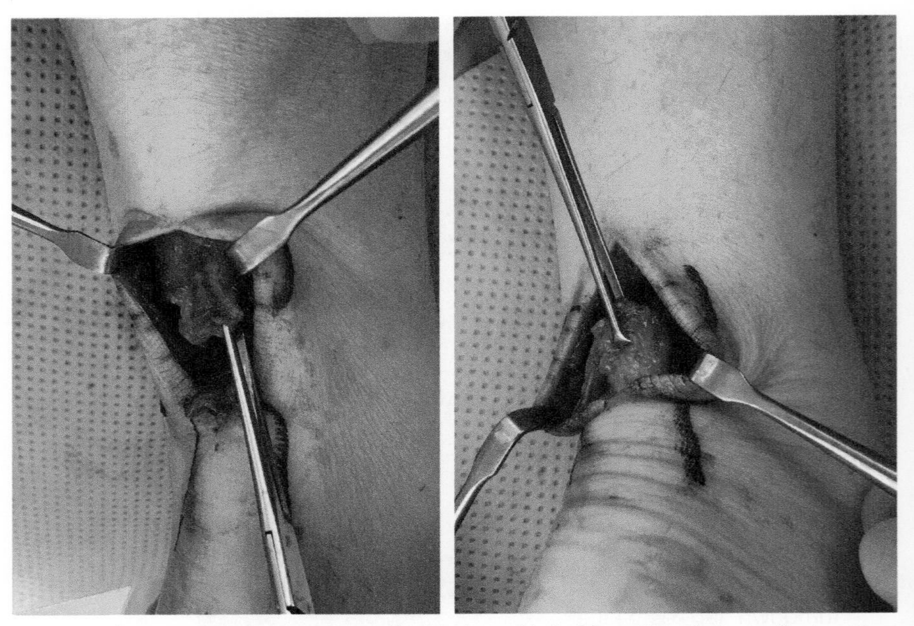

Fig. 2. Tendon stumps are approximated with the ankle in 20° to 30° of plantarflexion. Proximal (*left*) and distal (*right*) tendon stumps are retrieved. Adhesions are released between the tendon and sheath to ensure that the triceps surae moves freely after repair.

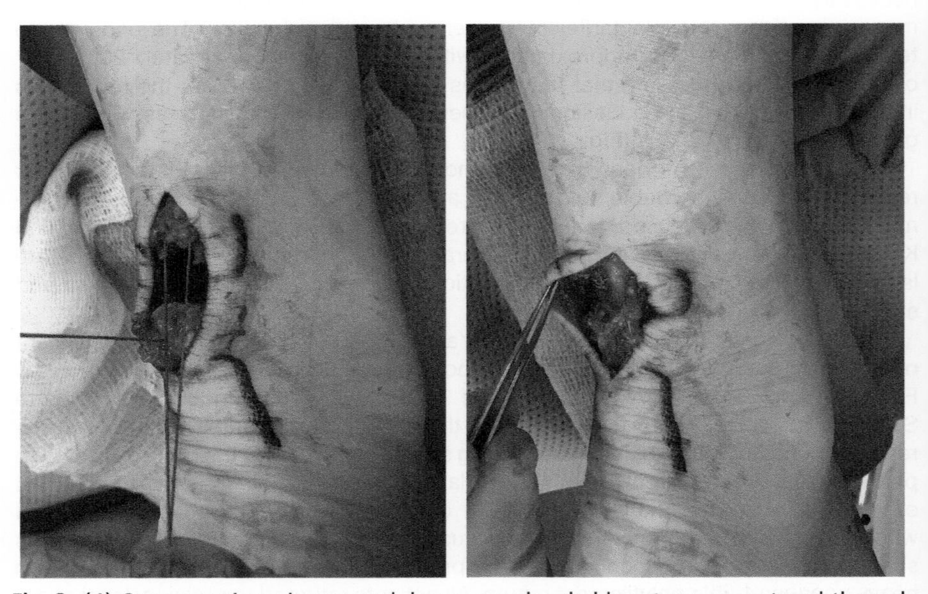

Fig. 3. (*A*) Once scar tissue is removed, heavy nonabsorbable sutures are sutured through the tendon ends in a modified Krackow technique. (*B*) The proximal and distal strands of suture are then tied together to approximate the proximal and distal tendon stumps.

V-Y TENDON ADVANCEMENT

The V-Y tendinous flap was first described by Abraham and Pankovich[5] in 1975 to achieve end-to-end anastomosis of tendon ends in neglected ruptures. Many variations of this technique exist, and this technique often is performed in combination with other tendon transfer procedures and fascial flaps.[6–8] An inverted V-shaped incision is made at the proximal part of the Achilles tendon near the musculotendinous junction. Each arm of the V should measure at least 1.5-times to 2-times the size of the gap, with a larger arm for larger defects.[6] The distal portion of the cut tendon then is advanced until the proximal and distal tendon stump are approximated, without separating the tendon from the underlying muscle. Repair of the tendon stumps is performed using Krackow sutures and no. 5 nonabsorbable polyfilament suture, followed by repair of the proximal tendon in a Y-shaped fashion with no. 0 braided suture. In the original small series of 4 patients with follow-up from 9 months to 15 months, 3 patients regained full strength of the triceps surae and were able to perform a straight leg raise, whereas 1 patient experienced continued weakness. It is difficult to compare this with subsequent studies, because most subsequent techniques have incorporated the V-Y advancement technique with some other additional method of augmentation, such as fascial turndowns or tendon transfers.

TURNDOWN FLAP

The turndown flap technique is useful for reconstruction of moderate-sized defects as well as for reinforcement of attempted primary repairs in which small defects still remain after approximation of tendon ends. Since the technique was introduced by Christensen in 1956,[9] several variations of the technique have been described, either performed independently or in combination with other reconstructive techniques.[7,10,11] This technique involves using a distally based flap, or in some cases 2 adjacent flaps, to span or reinforce the gap in the Achilles tendon.

A posterior longitudinal incision is made centered over the Achilles tendon. The tendon defect is exposed through sharp dissection of the paratenon. If a turndown flap is deemed necessary after inspection of the tendon gap, the length of the flap is determined by measuring the size of the defect. Although there is no standardized technique for determining the exact graft length, Sanada and colleagues[12] suggest preoperatively assessing the contralateral unaffected lower extremity to determine resting gravity ankle plantarflexion with the knee flexed at 90°. By performing the same maneuver on the injured extremity, the true gap distance and thus, length of flap harvest, then can be determined.[12] Depending on the length of the defect, either native Achilles tendon (for shorter defects) or gastrocnemius fascia (for longer defects) may be used. Most techniques describe a distally based flap with a 1-cm to 2-cm cuff left attached, measuring 1 cm to 3 cm in width and up to 12 cm in length.[7,8,12] Alternatively, 2 separate flaps measuring 1 cm each also can be harvested separately as medial and lateral flaps and similarly turned down.[10,11] The proximal aspect of the flap then is sutured with nonabsorbable braided suture into the distal stump, with or without overlap (**Fig. 4**). The proximal harvest defect and the paratenon then typically are sutured closed with a side-to-side repair. Postoperatively, patients typically are splinted or casted in equinus to protect the repair.

Several investigators have reported success with the turndown technique, either performed in isolation or in combination with other procedures. In a retrospective case series of 21 patients who underwent a split medial and lateral flap turndown, Seker and colleagues[10] reported excellent outcomes at 10-year follow-up. There were no reruptures and no significant difference in calf size, ankle range of motion,

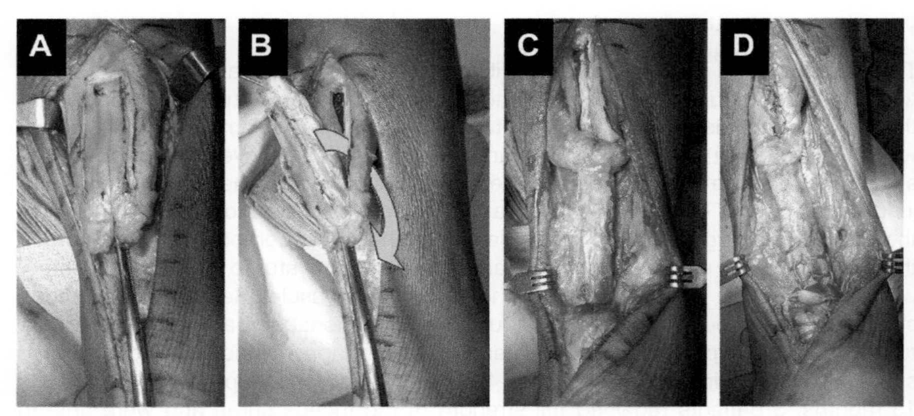

Fig. 4. (*A*) A distally based flap with a 1-cm to 2-cm cuff left attached, measuring 1 cm to 3 cm in width and up to 12 cm in length, is made. (*B*) The flap is then mobilized and turned down through the remaining tendon. (*C*) The turn down flap is able to span the large defect between the proximal and distal stump. (*D*) The proximal harvest defect and the paratenon are sutured closed with a side to side repair. The turned down flap and distal stump are repaired using proximal and distal modified Krackow sutures.

and dynamometric evaluations of peak torque at 30° and 120° using Cybex isokinetic dynamometer device (Cybex International, Medway, Massachusetts) between the injured and uninjured extremity. Furthermore, mean AOFAS scores and Foot and Ankle Disability Index scores were 98.5 (range 90–100) and 98.9 (96.2–100), respectively, and all patients reported a visual analog scale (VAS) score of 0.

Us and colleagues[7] reported a case series of 6 patients who underwent combined V-Y plasty and gastrocnemius turndown with 11-month to 16-month follow-up. Although isokinetic strength testing demonstrated peak torque deficiencies between 2.5% and 22%, there was no observed clinical or functional deficiency. All patients were able to return to their preinjury level of activity, with normal ability to walk, run, jump, and climb stairs. All patients had symmetric and propulsive gaits and were able to walk on their toes and perform single-leg heel raises. Guclu and colleagues[13] reported a case series of 17 patients with mean follow-up of 16 years (13–18 years), with similar results. Mean calf atrophy was 3.4 cm, and mean plantarflexion peak torque at 30° and 120° and was 16% and 17% deficient, respectively. Mean AOFAS score was 95, and no patients sustained rerupture.

TENDON TRANSFERS

Flexor Hallucis Longus

Multiple tendon transfers have been described for the treatment of chronic Achilles tendon ruptures. In 1993, Wapner and colleagues[14] described transferring the flexor hallucis longus (FHL) tendon through a medial midfoot incision to the calcaneus, anterior to the Achilles insertion with satisfactory results. Since then, the technique has been modified and can be performed through either 2 incisions or a single posterior incision.[15] The FHL tendon is the most commonly used donor for tendon transfer due to due to its biomechanical strength, phase of action, and line of pull.[16]

To perform this technique, a second incision can be made over the knot of Henry, and the FHL is transected and pulled through the proximal incision. The distal stump of FHL then is tenodesed to the flexor digitorum longus. Alternatively, the FHL tendon can be approached through the posterior longitudinal incision without a second incision.[6] With the Achilles tendon reflected, the deep posterior compartment may be incised and released, gaining access to the FHL muscle (beef of the heel). The FHL is confirmed by digital retraction of the tendon, watching for flexion of the hallux. Dissection of the FHL tendon is followed to the posterior talus and FHL tunnel, remaining lateral to avoid the neurovascular bundle. Release of the fibro-osseous tunnel along the posterior talus is necessary to gain length. With the hallux and ankle plantar flexed, the FHL tendon is transected as distally as possible. The tendon is fixed to the calcaneus just anterior to the Achilles stump insertion (**Fig. 5**). This approach has the theoretic disadvantage of hallux weakness, because a tenodesis of the distal FHL tendon is not performed. Although prior studies have identified weakness with hallux interphalangeal joint active flexion, patients do not seem to have any functional deficits, including toe-off or hyperextension deformities.[17,18] Once harvested, the FHL tendon is directly sutured to the distal Achilles stump, woven or sutured into the Achilles tendon and stump, or transfixed to the calcaneus. Multiple techniques for fixation of the tendon to the calcaneus are described, including the use of bone tunnels, suture anchors, or an interference screw.[6,14–17,19–21]

Although there are numerous technical variations for performing the FHL transfer, there remains a lack of studies comparing clinical results of different fixation and repair methods. A biomechanical study comparing the fixation of FHL tendon to calcaneus using interference screws versus bone tunnel fixation found no differences in ultimate strength, peak stress, and failure strain between the 2 groups.[22] Rahm and colleagues[20] retrospectively compared FHL transfer to the Achilles tendon using a

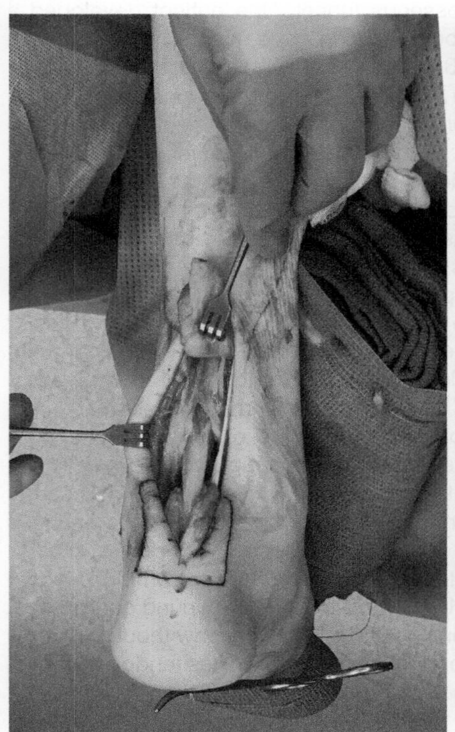

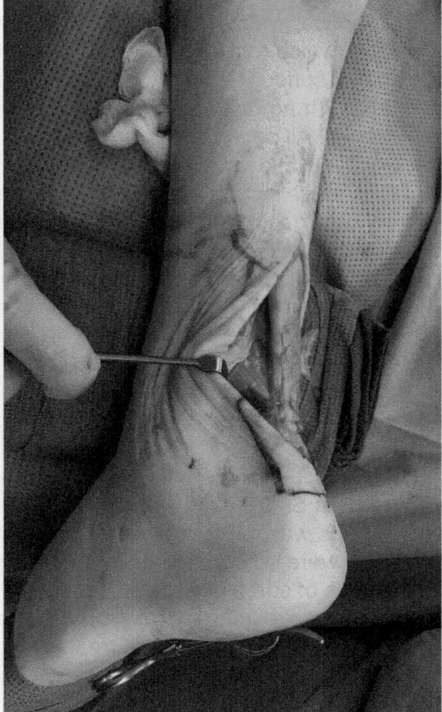

Fig. 5. (*Left*) The FHL tendon, which has been mobilized, is fixed to the calcaneus just anterior to the Achilles insertion. (*Right*) The transferred tendon then is incorporated and sutured into the available Achilles tendon tissue.

transtendinous technique versus a transosseous technique and found that both groups had excellent clinical and functional outcomes.[19] Due to the lack of comparative studies, there is no consensus for the best way to perform an FHL transfer.

Regardless of operative technique, most studies report excellent outcomes with FHL transfer, with or without additional treatment strategy, such as a flap turndown. Wegrzyn and colleagues[21] report a case series of 11 patients who underwent FHL transfer. A medial plantar incision was used to harvest the FHL, which then was passed through a 4.5-mm calcaneal drill hole. With average follow-up of 79 months, there were no major wound-healing complications, although 1 patient developed reflex sympathetic dystrophy, which resolved at the time of final follow-up. AOFAS score improved from 64 to 98. There was no difference in ankle range of motion, although with isokinetic testing, there was an average strength deficit of 28% $\pm$ 11% at 30° and 36% $\pm$ 4% at 120°. On average, there was 1.7 cm of calf atrophy compared with the uninjured size. All patients were able to tiptoe stand and demonstrated no functional hallux weakness with athletic activities or daily life.

Another case series of 3 patients examined the treatment of chronic AT ruptures that were neglected for at least 2 years.[19] At final follow-up, between 18 months and 24 months, average AOFAS score was 96.5, and ATRS improved from 23.5 to 83. All patients were able to perform a heel raise and there were no appreciable functional deficits from FHL harvest. Elgohary and colleagues[23] reported on 19 patients who underwent combined FHL transfer with gastrocnemius recession who were followed for an average of 29 months (range 13–52 months). FHL transfer was performed with either a transtendinous weave or a transosseous tunnel. One patient developed a deep infection, which required a myofasciocutaneous flap; 1 patient developed skin sloughing, which required a skin graft; and 3 patients developed superficial infections. No patients suffered from reruptures. Mean AOFAS score improved significantly, from 65 to 94, with no difference in outcome for transosseous tunnels versus transtendinous weave. All patients returned to sport, although none to the level of activity prior to injury. No patients complained of functional hallux dysfunction at final follow-up. Based on these results, the investigators concluded that FHL tendon transfer in combination with gastrocnemius recession was a safe and reliable treatment option for chronic Achilles tendon ruptures with gaps measuring 5 cm to 8 cm.

A recent retrospective cohort study compared 29 patients who underwent isolated FHL tendon transfer versus 20 patients who underwent combined FHL tendon transfer and turndown flap.[24] FHL transfer was performed through a 1-incision approach, transecting the tendon at the medial malleolus, and the tendon was transfixed to the calcaneal tunnel with a bioabsorbable screw. A 2-flap turndown technique was used. At 12-month follow-up, both groups of patients had excellent results, with AOFAS score of 90 $\pm$ 11 for the isolated tendon transfer group and 95 $\pm$ 10 for the combined group. There were no significant differences in VAS score, AOFAS score, 3 and 6-Item Short Form Health Survey, and the only significant difference between the 2 groups was longer operative time for the combined procedures group. In addition, there were no complications in the FHL transfer group, but the combined group had 2 cases of soft tissue complications—1 stitch abscess and 1 wound dehiscence. Based on these results, the investigators conclude that FHL transfer without additional procedure is a safe and reliable treatment option for chronic Achilles tendon ruptures.

Peroneus Brevis

The peroneus brevis tendon transfer was described in 1974 by Teuffer[25] for acute Achilles tendon ruptures and has since been adapted for treatment of chronic Achilles tendon ruptures.

To perform this technique, as described by Maffulli and colleagues,[26] a 10-cm to 12-cm skin incision is made over the lateral border of the Achilles tendon. The sural nerve is identified and protected. The paratenon is incised in the midline and the stumps of the Achilles tendon are exposed. Scar tissue is excised to healthy tendon, and the gap is measured while maximally plantarflexing the ankle and pulling traction on the proximal tendon stump. Next, a small longitudinal incision is made in the lateral aspect of the floor of the Achilles tendon compartment to expose the distal portion of the peroneal muscle belly. The proximal peroneus brevis tendon is identified. A separate 2.5-mm longitudinal incision is made over the lateral base of the fifth metatarsal to identify the distal portion of the tendon. The tendon is detached from the base of the metatarsal and pulled through the proximal wound. The tendon then is passed through the distal stump of the Achilles tendon from lateral to medial and then passed through the proximal stump from medial to lateral. The repair then is sutured in place at each entry and exit point and reinforced with sutures between the musculotendinous junction of the peroneus brevis and the adjacent portion of the Achilles tendon. Interrupted sutures are used to approximate the ascending and descending limb of the peroneus brevis tendon. To minimize disruption of the soft tissue envelope, the same repair also can be performed through a minimally invasive approach through 3 separate smaller incisions, over the proximal stump, distal stump, and peroneus brevis insertion.[27] If the plantaris tendon is encountered, it also can be used to augment the repair.[28] A biomechanical study by Sebastian and colleagues[29] compared FHL tendon and peroneus brevis tendon transfers. They reported no significant difference in stiffness and energy-to-peak load between the 2 groups but did note a significantly higher mean failure load for the peroneus brevis group. Due to the very high magnitude of mean failure load in both groups, however, these findings are likely to have little clinical significance. Based on these observations, the investigators suggest that both FHL tendon and peroneus brevis tendon are appropriate treatment options for chronic AT ruptures.

Maffulli and colleagues[26] reported on the long-term outcomes of 16 patients who underwent peroneus brevis tendon for Achilles tendon defects up to 6.5 cm, with average follow-up of 15.5 years. No patients sustained a rerupture. The maximum calf circumference and isometric plantarflexion strength with the ankle in neutral were both significantly decreased, although patients did not perceive any weakness in strength in daily and leisurely activities. Complications reported included superficial infection, contralateral Achilles tendinopathy, hypersensitive surgical wounds, and hypertrophic scar.

AUTOGRAFT

Multiple autograft reconstruction techniques for chronic Achilles tendon rupture have been described, including hamstring[30–32] and quadriceps tendon autograft.[33] A tendon autograft may be useful in patients with very large defects of greater than 6 cm, in which an isolated tendon transfer is insufficient to fill the gap. In addition, autograft may be considered when FHL or peroneus brevis tendon cannot be transferred. The technique for performing a semitendinosus autograft is outlined below.

The approach to the Achilles tendon can be made with 1 large longitudinal incision[32] or using separate smaller incisions over the proximal and distal stump of the Achilles tendon.[30,31] A separate 2-cm transverse incision is made in the popliteal fossa, directly over the semitendinosus tendon. The tendon is carefully dissected and harvested using a tendon stripper, with the knee flexed at 30° to reduce tension on the tendon.

Each end of the harvested tendon then is prepared with a whipstitch. After careful dissection and exposure of the proximal tendon stump with excision of nonviable tissue, the semitendinosus tendon then is passed transversely through the substance to the proximal stump in the medial to lateral direction and sutured to the stump at the entry and exit points. The 2 ends of the autograft are secured to the calcaneus anterior to the insertion of the Achilles tendon and secured at maximal tension with an interference screw. Finally, the autograft is sutured to the distal stump of the tendon.

Maffulli and colleagues[31] report excellent results for this technique in a case series of 28 patients who underwent free semitendinosus graft reconstruction for Achilles tendon defects greater than 6 cm, with mean follow-up of 31.4 months. A minimally invasive technique was used to minimize soft tissue disruption. Overall, ATRS improved from 42 (range 29–45) to 86 (78–95). Maximum calf circumference and isometric plantarflexion strength significantly improved after surgery but remained significantly weaker than the unaffected side. All patients were able to walk on their tiptoes and return to their preinjury occupation.

Dumbre Patil and colleagues[32] reported results for 35 patients who underwent semitendinosus reconstruction for defects ranging between 5 cm and 9 cm. All patients had satisfactory outcomes, good soft tissue healing, and no reruptures. Manual muscle testing, preoperatively to postoperatively, improved from 2/5 to 4/5 or 5/5 in all patients. In addition, all patients returned to prerupture daily activity.

OTHER GRAFT OPTIONS

Allograft, xenograft, and synthetic graft reconstruction techniques also have been described for chronic Achilles tendon ruptures.[34–36] These techniques allow for bridging of large defects without potential donor site morbidity. There are few published reports, however, on the use of allografts, xenografts, and synthetic grafts, and most studies are limited to case reports and small case series. A recent publication by the senior author demonstrates the allograft technique.[37]

Ofili and colleagues[34] report results of 14 patients who underwent frozen Achilles tendon allograft reconstruction for gaps ranging between 4 cm and 5 cm. A standard posterior approach was used to expose the tendon stumps and excise fibrotic tissue. Allograft was secured to the distal tendon stump with modified Krackow or Kessler stitch or with a calcaneal bone block if not enough healthy tendon stump was present distally. The graft then was tensioned and sutured to the remaining proximal stump. At final follow-up (mean 16.1 months), all patients were able to perform a single-leg heel raise, and no patients experienced infections, wound healing issues, or reruptures. One patient treated with a calcaneal bone block was treated with prolonged immobilization until radiographic union at 12 weeks.

Hollawell and Baione[36] describe a technique in which interposition Achilles tendon allograft and simultaneous xenograft augmentation were performed. In this case series of 4 patients, the median gap length was 4.75 cm. After débridement of the proximal and distal stumps, the stumps were incised transversely to create a separation of anterior and posterior ends. Achilles tendon allograft then was seated intrasubstance between the anterior and posterior flaps, and sutured with 2-0 FiberWire (Arthrex, Naples, Florida). Inforce Reinforcement Matrix (Integra LifeSciences, Plainsboro, New Jersey) xenograft was cut to approximately 3 cm^2 and sutured to the proximal and distal repair sites using 4-0 looped FiberWire in a running, locking fashion. At median follow-up of 37 months, mean Foot and Ankle Outcomes Instrument core scale score was 97 and Foot and Ankle Outcomes Instrument shoe comfort core scale was 100. All patients returned to preinjury activity.

Shoaib and Mishra[35] used a combined V-Y plasty and synthetic graft augmentation technique for treatment of 7 patients with Achilles tendon gap of 6 cm to 7 cm. In all 7 cases, V-Y plasty was performed first, but the end-to-end repair was deemed unsatisfactory due to poor quality of tissue; 2 narrow strips of Artelon (Artimplant, Västra Frölunda, Sweden), a synthetic bioabsorbable urethane graft, measuring 4 cm × 0.5 cm, then were used to augment the medial and lateral aspects of the tendon graft. This then was sutured to the tendon using nonabsorbable polyfilament suture using Krackow suture technique. At mean follow-up of 29 months, AOFAS score improved from 59 to 91, and mean ATRS score was 92. No reruptures occurred, and all patients returned to satisfactory daily activity, with 4 of 7 patients returning to sports; 6 of the 7 patients were able to perform a single-leg heel raise, and maximum calf diameter difference was less than 2 cm in all patients. Based on their results, the investigators conclude that synthetic graft augmentation is a safe, simple, and effective alternative to tendon transfer procedures.

DEEP VEIN THROMBOSIS PROPHYLAXIS

Regardless of technique used for reconstruction of chronic Achilles tendon ruptures, pharmaceutical anticoagulation should be considered after surgical intervention. In a retrospective review of surgically treated acute and chronic Achilles tendon ruptures, there was a significantly higher rate of deep vein thrombosis (DVT) and pulmonary embolism in patients with chronic ruptures. The incidence of DVT and of pulmonary embolism were 17.6% and 11.8%, respectively.[38] The risks and benefits of pharmaceutical anticoagulation should be considered for each individual patient. Patients with inherent risk factors, such as inherited hypercoagulable conditions, pregnancy, oral contraceptive use, smoking, cancer, acute infection, diabetes mellitus, age, and body mass index, may be at increased risk of developing DVT. Anticoagulation, however, also may carry a risk of bleeding, wound necrosis, wound dehiscence, and hematoma formation. To minimize the risk of complication, meticulous hemostasis should be achieved after tourniquet deflation.

SUMMARY

In conclusion, multiple reconstructive strategies exist for the treatment of chronic Achilles tendon rupture. Choosing a treatment strategy typically depends on the quality of the existing tendon, size of the gap, and surgeon's comfort with each technique. In general, the treatment strategies, outlined previously, achieve similar functional outcomes, as evidenced by the drastic improvement in functional outcome scores in almost every study. Regardless of treatment strategy, patients should be counseled on the likelihood of generalized calf atrophy, ankle plantar flexion strength deficits compared with the uninjured side, and the possibility of weakened donor tendon function (eg, hallux interphalangeal flexion strength in FHL transfer). Patients should still expect to return to leisure and athletic activities however, without functional deficits. Finally, patients should be counseled on the risk of thromboembolic events, and pharmaceutical anticoagulation should be considered.

REFERENCES

1. Myerson MS. Achilles tendon ruptures. Instr Course Lect 1999;48:219–30.
2. Porter DA, Mannarino FP, Snead D, et al. Primary repair without augmentation for early neglected Achilles tendon ruptures in the recreational athlete. Foot Ankle Int 1997;18(9):557–64.

3. Yasuda T, Shima H, Mori K, et al. Direct repair of chronic Achilles tendon ruptures using scar tissue located between the tendon stumps. J Bone Joint Surg Am 2016;98:1168–75.
4. Lee DK. Achilles tendon repair with acellular tissue graft augmentation in neglected ruptures. J Foot Ankle Surg 2007;46(6):451–5.
5. Abraham E, Pankovich AM. Neglected ruptures of the Achilles tendon. Treatment by V-Y tendinous flap. J Bone Joint Surg Am 1975;57(2):253–5.
6. Elias I, Besser M, Nazarian LN, et al. Reconstruction for missed or neglected Achilles tendon rupture with V-Y lengthening and flexor hallucis longus transfer through one incision. Foot Ankle Int 2007;28(12):1238–48.
7. Us AK, Bilgin SS, Aydin T, et al. Repair of neglected Achilles tendon ruptures: procedures and functional results. Arch Orthop Trauma Surg 1997;116:408–11.
8. Ponnapula P, Aaranson RR. Reconstruction of Achilles tendon rupture with combined V-Y plasty and gastrocnemius-soleus fascia. J Foot Ankle Surg 2010;49(3): 310–5.
9. Christensen I. Rupture of the Achilles tendon; analysis of 57 cases. Acta Chir Scand 1953;106:50–60.
10. Seker A, Kara A, Armagan R, et al. Reconstruction of neglected Achilles tendon rupture with gastrocnemius flaps: excellent results in long term follow-up. Arch Orthop Trauma Surg 2016;136(10):1417–23.
11. Peterson KS, Hentges MJ, Catanzariti AR, et al. Surgical considerations for the neglected or chronic achilles tendon rupture: a combined technique for reconstruction. J Foot Ankle Surg 2014;53(5):664–71.
12. Sanada T, Uchiyama E. Gravity equinus position to control the tendon length of reversed tendon flap reconstruction for chronic Achilles tendon rupture. J Foot Ankle Surg 2017;56(1):37–41.
13. Guclu B, Basat HC, Yildirim T, et al. Long-term results of chronic Achilles tendon ruptures repaired with V-Y tendon plasty and fascia turndown. Foot Ankle Int 2016;37(7):737–42.
14. Wapner KL, Pavlock S, Hecht PJ, et al. Repair of chronic Achilles tendon rupture with flexor hallucis longus tendon transfer. Foot Ankle 1993;14(8):443–9.
15. Den Hartog BD. Flexor hallucis longus transfer for chronic Achilles tendonosis. Foot Ankle Int 2003;24(3):233–7.
16. Neufeld SK, Farber DC. Tendon transfers in the treatment of Achilles' tendon disorders. Foot Ankle Clin 2014;19(1):73–86.
17. Coull R, Flavi R, Stephens MM. Flexor hallucis longus tendon transfer: evaluation of postoperative morbidity. Foot Ankle Int 2003;24(12):931–4.
18. Schon LC, Shores JL, Faro FD, et al. Flexor hallucis longus tendon transfer in treatment of Achilles tendinosis. J Bone Joint Surg Am 2013;95(1):54–60.
19. Lee KB, Park YH, Yoon TR, et al. Reconstruction of neglected Achilles tendon rupture using the flexor hallucis tendon. Knee Surg Sports Traumatol Arthrosc 2009;17:316–20.
20. Rahm S, Spross C, Gerber F, et al. Operative treatment of chronic irreparable Achilles tendon ruptures with large flexor hallucis longus tendon transfers. Foot Ankle Int 2003;34(8):1100–10.
21. Wegrzyn J, Luciani JF, Philippot R, et al. Chronic Achilles tendon rupture reconstruction using a modified flexor hallucis longus transfer. Int Orthop 2010;34(8): 1187–92.
22. Liu GT, Balldin BC, Zide JR, et al. A biomechanical analysis of interference screw versus bone tunnel fixation of flexor hallucis longus tendon transfers to the calcaneus. J Foot Ankle Surg 2017;56(4):813–6.

23. Elgohary HEA, Elmoghazy NA, Abd Ellatif MS. Combined flexor hallucis longus tendon transfer and gastrocnemius recession for reconstruction of gapped chronic Achilles tendon ruptures. Injury 2016;47(12):2833–7.
24. Koh D, Lim J, Chen JY, et al. Flexor hallucis longus transfer versus turndown flaps augmented with flexor hallucis longus transfer in the repair of chronic Achilles tendon rupture. J Foot Ankle Surg 2017;25(2):221–5.
25. Perez Teuffer A. Traumatic rupture of the Achilles tendon. Reconstruction by transplant and graft using the lateral peroneus brevis. Orthop Clin North Am 1974;5:89–93.
26. Maffulli N, Spiezia F, Pintore E, et al. Peroneus brevis tendon transfer for reconstruction of chronic Achilles tendon: a long-term follow-up study. J Bone Joint Surg Am 2012;94(10):901–5.
27. Maffulli N, Spiezia F, Long UG, et al. Less-invasive reconstruction of chronic Achilles tendon rupture using a peroneus brevis tendon transfer. Am J Sports Med 2010;38(11):2304–12.
28. McClelland D, Maffulli N. Neglected rupture of the Achilles tendon: reconstruction with peroneus brevis tendon transfer. Surgeon 2004;2:209–13.
29. Sebastian H, Datta B, Maffulli N, et al. Mechanical properties of reconstructed Achilles tendon with transfer of peroneus brevis or flexor hallucis longus tendon. J Foot Ankle Surg 2007;46(6):424–8.
30. Maffulli N, Longo UG, Gougoulias N, et al. Ipsilateral free semitendinosus tendon graft transfer for reconstruction of chronic tears of the Achilles tendon. BMC Musculoskelet Disord 2008;9:100.
31. Maffulli N, Loppini M, Long U, et al. Minimally invasive reconstruction of chronic Achilles tendon ruptures using the ipsilateral free semitendinosus tendon graft and interference screw fixation. Am J Sports Med 2013;41(5):1100–7.
32. Dumbre Patil SS, Dumbre Patil VS, Basa VR, et al. Semitendinosus tendon autograft for reconstruction of large defects in chronic Achilles tendon ruptures. Foot Ankle Int 2014;35(7):699–705.
33. Mudgal CS, Martin TL, Wilson MG. Reconstruction of Achilles tendon defect with a free quadriceps bone-tendon graft without anastomosis. Foot Ankle Int 2000; 21(1):10–3.
34. Ofili KP, Pollard JD, Schuberth JM. The neglected Achilles tendon rupture repaired with allograft: a review of 14 cases. J Foot Ankle Surg 2016;55(6):1245–8.
35. Shoaib A, Mishra V. Surgical repair of symptomatic chronic Achilles tendon rupture using synthetic graft augmentation. Foot Ankle Surg 2017;23(3):179–82.
36. Hollawell S, Baione W. Chronic Achilles tendon rupture reconstructed with Achilles tendon allograft and xenograft combination. J Foot Ankle Surg 2015;54(6): 1146–50.
37. Kraeutler MJ, Purcell JM, Hunt KJ. Chronic achilles tendon ruptures. Foot Ankle Int 2017;38(8):921–9.
38. Bullock MJ, DeCarbo WT, Hofbauer MH, et al. Repair of chronic Achilles rupture has a high incidence of venous thrombosis. Foot Ankle Spec 2017;10(5):415–20.

Maximizing Return to Sports After Achilles Tendon Rupture in Athletes

Jon-Michael E. Caldwell, MD, J. Turner Vosseller, MD*

KEYWORDS

• Achilles tendon rupture • Return to play • Athlete • Sports injury • Tendonitis • Sports medicine

KEY POINTS

- Achilles tendon ruptures are devastating injuries to the athlete with return-to-sport rates around 70% and some risk for diminished performance postinjury.
- Surgical management is often favored for athletes, but evidence is limited in this population.
- Functional rehabilitation protocols are critical regardless of operative or nonoperative management.
- Return-to-play protocols are sparse and varied because of ambiguous definitions of return-to-sport criteria in the literature.
- Optimal sport-specific return-to-play milestones should be defined to guide the rehabilitation of injured athletes.

INTRODUCTION

Achilles tendon ruptures (ATR) are common injuries that can affect those not only at the apex of athleticism, but also those that only irregularly engage in athletic endeavor. Generally speaking, frequent athletic activity is a risk factor for ATR.[1] Historically, most of these injuries occurred in young (25–35 years) active men. However, it seems that the mean age at which patients rupture their Achilles tendons has increased with time, as has the proportion of women sustaining these injuries.[2] Although the optimal

Disclosure Statement. J.M. Caldwell: nothing to disclose. J.T. Vosseller: AAOS, board or committee member; American Orthopaedic Foot and Ankle Society, board or committee member; DJ Orthopaedics, paid consultant; Foot and Ankle Orthopaedics, editorial or governing board; New Clip Technics, IP royalties; Saunders/Mosby-Elsevier, publishing royalties, financial, or material support.
Department of Orthopedic Surgery, Columbia University Irving Medical Center/NewYork-Presbyterian Hospital, 622 West 168th Street, PH11–Center Wing, New York, NY 10032, USA
* Corresponding author.
E-mail address: turner.vosseller@gmail.com

Foot Ankle Clin N Am 24 (2019) 439–445
https://doi.org/10.1016/j.fcl.2019.04.003
1083-7515/19/

treatment of an ATR has been and continues to be a subject of some debate, a consistent truth is that, irrespective of how the rupture is treated, patients can take upward of a year to return to preinjury levels of function.

In higher level athletes and certainly in professional athletes, the bias continues to be toward surgical treatment. This trend is most likely because with surgical repair the tension of the tendon is directly restored and most of these patients are young and healthy, perhaps minimizing the risk of surgical treatment, namely wound healing issues. Moreover, these patients are likely to have every facet of treatment optimized postoperatively in terms of rehabilitation. However, even in this setting, it often takes professional athletes 6 months or longer to return to preinjury function, if they are even able to attain that level. Therefore, these injuries in any patient constitute a significant blow to physical capability that necessitates a long period of functional recovery.

Formal return to play (RTP) criteria have been developed for some orthopedic injuries, most notably anterior cruciate ligament reconstruction, although many of these guidelines are still being developed.[3] However, objective criteria for RTP still do not exist for many injuries, which can make decisions regarding RTP difficult. The higher the level of sport, the higher are the stakes, and the pressure on medical professionals to get athletes back to play as quickly as possible. In this review we look at the current state of ATR treatment and assess expected outcomes after Achilles rupture in athletes, and what data exist with regards to RTP for ATRs.

OPERATIVE VERSUS NONOPERATIVE MANAGEMENT IN THE ATHLETE

Any discussion of ATR treatment has traditionally been framed by the balance between the risk of rerupture with nonoperative treatment on the one side versus the risk of wound issues with operative treatment on the other. In athletes, operative treatment is often favored because, given the long recovery with these injuries, a rerupture would be a disaster for an athlete. Although it could be reasonably argued that a wound complication would be no less a disaster, the reality is that most athletes and certainly most professional athletes are in excellent health, potentially mitigating the risk of wound issues. A second concept may play some role in treatment decisions. There is some evidence to suggest that strength is better after surgical repair of an ATR. Perhaps the most influential recent article on Achilles rupture treatment is that by Willits and colleagues[4] This study supported nonoperative treatment, noting no significant difference in rerupture rate between operative and nonoperative treatment arms. However, these authors did note that the surgical patients were significantly stronger than the nonoperative ones at final follow-up. Some other authors have noted this trend as well,[5] although the literature suffers from a lack of consistent means of reporting strength data in follow-up of these patients. A large meta-analysis found that surgical and nonsurgical treatment had equivalent rates of rerupture when the nonsurgical treatment included functional rehabilitation.[6] However, the authors noted that when such early range of motion was not used, surgery reduced the rerupture rate by more than 8%. It should be noted this study did not differentiate between athletes and nonathletes. A final reason that may influence why most athletes are treated surgically is simply that there is an assumption among these patients that surgical treatment is most appropriate and "better." Although it is no doubt the job of the physician to educate the patient as to his or her options, a patient that has decided on surgery will likely ultimately find a surgeon that will do it.

EARLY FUNCTIONAL REHABILITATION

One aspect of treatment that seems to lower the rate of rerupture among patients with this injury without regard to whether the patient is treated operatively or nonoperatively is early functional rehabilitation. There are now reams of data showing that early weight-bearing and early functional rehabilitation leads to stronger new tendon formation and better ultimate functional outcomes.[7–11] Many treatment protocols do not differentiate much between operative and nonoperative treatment when it comes to the rehabilitation progression. As a gross simplification, rehabilitation focuses on motion for roughly the first 2 months and then strengthening thereafter.

RETURN TO PLAY PROTOCOLS

Clearly, these injuries are significant ones that severely affect an athlete's ability to function at a high level. However, the goal of surgeon and athlete alike is to try to minimize this impact. To that end, some authors have suggested optimal RTP protocols for these patients. Grävare Silbernagel and Crossley[12] offered a starting point with their proposed program for RTP with noninsertional Achilles tendinopathy by codifying a protocol and a proposed progression. However, they did not precisely define what return to sport means nor did they provide exact criteria for determining if that occurred. The lack of an explicit definition for "return to sport" and measurable criteria for tracking progress pervades the literature as noted in a recent systematic review, making interpretation and comparison of outcomes difficult.[13] Furthermore, the application of programs for tendinopathy is limited because of the obvious fact that Achilles tendinopathy, although on the same continuum of disease, is not the same as an Achilles rupture.

Any proposed RTP protocols should include some ability to assess where a patient is in their recovery relative to where they should (or want to) be. Return to sport should be defined in the context of the athlete's sport and level of participation. As described by the consensus statement by Ardern and colleagues,[14] RTP can be thought of as a continuum progressing sequentially from return to participation, return to sport, and finally, return to performance. Objective criteria should be used when possible. In the context of Achilles rupture, the Achilles tendon Total Rupture Score has been used widely as an outcome measure. This score is a patient-reported outcome instrument consisting of 10 questions that has demonstrated clinical utility for measuring outcomes after ATRs.[15] Hansen and colleagues[16] noted that a patient's Achilles tendon Total Rupture Score at 3 months after injury could predict a patient's ability to return to sports at 1 year. Establishing these objective benchmarks is a critical step toward being able to provide the most useful criteria for RTP. Others have noted that males, patients with Achilles pain at rest at 3 months, and patients with lower physical functioning and calf endurance at 6 months all have delayed recovery of calf endurance at 1 year.[17] Although these data may be skewed slightly given the relative infrequence of ATRs in females, Achilles pain at rest at 3 months could identify those patients at risk for slower recovery so that some intervention could be made to try to fortify their recovery.

Explicit criteria and protocols for RTP are generally lacking at this point for ATR. Time-based guidelines have suggested resumption of noncontact sports 16 weeks after injury and contact sports 20 weeks after injury, but these recommendations are not evidence based.[14] Fanchini and colleagues[18] offered a case report of an Italian professional soccer player in an effort to provide a potential protocol. Indeed, this report mainly highlights the vast difference between the resources at the disposal of a professional athlete versus almost anyone else, because the attention paid to this one athlete is likely not possible for most of the public and most amateur athletes. Despite that, it does provide for some sense of how the progression should work and what the stages of recovery are. A similar case report with a graduated RTP program was published with a case report of an Olympic bobsled athlete who competed in the Winter Olympics 29 weeks following injury with good results at 2-year follow-up.[19] Finally, there has been one systematic review with meta-analysis on this topic. The mean RTP rate across all included studies was about 80%. However, the authors noted that those studies that were more objective about how RTP was defined were generally associated with lower RTP rates, and perhaps unsurprisingly, measures that evaluate RTP are variable and inconsistent.[20]

PERFORMANCE FOLLOWING ACHILLES TENDON RUPTURE

Many authors have looked at the effect of an ATR on professional athletes in various sports. Parekh and colleagues[21] assessed the epidemiology and outcomes of ATRs in the National Football League (NFL), retrospectively reviewing 31 ATRs over a 5-year period (1997–2002). In this cohort, only 68% of athletes were able to return to sport and those that did generally returned at a lower level of efficacy compared with preinjury. Another study used the NFL Orthopedic Surgery Outcomes Database looking specifically at all injuries over a 10-year period (2003–2013). Achilles tendon repair, along with patellar tendon repair, led to significantly fewer games played postinjury than other injuries. Moreover, Achilles repair along with anterior cruciate ligament reconstruction, patellar tendon repair, and tibia intramedullary nail led to significant decreases in performance in the first year after injury, although the Achilles repair patients returned to preinjury performance levels in the second and third year postinjury.[22] Jack and colleagues[23] most recently and comprehensively assessed ATRs in the NFL using publicly available performance data. A total of 71 of 95 players included in the study were able to return to competition (72.4%) and those that returned had shorter postoperative careers than matched control subjects. The authors also noted a player's ability to return to a certain level of performance depended in large part on the player's position, with running backs and linebackers performing significantly worse than their preoperative levels.

Achilles ruptures have also been assessed in other sports. Amin and colleagues[24] assessed 18 players from the National Basketball Association that had ATRs over a 23-year period (1988–2011). The injuries had a profound negative impact on the athletes, because only 61% were able to return to competition and those that did return showed a significant decrease in playing time and performance. Further data have shown that Achilles tendon repair is associated with the lowest RTP rates of any orthopedic surgical procedure among National Basketball Association players.[25] Other authors have assessed ATRs in Major League Baseball. Given the nature of the sport, the incidence of ATRs is significantly less than in sports, such as basketball and football, that require frequent eccentric contractures. However, only 62% of position players that sustained ATRs were able to RTP.[26]

A few studies from Europe have assessed athletes from other sports. Maffulli and colleagues[27] compiled data on 17 elite athletes from sports as diverse as badminton and martial arts, although most of the athletes were soccer players. All athletes were able to return to competition, although one was not able to compete at the same level as before the injury and one other had to make permanent adaptations to their technique to compensate after injury. The authors did not assess performance capacity objectively and return to competition was ultimately a binary variable. ATRs have been found to be uncommon in soccer, a somewhat unexpected finding, although there are little data on postinjury performance in these patients.[28]

Less severe Achilles pathology has been shown to negatively impact performance. In a related study, Amin and colleagues[29] found that Achilles tendinopathy without rupture also resulted in fewer minutes of playing time and decreased performance metrics, although the difference was not as profound as with complete rupture. Similarly, Hardy and colleagues[30] found only 71% of patients were able to return to their prior level of sports participation 1 year following calcaneal debridement with or without detachment/reattachment of the Achilles for insertional tendinopathy.

Synthesizing much of this data, Trofa and colleagues[31] assessed the major professional sports in the United States for ATRs over a 24-year period. Only established professional athletes were included and matched control players were used to assess the effect of the injury on the player's estimated career trajectory. Only 70% of athletes were able to RTP and those that did return played at a lower level than matched control subjects at 1 year after injury. Performance normalized relative to control subjects by 2 years after injury. This finding suggests that, if an athlete can continue as a professional into the second year after injury, his or her statistics would not be different from what would have been expected had they not suffered the injury.

SUMMARY

ATRs are devastating injuries for athletes that require a long recovery and may not allow athletes to achieve the heights of athletic ability that they had before the injury. The understanding of RTP in these injuries is in its infancy. Currently, there are no validated guidelines for returning an athlete to sport and the decision rests on clinical judgment and collaboration between the clinician, physical therapist, trainer, and the athlete. As the understanding of this injury and its management in the athlete expands, the negative impact of these injuries may be lessened to some degree.

REFERENCES

1. Noback PC, Jang ES, Cuellar DO, et al. Risk factors for Achilles tendon rupture: a matched case control study. Injury 2017;48(10):2342–7.
2. Ho G, Tantigate D, Kirschenbaum J, et al. Increasing age in Achilles rupture patients over time. Injury 2017;48(7):1701–9.
3. Davies GJ, McCarty E, Provencher M, et al. ACL return to sport guidelines and criteria. Curr Rev Musculoskelet Med 2017;10(3):307–14.
4. Willits K, Amendola A, Bryant D, et al. Operative versus nonoperative treatment of acute Achilles tendon ruptures. J Bone Joint Surg Am 2010;92(17):2767–75.
5. Barfod KW, Bencke J, Lauridsen HB, et al. Nonoperative dynamic treatment of acute Achilles tendon rupture: the influence of early weight-bearing on clinical outcome. J Bone Joint Surg Am 2014;96(18):1497–503.
6. Soroceanu A, Sidhwa F, Aarabi S, et al. Surgical versus nonsurgical treatment of acute Achilles tendon rupture: a meta-analysis of randomized trials. J Bone Joint Surg Am 2012;94(23):2136–43.
7. Enwemeka CS. Functional loading augments the initial tensile strength and energy absorption capacity of regenerating rabbit Achilles tendons. Am J Phys Med Rehabil 1992;71(1):31–8.
8. Lin TW, Cardenas L, Soslowsky LJ. Biomechanics of tendon injury and repair. J Biomech 2004;37(6):865–77.

9. Schepull T, Aspenberg P. Early controlled tension improves the material properties of healing human Achilles tendons after ruptures. Am J Sports Med 2013; 41(11):2550–7.
10. Suchak AA, Bostick GP, Beaupré LA, et al. The influence of early weight-bearing compared with non-weight-bearing after surgical repair of the Achilles tendon. J Bone Joint Surg Am 2008;90(9):1876–83.
11. Kangas J, Pajala A, Ohtonen P, et al. Achilles tendon elongation after rupture repair. Am J Sports Med 2007;35(1):59–64.
12. Grävare Silbernagel K, Crossley KM. A proposed return-to-sport program for patients with midportion Achilles tendinopathy: rationale and implementation. J Orthop Sports Phys Ther 2015;45(11):876–86.
13. Habets B, van den Broek AG, Huisstede BMA, et al. Return to sport in athletes with midportion Achilles tendinopathy: a qualitative systematic review regarding definitions and criteria. Sports Med 2018;48(3):705–23.
14. Ardern CL, Glasgow P, Schneiders A, et al. 2016 Consensus statement on return to sport from the First World Congress in Sports Physical Therapy, Bern. Br J Sports Med 2016;50(14):853–64.
15. Nilsson-Helander K, Thomeé R, Grävare-Silbernagel K, et al. The Achilles tendon total rupture score (ATRS). Am J Sports Med 2007;35(3):421–6.
16. Hansen MS, Christensen M, Budolfsen T, et al. Achilles tendon total rupture score at 3 months can predict patients' ability to return to sport 1 year after injury. Knee Surg Sports Traumatol Arthrosc 2016;24(4):1365–71.
17. Bostick GP, Jomha NM, Suchak AA, et al. Factors associated with calf muscle endurance recovery 1 year after Achilles tendon rupture repair. J Orthop Sports Phys Ther 2010;40(6):345–51.
18. Fanchini M, Impellizzeri FM, Silbernagel KG, et al. Return to competition after an Achilles tendon rupture using both on and off the field load monitoring as guidance: a case report of a top-level soccer player. Phys Ther Sport 2018;29:70–8.
19. Byrne PA, Hopper GP, Wilson WT, et al. Knotless repair of Achilles tendon rupture in an elite athlete: return to competition in 18 weeks. J Foot Ankle Surg 2017; 56(1):121–4.
20. Zellers JA, Carmont MR, Grävare Silbernagel K. Return to play post-Achilles tendon rupture: a systematic review and meta-analysis of rate and measures of return to play. Br J Sports Med 2016;50(21):1325–32.
21. Parekh SG, Wray WH, Brimmo O, et al. Epidemiology and outcomes of Achilles tendon ruptures in the National Football League. Foot Ankle Spec 2009;2(6): 283–6.
22. Mai HT, Alvarez AP, Freshman RD, et al. The NFL orthopaedic surgery outcomes database (NO-SOD). Am J Sports Med 2016;44(9):2255–62.
23. Jack RA, Sochacki KR, Gardner SS, et al. Performance and return to sport after Achilles tendon repair in National Football League players. Foot Ankle Int 2017; 38(10):1092–9.
24. Amin NH, Old AB, Tabb LP, et al. Performance outcomes after repair of complete Achilles tendon ruptures in National Basketball Association players. Am J Sports Med 2013;41(8):1864–8.
25. Minhas SV, Kester BS, Larkin KE, et al. The effect of an orthopaedic surgical procedure in the National Basketball Association. Am J Sports Med 2016;44(4): 1056–61.
26. Saltzman BM, Tetreault MW, Bohl DD, et al. Analysis of player statistics in Major League Baseball players before and after Achilles tendon repair. HSS J 2017; 13(2):108–18.

27. Maffulli N, Longo UG, Maffulli GD, et al. Achilles tendon ruptures in elite athletes. Foot Ankle Int 2011;32(1):9–15.
28. Gajhede-Knudsen M, Ekstrand J, Magnusson H, et al. Recurrence of Achilles tendon injuries in elite male football players is more common after early return to play: an 11-year follow-up of the UEFA Champions League injury study. Br J Sports Med 2013;47(12):763–8.
29. Amin NH, McCullough KC, Mills GL, et al. The impact and functional outcomes of Achilles tendon pathology in National Basketball Association players. Clin Res Foot Ankle 2016;4(3). https://doi.org/10.4172/2329-910X.1000205.
30. Hardy A, Rousseau R, Issa S-P, et al. Functional outcomes and return to sports after surgical treatment of insertional Achilles tendinopathy: surgical approach tailored to the degree of tendon involvement. Orthop Traumatol Surg Res 2018. https://doi.org/10.1016/j.otsr.2018.05.003.
31. Trofa DP, Miller JC, Jang ES, et al. Professional athletes' return to play and performance after operative repair of an Achilles tendon rupture. Am J Sports Med 2017;45(12):2864–71.

Management of Complications of Achilles Tendon Surgery

Jordan Liles, MD[a,*], Samuel B. Adams Jr, MD[b]

KEYWORDS

• Achilles tendon graft • Reconstruction • Augmentation

KEY POINTS

- Complications after surgical repair of Achilles tendon rupture or débridement for Achilles tendinopathy can be broken down into these main categories: wound breakdown, infection, and rerupture/tendon gap.
- There are multiple techniques to treat tendon defects in the event end-to-end repair cannot be achieved after débridement. In general, the choice of treatment technique is based on size of the resultant gap.
- Treatment options include negative-pressure therapy and skin grafting, bipedicle tissue transfer and graft, flexor hallucis augmentation, flexor digitorum longus transfer, peroneus brevis tendon transfer, V-Y lengthening, gastrocnemius turndown, and allograft.
- Although each treatment technique has literature to support its use, there are no data to support the use of 1 technique over another. Treatment should be based on the experience and discretion of the treating surgeon.
- This article proposes an algorithm for wound breakdown, infection, and rerupture after Achilles tendon surgery. This algorithm should be used as a guide.

INTRODUCTION

Achilles tendon ruptures can be debilitating for patients, affecting ankle stability, strength, and proper gait mechanics. Over the past 40 years, incidence of Achilles tendon ruptures has continually risen, especially in so-called weekend warriors.[1] Although debate still exists among surgeons as to the best treatment of acute ruptures, primary repair is associated with good outcomes, a decreased rerupture rate, and increased strength compared with nonoperative treatment.[2] Despite these benefits of operative treatment of Achilles tendon ruptures, surgical complications exist.

Disclosure Statement: No disclosures.
[a] Department of Orthopaedic Surgery, Duke University Medical Center, Box 3000, Durham, NC 27710, USA; [b] Duke University Medical Center, 40 Duke Medicine Circle, Room 5309 (Orange), Durham, NC 27710, USA
* Corresponding author.
E-mail address: Jordan.liles@duke.edu

Foot Ankle Clin N Am 24 (2019) 447–457
https://doi.org/10.1016/j.fcl.2019.04.008
1083-7515/19/

Complications after surgical repair of Achilles tendon rupture or débridement for Achilles tendinopathy can be broken down into these main categories: wound breakdown, infection, and rerupture/tendon gap. These are not mutually exclusive problems, meaning often untreated wound breakdown leads to surgical site infection and tendon débridement and the treating surgeon must find resolution for all 3 problems. Additional complications can include decreased strength, sural nerve injury, venous thrombosis, and loss of ankle dorsiflexion among others. This article focuses on the management of wound breakdown, infection, and rerupture/tendon gap.

Although there is a plethora of case studies and small retrospective studies outlining single-episode success with Achilles surgery complications, there are few long-term, prospective data to help guide surgeons as to which surgery provides the best option for postsurgical complications. This article reviews the literature for the treatment of complications after Achilles tendon surgery. Although the pathology and surgical treatment of acute Achilles tendon rupture and Achilles tendinosis are different, the treatment of complications from these 2 surgeries are similar and are discussed as 1 throughout this text.

RISK FACTORS FOR COMPLICATIONS

The complication rate after open Achilles tendon surgery is low. Rensing and colleagues[3] used the National Surgical Quality Improvement Program database to review 1626 Achilles tendon surgeries for complications. They found a 1.7% perioperative complication rate. There were 0.7% superficial wound infections and 0.4% wound disruptions. There were no reported cases of nerve injury or repair failure, although this was a large database study likely lacking some of this information. Systemic complications occurred in 0.4% of patients, most commonly with deep vein thrombosis or nonfatal pulmonary embolism.

The complications after Achilles tendon surgery can be devastating and, therefore, it is important to understand the potential risk factors implicated in these complications so that they can be mitigated. Traditionally theorized risk factors leading to infection and rerupture include steroids, smoking, diabetes, and treatment delay. Pajala and colleagues[1] reviewed 409 operatively treated Achilles tendon ruptures and found a rerupture rate of 5.6% and a deep infection rate of 2.2%. Patients with deep infections were significantly older and had received steroid medication more often, had sustained tendon injury during everyday activities more often, and had a longer delay before treatment than patients without reruptures and patients with simple rerupture. They also reported a staggering increasing incidence of infection with time.

Similarly, Jildeh and colleagues[4] retrospectively reviewed 423 patients who underwent operative treatment of Achilles tendon rupture. They found that that the incidence of rerupture was 1% and the infection rate was 2.8%. The median time between surgery and rerupture was 38 days and the median time between surgery and infection was 30 days. Bruggeman and colleagues[5] retrospectively reviewed 164 open Achilles repairs and found a 10.4% incidence of wound complications. Tobacco use, steroids, and female gender are statistically significant independent risk factors for wound complication.

There also are risk factors at the time of surgery that can be mitigated. Meticulous hemostasis and careful wound handling technique, such as limited wound grabbing and avoidance of superficial self-retainer retractors, can help avoid devastating complications. Unfortunately, the nature of the trauma and surgical repair lends to potential problems with wound closure. If a tenuous closure occurs, consideration should be given to increasing the amount of sutures, leaving the sutures in longer, and the use of an incisional negative-pressure wound dressing. Additionally, an anterior-based splint to avoid pressure on the wound can help avoid pressure on the wound but does leave the wound unprotected if a patient is supine.

In addition to surgical mindfulness of the soft tissues, the approach also can lead to complications. Wong and colleagues[6] reviewed complication rates between percutaneous repairs and open repairs. They found the wound complication rate 4.9% with percutaneous repairs and 12.3% with open repairs. Moreover, some investigators have reported no wound complications with percutaneous repairs. Lim and colleagues[7] reported a wound infection rate of 21% with open repair and 0% for percutaneous repair. Yang and colleagues[8] performed a meta-analysis of percutaneous repair versus open repair of acute Achilles tendon ruptures. They found that the sural nerve injury rate was significantly higher in percutaneous repairs but the deep infection rate was significantly higher with open repairs. There was no difference in rerupture rate between the 2 repair techniques.

Surgery increases the risk of infection, but it can reduce the risk of rerupture. Bhandari and colleagues[9] published a meta-analysis of Achilles tendon ruptures and found that the risk of rerupture was 13% for nonoperatively treated patients and only 3.1% for patients treated with surgery. Similarly, Khan and colleagues[10] published a meta-analysis and found the rerupture rate with conservative treatment was 12.6% and only 3.5% for operatively treated patients.

TREATMENT OF WOUND BREAKDOWN AND DEEP INFECTION

A deep infection after surgical repair of an Achilles tendon rupture is a relatively rare but devastating problem, because the skin and soft tissue defects associated with Achilles tendon loss constitute a major challenge for the surgeon. Although wound breakdown and deep infection do not necessarily occur together, the treatment of both is similar.

The authors recommend aggressive early treatment of wound breakdown to prevent deep infection (**Fig. 1**). Although nonoperative wound care can be appropriate in certain settings, such as unexposed tendon, the authors believe that aggressive early operative intervention is important because deep infection necessitates the removal of the braided nonabsorbable sutures used in the Achilles tendon repair or Achilles tendon attachment to the calcaneus. Most likely, early débridement and wound management can prevent deep infection after wound breakdown. If deep infection occurs and removal of the tendon is required, the resultant tendon deficit can be treated like a chronic tendon rupture (discussed later). There are few data describing the outcome after débridement for infection.

In the setting of deep infection, the patient should be returned to the operating room until the infection is under control and the tendon is appropriately débrided. All foreign material used for the repair should be removed. An infectious disease consult should be obtained for antibiotic treatment. A negative-pressure wound device should be placed after each débridement. Pajala and colleagues[1] treated 9 infections with operative intervention, including débridement, necrotic Achilles tendon débridement, and wound revision. Three patients necessitated only 1 surgery. Six patients required serial débridement and ultimately split-thickness skin grafting. Four of these 6 patients lost the Achilles tendon in its entirety.

Once the wound bed has been adequately débrided and the infection is under control, coverage is provided with split-thickness skin grafts, local transposition flaps, or free tissue transfers with use of a microvascular anastomosis. These techniques all have demonstrated success but the literature supporting the treatment of 1 technique over another is sparse. Therefore, it is important to consult plastic surgery early in this process. The

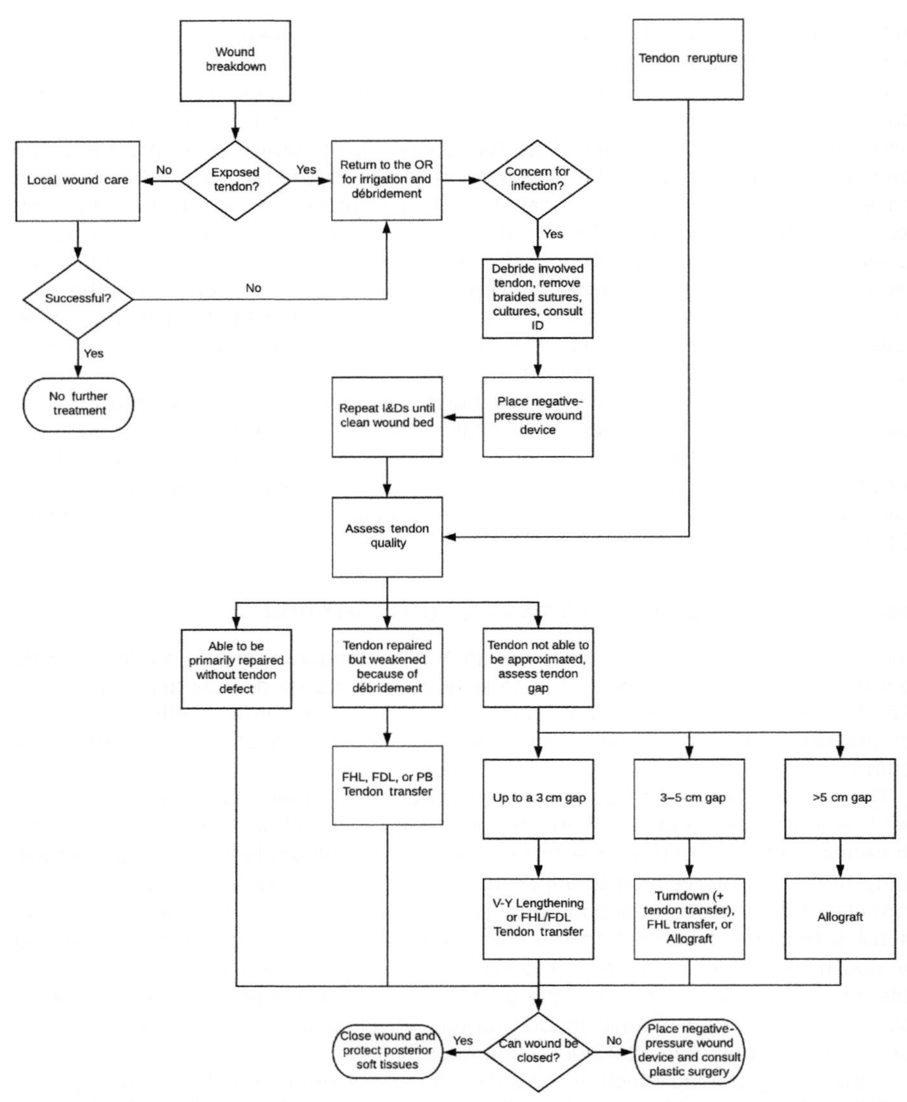

Fig. 1. Algorithm for wound breakdown, infection, and rerupture after Achilles tendon surgery. This is algorithm should be used as guide. I&D, Incision and Debridement; OR, Operating Room.

authors' plastic surgery colleagues have a reconstructive ladder that ranks reconstruction techniques by progressive complexity and wound characteristics. Techniques include secondary intention, skin grafting, and flaps. The literature on this topic is full of case reports and small case series demonstrating the effectiveness of flaps, and, therefore, flaps are the currently accepted treatment to repair wounds to this area. Numerous kinds of flaps are available, including local, perforator, and free flaps.

Although a majority of these techniques necessitate plastic surgery involvement, there are a few techniques that can be used by the orthopedic surgeon. These are discussed later.

Negative-pressure Therapy and Skin Grafting

Negative-pressure therapy, although potentially suited for definitive treatment of Achilles wounds, mostly has been used as temporary coverage between débridement surgeries and/or until such time that definitive coverage occurs. In instances where plastic surgery support is not available, however, negative-pressure therapy and skin grafting are available for the orthopedic surgeon to initiate. Its most common reported usage has been for wound bed preparation prior to skin grafting. Heugel and colleagues[11] reported the case of successful negative-pressure wound therapy used on an Achilles wound prior to skin grafting. In a case series of 3 patients with Achilles wounds, Repta and colleagues[12] successfully used negative-pressure therapy followed by skin grafting. Their protocol involved negative-pressure therapy placed in the operating room with subsequent home health care vacuum changes. Patients are allowed activity as tolerated. Once sufficient granulation tissue was evident in the wound bed, the patients underwent split-thickness skin grafting. The time from wound vacuum placement to skin grafting was 4 weeks, 7 weeks, and 12 weeks in these 3 patients.

The reports, discussed previously, used this technique in the setting of a clean wound bed. Mosser and colleagues[13] used wound vacuum and skin grafting to treat 6 patients with deep infections after open Achilles tendon surgery. After adequate débridement, the wound vacuum was used for wound bed preconditioning and then a split-thickness skin graft was placed. Unlike in the study by Repta and colleagues,[12] the duration of wound vacuum therapy for these 6 patients was an average of 13.6 days. There were no further wound breakdowns or infection persistence at a mean of 30 months.

Although a potentially long time for wound healing is needed, negative-pressure therapy has an advantage over free flaps because there is no donor site morbidity. Negative-pressure therapy and skin grafting also should be considered in patients with medical comorbidities precluding them from successful flap coverage.

Bipedicle Tissue Transfer and Skin Graft

Dekker and colleagues[14] described a simple, local tissue transfer, a bipedicle fasciocutaneous flap that uses a dissection that can be performed by a community surgeon without resources of tertiary/specialized care or microvascular support. The report was a case series of 3 patients successfully treated with this technique. The technique involves a longitudinal incision directly posterior to the lateral malleolus and anterior to the peroneal artery and sural nerve. The incision is made to the depth of the fascia and the dissection is performed posteriorly to the posterior wound. The flap then is mobilized posteriorly to close the posterior wound. The resultant lateral wound is skin grafted.

TREATMENT OF RERUPTURE/TENDON GAP

Although reruptures in the setting of no wound problem can be treated nonoperatively, typically, defects created from débridement for infection are treated operatively, including simple repair, Achilles lengthening procedure, and/or augmentation, depending on the chronicity and tendon gap. There is a lack of literature to determine an algorithm for tendon reconstruction. Pajala and colleagues[1] treated 23 reruptures with 6 weeks of immobilization (4) and various surgical procedures (19) and found that only 2 patients had a second rerupture. Both of these patients had previous Achilles surgery. Unfortunately, with the numbers provided, there was no way to tell superiority of 1 treatment method. The size of the tendon defect after débridement is an important determinate of the reconstruction technique (see **Fig. 1**). The authors' algorithm is simply a guide but in general favors more aggressive options for a certain sized defect than what previously has been published. This article reviews the treatment options for treating tendon gaps.

Flexor Hallucis Longus Augmentation

The flexor hallucis longus (FHL) tendon transfer has become popular in the management of Achilles tendon disorders. It can be used independently or in conjunction with other techniques. Therefore, there are many variations in techniques for harvesting the FHL and securing it to either the calcaneus, the Achilles tendon, or itself. This article describes the basic techniques and relevant literature.

The FHL tendon can be harvested from the Achilles tendon wound or from the midfoot for a longer tendon harvest. When harvested from the posterior wound, the Achilles tendon is retracted to reveal the anterior paratenon and underlying fascia over the posterior compartment. This fascia is subsequently excised to reveal the FHL muscle belly. A traction suture or clamp is used to pull the tendon proximally whereas plantar flexion of the great toe and ankle expose more tendon length. Distally, at the entrance of the tarsal tunnel, the tendon is sharply cut and then pulled proximally out of the surgical incision. The tendon then is secured with thick braided suture and pulled through a tunnel in the calcaneus placed just anterior to the native Achilles tendon insertion. With tension preserved, an interference screw is placed in the tunnel to secure the tendons insertion at the calcaneus.

Alternatively, the FHL can be harvested from the midfoot through an incision from the inferior navicular distally along the dorsal border of the abductor hallucis muscle toward the first metatarsophalangeal joint. After reflecting the abductor hallucis muscle, the flexor digitorum longus (FDL) and FHL tendons can be visualized. The FHL tendon is transected as far distally as possible. The remaining distal stump of the FHL is sutured to the FDL with all 5 toes in neutral position. The FHL is retrieved through the posterior wound and can be looped through a drill hole in the calcaneus and back onto itself and the Achilles tendon. Although this technique provides for more tendon length, there is a theoretic increased risk of nerve injury. Mulier and colleagues,[15] in a cadaver study of FHL harvests from the midfoot, found a 33% incidence of medial or lateral plantar nerve injury and 2 complete transections of medial plantar nerve.

The outcomes of FHL transfer generally are good. A recent retrospective study of 21 patients treated with FHL transfer harvested from the midfoot demonstrated no difference in concentric strength between the operative and nonoperative sides.[16] The FHL transfer side, however, had diminished endurance and total work energy. Similarly, Lever and colleagues[17] reported a mean reduction in dynamometer-measured strength of ankle plantar flexion, in comparison to the nonoperative side, of 24% after midfoot harvest of the FHL tendon. The hallux had a mean of 40% reduction in plantar flexion strength compared with the nonoperative side. A similar retrospective review of 40 patients (42 ankles) demonstrated significant improvement in the American Orthopaedic Foot and Ankle Society (AOFAS) hindfoot score.[18]

FHL transfer has been combined with other augmentation techniques. Koh and colleagues[19] compared FHL transfer to midsubstance turndown plus FHL transfer for chronic ruptures. The investigators followed the patients for 1 year and found significant improvement and minimal pain in both groups. This study also demonstrated that the FHL transfer alone can be used for large gaps. The mean gap length in this study for FHL transfer was 5 cm. Similarly, another study evaluated a combined proximal stump turndown combined with an FHL transfer in 32 patients with 6 cm or larger defects.[20] They found full healing in all patients by 5 months and significant improvement in the Foot and Ankle Ability Measure and visual analog scale for pain.

Comparisons between calcaneus fixation techniques have been reported. Benca and colleagues[21] compared the transosseus calcaneus tunnel technique to the tenodesis screw technique in cadavers. The tenodesis screw group demonstrated significantly less displacement (loosening) and higher load than the transosseus group. A similar study by Liu and colleagues,[22] however, found no differences in ultimate strength, peak stress, or failure strain between the groups.

The authors typically use the FHL tendon transfer as an augment to end-to-end repairs or other repair techniques or by itself for tendon gaps of up to 3 cm (see **Fig. 1**).

Flexor Digitorum Longus Tendon Transfer

The FDL tendon can be harvested as an alternative to the FHL tendon. The FDL typically is harvested from the midfoot as described for FHL tendon transfer. The FDL is transected proximal to the division into digital branches. The distal stump should then be sutured to the FHL. The FDL then can be retrieved through the posterior wound and can be looped through a drill hole in the calcaneus, similar to securing the FHL. Mann and colleagues[23] reported on 7 patients with and FDL transfer. At a mean of 39 months, 6 patients were doing good or excellent.

If less FDL length is needed and less morbid dissection is required, the FDL can be harvested through a small incision over the talonavicular joint.[24] With a shorter FDL using this technique, the FDL was attached to the calcaneus with an anchor. Although this study was performed in chronic Achilles tendinopathy and not necessarily Achilles tendon defects, the investigators found significant improvement in pain and 36-Item Short Form Health Survey function in 15 patients. Although not directly comparing to FHL transfer, the investigators propose the use of FDL transfer in a more active population. It is important to understand, however, that there was some native Achilles tendon intact in all cases with the use of FDL transfer. Therefore, the authors do not use this technique alone, only to supplement other techniques. Unfortunately, the authors are unaware of a direct comparison between FHL and FDL transfers.

Peroneus Brevis Tendon Transfer

Although less common than FHL or FDL transfer, the peroneus brevis (PB) transfer has demonstrated promise in Achilles defect repair. Although not supported by data, the authors prefer to preserve the PB whenever possible and favor FHL and FDL transfer over PB transfer whenever possible because of the important eversion function of the PB. Although, as described later, studies show that PB harvest does not cause appreciable weakness. The authors believe that if used, the PB should be used in conjunction with another treatment technique, either direct repair, V-Y advancement, gastrocnemius turndown, or allograft. PB transfer originally was described in 1974.[25] The technique is as follows. The insertion point of the PB then is identified at the base of the fifth metatarsal through a minitransverse incision. The PB tendon then is brought through the posterior wound and is looped through a drill hole in the calcaneus and fixed to itself and/or the Achilles tendon.

Transfer of the PB does not seem to cause noticeable weakness. Gallant and colleagues[26] evaluated eversion and plantar flexion strength after PB transfer. They found mild eversion weakness and no plantar flexion weakness in 8 patients. Tawari and colleagues[27] reported good or excellent results in 85% of patients using a PB tendon to augment a direct repair in the acute setting by using a transverse bone tunnel through the calcaneus. The Achilles tendon was repaired directly and the PB tendon was passed through the tunnel and sutured to itself. Sebastian and colleagues[28] performed a cadaveric study comparing PB with FHL tendon transfer for Achilles tendon augmentation and found that failure load with the PB transfer was significantly higher than with transfer of the FHL; however, all failures were related to pullout of the transferred tendon and not direct tendon failure.

V-Y Lengthening

For defects up to 3 cm in length, a V-Y lengthening is considered by the authors. Proximally, each arm of the V should be at least twice the length of the measured defect to allow for as little tension as possible on the repair. Once the arms are marked, incision is made through the gastrocnemius fascia but not carried anteriorly through the muscle. The distal aspect of the tendon then is stretched over time until the correct length is obtained using either suture tags or a clamp. The proximal inverted V is repaired with nonabsorbable braided suture to create a Y repair. Distally, there is direct end-t- end repair of the tendon using nonabsorbable suture.

The authors believe this technique was first in 1975 by Abraham and Pankovich.[29] They reported on the successful use of this technique in 4 patients with the only complication sural nerve injury in 1 patient. Zayda retrospectively studied 9 patients with large (range 5–7 cm), chronic defects of the Achilles tendon, which were repaired with V-Y lengthening and plantaris tendon augmentation and reported this technique as an "adequate surgical option with no major complications and no rerupturing."[30] Of the 9 patients, 3 developed superficial infection, which was treated with wound care and antibiotics for 2 and surgical débridement for the third.

Augmentation of the V-Y lengthening has been described. The close proximity of the plantaris tendon to the Achilles tendon makes it an obvious choice for augmentation but there is no biomechanical study to the authors' knowledge studying strength of repair by using a V-Y lengthening with plantaris augmentation. Nevertheless, there are case reports describing its technique with good outcomes and no rerupture. Elias and colleagues[31] reported on the use of V-Y lengthening and FHL transfer for neglected Achilles tendon rupture in 15 patients with 5 cm or larger gaps. All patients had good to excellent AOFAS scores and were satisfied with the surgery. Although this report demonstrates successful use of this technique in greater than 5 cm defects, the authors find it difficult to reliably achieve more than 3 cm of length with V-Y lengthening.

Gastrocnemius Turndown

With defects ranging from 3 cm to 5 cm and adequate gastrocnemius fascia distally in proximity to the tear, a gastrocnemius turndown may be considered. Typically, this technique is supported by a tendon transfer. Using this technique, 2 longitudinal incisions separating the gastrocnemius fascia into thirds are made 1 cm proximal to the proximal end of the defect and carried proximally until the incisions are 2 cm longer than the defect. The fascia then is dissected from the underlying gastrocnemius muscle and turned distally over the defect until it contacts the distal stump. The turndown then is reinforced on both ends proximally with nonabsorbable suture, to prevent propagation of tears in the fascia proximally, and distally with a direct end-to-end repair with nonabsorbable suture.

Koh and colleagues[19] reported on mean 5.5-cm defects treated with turndown flaps supplemented with FHL transfer. They reported significant improvement in outcome scores at 1 year. Another study performed turndown and V-Y lengthening in 17 patients with a mean defect length of 6 cm. The mean AOFAS score improved from 64 to 95.[32]

Achilles Tendon Allograft

Achilles tendon allograft with or without a bone block attached to the calcaneus is an underreported but viable treatment option for large defects. The authors have found this technique reliable in repairing defects of greater than 5 cm. The distal Achilles stump must be inspected carefully. If there is any degeneration, then an Achilles allograft with a bone block into the calcaneus should be used. The graft is inspected and the calcaneus bone block is measured. The corresponding size and shape are removed from a patient's calcaneus and secured with a screw. The leg is plantarflexed and the allograft is secured to the proximal stump. The authors typically use a Krackow suture in the allograft and proximal native tendon to secure.

Song and Hua[33] performed a systematic review of allograft treatment of chronic Achilles tendon ruptures. They found 34 patients in 9 publications who met their inclusion criteria. All patients experienced good clinical and functional results. Deese and colleagues[34] retrospectively reviewed 8 patients who had tendon allograft with calcaneal bone block. All patients had good function at most recent follow-up.

SUMMARY

Operative treatment of Achilles tendon rupture can be treated successfully with surgery. Surgical repair is not without complications, mainly wound breakdown and rerupture. The literature addressing these complications is sparse and a universally accepted treatment protocol has not been established. Wound breakdown should be treated aggressively to prevent deep infection if not already present. Wound breakdown that is unable to be closed can be treated with local tissue rearrangement or flaps, potentially under the direction of a plastic surgeon. Deep infection should be treated with serial irrigations and tendon repair or reconstruction. There are multiple techniques to treat tendon defects in the event end-to-end repair cannot be achieved after débridement. In general, the choice of treatment technique is based on size of the resultant gap. Although each treatment technique has literature to support its use, there are no data to support the use of 1 technique over another. Treatment should be based on the experience and discretion of the treating surgeon.

REFERENCES

1. Pajala A, Kangas J, Ohtonen P, et al. Rerupture and deep infection following treatment of total Achilles tendon rupture. J Bone Joint Surg Am 2002;84-A(11): 2016–21.
2. Erickson BJ, Mascarenhas R, Saltzman BM, et al. Is operative treatment of Achilles tendon ruptures superior to nonoperative treatment?: A systematic review of overlapping meta-analyses. Orthop J Sports Med 2015;3(4). 2325967115579188.
3. Rensing N, Waterman BR, Frank RM, et al. Low risk for local and systemic complications after primary repair of 1626 achilles tendon ruptures. Foot Ankle Spec 2017;10(3):216–26.
4. Jildeh TR, Okoroha KR, Marshall NE, et al. Infection and rerupture after surgical repair of achilles tendons. Orthop J Sports Med 2018;6(5). 2325967118774302.
5. Bruggeman NB, Turner NS, Dahm DL, et al. Wound complications after open Achilles tendon repair: an analysis of risk factors. Clin Orthop Relat Res 2004;(427):63–6.
6. Wong J, Barrass V, Maffulli N. Quantitative review of operative and nonoperative management of achilles tendon ruptures. Am J Sports Med 2002;30(4):565–75.
7. Lim J, Dalal R, Waseem M. Percutaneous vs. open repair of the ruptured Achilles tendon–a prospective randomized controlled study. Foot Ankle Int 2001;22(7): 559–68.

8. Yang B, Liu Y, Kan S, et al. Outcomes and complications of percutaneous versus open repair of acute Achilles tendon rupture: A meta-analysis. Int J Surg 2017;40: 178–86.
9. Bhandari M, Guyatt GH, Siddiqui F, et al. Treatment of acute Achilles tendon ruptures: a systematic overview and metaanalysis. Clin Orthop Relat Res 2002;(400): 190–200.
10. Khan RJ, Fick D, Keogh A, et al. Treatment of acute achilles tendon ruptures. A meta-analysis of randomized, controlled trials. J Bone Joint Surg Am 2005; 87(10):2202–10.
11. Heugel JR, Parks KS, Christie SS, et al. Treatment of the exposed Achilles tendon using negative pressure wound therapy: a case report. J Burn Care Rehabil 2002;23(3):167–71.
12. Repta R, Ford R, Hoberman L, et al. The use of negative-pressure therapy and skin grafting in the treatment of soft-tissue defects over the Achilles tendon. Ann Plast Surg 2005;55(4):367–70.
13. Mosser P, Kelm J, Anagnostakos K. Negative pressure wound therapy in the management of late deep infections after open reconstruction of achilles tendon rupture. J Foot Ankle Surg 2015;54(1):2–6.
14. Dekker TJ, Avashia Y, Mithani SK, et al. Single-stage bipedicle local tissue transfer and skin graft for achilles tendon surgery wound complications. Foot Ankle Spec 2017;10(1):46–50.
15. Mulier T, Rummens E, Dereymaeker G. Risk of neurovascular injuries in flexor hallucis longus tendon transfers: an anatomic cadaver study. Foot Ankle Int 2007; 28(8):910–5.
16. Alhaug OK, Berdal G, Husebye EE, et al. Flexor hallucis longus tendon transfer for chronic Achilles tendon rupture. A retrospective study. Foot Ankle Surg 2018. [Epub ahead of print].
17. Lever CJ, Bosman HA, Robinson AHN. The functional and dynamometer-tested results of transtendinous flexor hallucis longus transfer for neglected ruptures of the Achilles tendon at six years' follow-up. Bone Joint J 2018;100-B(5):584–9.
18. Rahm S, Spross C, Gerber F, et al. Operative treatment of chronic irreparable Achilles tendon ruptures with large flexor hallucis longus tendon transfers. Foot Ankle Int 2013;34(8):1100–10.
19. Koh D, Lim J, Chen JY, et al. Flexor hallucis longus transfer versus turndown flaps augmented with flexor hallucis longus transfer in the repair of chronic Achilles tendon rupture. Foot Ankle Surg 2017;25(2):221–5.
20. Ahmad J, Jones K, Raikin SM. Treatment of chronic Achilles tendon ruptures with large defects. Foot Ankle Spec 2016;9(5):400–8.
21. Benca E, Willegger M, Wenzel F, et al. Biomechanical evaluation of two methods of fixation of a flexor hallucis longus tendon graft. Bone Joint J 2018;100-B(9): 1175–81.
22. Liu GT, Balldin BC, Zide JR, et al. A Biomechanical analysis of interference screw versus bone tunnel fixation of flexor hallucis longus tendon transfers to the calcaneus. J Foot Ankle Surg 2017;56(4):813–6.
23. Mann RA, Holmes GB Jr, Seale KS, et al. Chronic rupture of the Achilles tendon: a new technique of repair. J Bone Joint Surg Am 1991;73(2):214–9.
24. de Cesar Netto C, Chinanuvathana A, Fonseca LFD, et al. Outcomes of flexor digitorum longus (FDL) tendon transfer in the treatment of Achilles tendon disorders. Foot Ankle Surg 2017 [pii:S1268-7731(17)31364-4].

25. Perez Teuffer A. Traumatic rupture of the Achilles Tendon. Reconstruction by transplant and graft using the lateral peroneus brevis. Orthop Clin North Am 1974;5(1):89–93.
26. Gallant GG, Massie C, Turco VJ. Assessment of eversion and plantar flexion strength after repair of Achilles tendon rupture using peroneus brevis tendon transfer. Am J Orthop (Belle Mead NJ) 1995;24(3):257–61.
27. Tawari AA, Dhamangaonkar AA, Goregaonkar AB, et al. Augmented repair of degenerative tears of tendo achilles using peroneus brevis tendon: early results. Malays Orthop J 2013;7(1):19–24.
28. Sebastian H, Datta B, Maffulli N, et al. Mechanical properties of reconstructed achilles tendon with transfer of peroneus brevis or flexor hallucis longus tendon. J Foot Ankle Surg 2007;46(6):424–8.
29. Abraham E, Pankovich AM. Neglected rupture of the Achilles tendon. Treatment by V-Y tendinous flap. J Bone Joint Surg Am 1975;57(2):253–5.
30. El sayed AS, Zayda AI. V-Y plasty and plantaris tendon augmentation repair in treatment of chronic ruptured achilles tendon. Biomed J Sci Tech Res 2018; 2(5). https://biomedres.us/pdfs/BJSTR.MS.ID.000823.pdf.
31. Elias I, Besser M, Nazarian LN, et al. Reconstruction for missed or neglected Achilles tendon rupture with V-Y lengthening and flexor hallucis longus tendon transfer through one incision. Foot Ankle Int 2007;28(12):1238–48.
32. Guclu B, Basat HC, Yildirim T, et al. Long-term results of chronic Achilles tendon ruptures repaired with V-Y tendon plasty and fascia turndown. Foot Ankle Int 2016;37(7):737–42.
33. Song YJ, Hua YH. Tendon allograft for treatment of chronic Achilles tendon rupture: a systematic review. Foot Ankle Surg 2018 [pii:S1268-7731(18)30025-0].
34. Deese JM, Gratto-cox G, Clements FD, et al. Achilles allograft reconstruction for chronic achilles tendinopathy. J Surg Orthop Adv 2015;24(1):75–8.

Endoscopic Management of Chronic Achilles Tendon Rupture

Turab Arshad Syed, MBChB, MRCS, MFSEM, DipSEM, DipSICOT, FRCS (Orth), MSc, MFST (Ed)[a,*],
Anthony Perera, MBChB, MRCS, MFSEM, PG Dip (Med Law), FRCS (Orth)[b]

KEYWORDS

- FHL • Flexor hallucis longus • Endoscopic reconstruction • Tendoachilles • Achilles • Chronic • Rupture

KEY POINTS

- An endoscopic flexor hallucis tendon reconstruction for chronic rupture tendoachilles surgical technique is described.
- Endoscopic flexor hallucis tendon harvest and reconstruction of chronic Achilles tendon rupture allows less soft tissue dissection, avoids violation of the plantar surface of the foot, decreases the chance of fracture through the osseous tunnel, and deceases complications associated with open reconstruction.
- Tips and pitfalls for this technique are shared from these authors' personal experiences to improve this technique and reduce risks and complications.

INTRODUCTION

Chronic ruptures of the Achilles tendon are defined as a complete tear that has been untreated for more than 4 weeks.[1,2] They often occur after missed injuries, but can also be seen after managed neglect, for instance when other medical complications have precluded surgical and or even conservative treatment. They present primarily with weakness of push-off because they are rarely very painful, particularly when long-standing[3,4] This situation presents a considerable challenge to the surgeon because the complications from complex late reconstruction are a significant concern.[5]

Primary repair may be attempted up to 4 weeks after rupture, but this depends primarily on the gap size and mandates an open approach. The missed injury often presents later than this and thus the gap is may often be greater than 4 cm, thus

Disclosure Statement: None.
[a] Department of Trauma & Orthopaedic Surgery, Royal Free London Hospital NHS Foundation Trust, Level 7, Pond Street, Hampstead, London NW3 2QG, UK; [b] University Hospital Llandough (UHL), Penlan Road, Llandough, CF64 2XX, UK
* Corresponding author.
E-mail address: Turab.syed@gmail.com

Foot Ankle Clin N Am 24 (2019) 459–470
https://doi.org/10.1016/j.fcl.2019.04.010 foot.theclinics.com

necessitating more complex reconstructions using local tissues such as turn-down flaps[6] and gastrocnemius VY plasty.[7] However, even these techniques are insufficient if the gap is greater than 6 cm[8] and this requires the use of tissues interposed in the gap such as a tendon graft (autograft or allograft)[9,10] or foreign material.[11] These surgeries are complex and require large incisions in an area of the body with a high rate of wound complications.[12]

HISTORY OF THE FLEXOR HALLUCIS LONGUS TRANSFER

The flexor hallucis longus (FHL) transfer was first proposed by Mann and associates[13] and has been used as an augment or on its own to take the place of the ruptured Achilles tendon. This strategy is particularly useful if the injury is chronic, because the gastrocsoleus muscles may already have undergone fatty atrophy and, therefore, cannot provide a useful motor. An MRI of the whole calf can demonstrate if this change has occurred, in which case the repaired Achilles will not restore the desired useful function and so an alternative motor has to be brought in.

Myerson[14] based his treatment guidance on the size of the tendon defect. For defects greater than 5 cm, he preferred the use of the FHL transfer. Although the FHL muscle generates a fraction of the power of the gastrocsoleus,[15] it is very useful because it is in close proximity, phasic, and also has a similar line of pull. This transfer has gained popularity because it has a good function with a low donor morbidity and low rate of complications.[16] The open technique has been used for a number of years and is associated with excellent outcomes.[17–19]

Different zones of the FHL are described[20]: zone 1 is posterior to the ankle; zone 2 is from the fibroosseous orifice of posterior talar tubercle, under the sustentaculum tali up to the master knot of Henry; and zone 3 extends from the master knot of Henry to the phalangeal insertion. The FHL is traditionally harvested in the distal part of zone 2 as a long graft from the master knot of Henry[18] when an open technique is used. The long graft has the advantage of giving a longer length of tendon for a tunneled tenodesis into the calcaneus. With modern interference screw fixation techniques, this advantage is no longer consider to be important. Moreover, harvesting at this level requires a significant midfoot dissection. Care must be taken to avoid injury to the lateral plantar nerve during harvesting. The lateral plantar nerve is on the lateral side of tibial nerve, which is compressed by scope if there is any dorsiflexion of ankle as it tenses up the nerve in tarsal tunnel.[21]

Lui[22] has described an endoscopic-assisted technique for the harvesting of a longer FHL graft (from zone 2) by introducing a Wissenger rod via the posterior ankle portal. The rod is then passed under sustentaculum to follow the FHL to just proximal of the knot of Henry. The tip of the rod is then palpated on the sole of the foot for a third plantar incision to be made and through which the tendon can be identified and released. Because this technique gives a very long graft, the FHL tendon can be tunneled through the bone and sutured back to itself and the remaining Achilles tendon. As a result, no interference screw is required with this technique.

Den Hartog[17] showed how the FHL could be harvested from a single posterior incision. Later Van Dijk and colleagues[23] described an endoscopic method for this procedure. These investigators described FHL tendoscopy using a 2-portal technique in conjunction with posterior ankle arthroscopy. Using this technique, the tendon can be harvested endoscopically under the sustentaculum tali in the proximal part of zone 2. This graft is slightly shorter, but still suitable for transfer to the posterior calcaneus.[24–26] Most important, it is technically easier to do and is done through the same posterior portal as the fixation.

Although an open posterior approach for harvesting of the graft allows a single incision, this technique does not avoid skin complications. This point is especially relevant in the case of chronic rupture, where the skin is often contracted owing to the gapping from the chronic retraction of the tendon (**Fig. 1**). Thus, the skin repair can be placed under tension and is a strong advantage of the endoscopic approach.

INDICATIONS

Consider this approach whenever surgery is indicated for a chronic Achilles rupture; however, it is an ideal salvage for gaps of more than 6 cm. This method can also be used for chronic Achilles tendinopathy, particularly when there are additional risk factors such as age, smoking, diabetes, vascular insufficiency, or soft tissue problems such as previous infection, surgery, lymphedema, or the presence of fatty atrophy of the gastrocsoleus muscle.

SETUP AND POSITIONING

The procedure can be performed in a lateral position with the patient lying on the affected side. However, this procedure is ideally done prone with the feet off the end of the table (see **Fig. 1**). In this position, the foot is often externally rotated making access to the medial side more difficult; therefore, the contralateral hip may need to be elevated to internally rotate the affected ankle to allow it to be vertical.

SURGICAL TECHNIQUE

The procedure is conducted with a 4.5-mm, 30° arthroscope. The classic posterior approach described by Van Dijk and coworkers[27] has been shown to be safe and

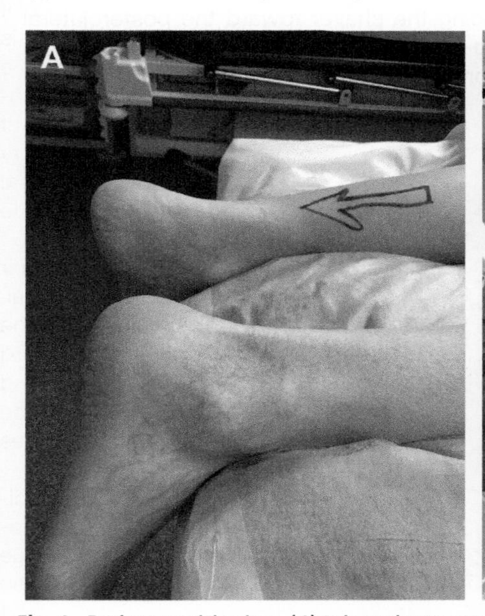

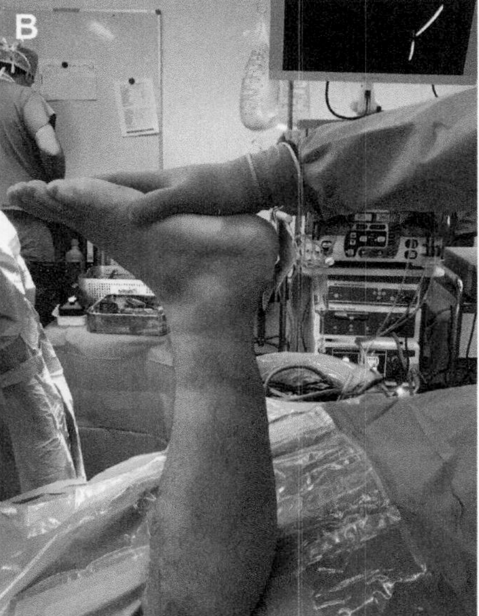

Fig. 1. Patient positioning. (*A*) It is easier to maneuver the foot for graft tensioning with the foot hanging off the end of the table. (*B*) Internally rotate the foot to gain the best possible access to the medial hindfoot. Note the lack of Achilles tendon in this patient with chronic wasting of the calf.

give good access to the FHL. The lateral portal is made adjacent to the Achilles tendon on a level with the tip of the lateral malleolus. The medial portal is made at the same level on the other side of the Achilles tendon.

Approach

The arthroscope is placed in the lateral portal aiming it toward the first web space. Then, a heavy clip is placed into the medial portal and once it contacts the scope it is drawn down the barrel of the scope until it comes into view. The clip is opened to create a working space. Once this triangulation is achieved, the clip is exchanged for a 4.0-mm shaver and dissection starts under direct vision with the shaver facing the scope.

Exposure of the Insertion

It is easiest to prepare the footprint of the insertion first. For this step, the shaving is directed plantarward onto the dorsal aspect of the calcaneus, always with the shaver facing the camera so that debridement is done under direct vision. With the camera facing back toward the Achilles tendon, the cortex directly in front of it is cleared (**Fig. 2**). A technique is described using a trans-Achilles tendon portal to allow the tunnel to be made even further back, but these authors have no experience with this approach.

Harvesting the Flexor Hallucis Longus Tendon

The medial neurovascular bundle is at risk during posterior ankle arthroscopy; fortunately, the FHL tendon itself is the key landmark to safely avoiding these structures. They lie on the medial side of the tendon and therefore the safe zone lies on the lateral/posterior side of the tendon. The approach thus begins on the lateral side dissecting the fat pad toward the FHL.

The FHL tendon is identified by advancing the shaver toward the posterolateral aspect of the talus with the shaver facing the scope and using suction to draw in and debride the fat. Once the posterior process is identified, the shaver is moved

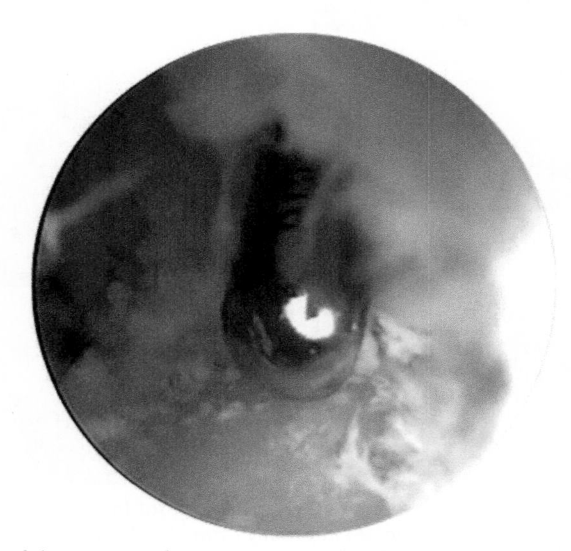

Fig. 2. Exposure of the FHL transfer insertion site. The chronic scarred and thickened Achilles stump lies to the right and the calcaneus anterior to this is exposed with a soft tissue shaver.

medially where the fibrous tissue, flexor retinaculum, and tendon sheath are debrided to expose the FHL tendon (**Fig. 3**). The surrounding tissue is cleared posteriorly to allow it to be released as distally as possible. Identification can be confirmed by moving the great toe.

Preparation of the Bony Tunnel

The ideal tunnel placement is still not clearly defined. The senior author (A.P.) aims to place this tunnel as far posteriorly as possible and thus near to the Achilles insertion. An entry point slightly medial to the midline is used to try and maintain the anatomic line of pull.

A guide wire is placed in calcaneus under direct vision and out through the plantar skin (**Fig. 4**A). The wire is then overdrilled with a 7-mm drill for approximately 2 cm, without the need to go all the way through to the plantar aspect. The periosteum and tissue around the tunnel is cleared using the soft tissue shaver to ensure that the tendon runs smoothly into it (**Fig. 4**B).

Harvesting and Preparation of the Flexor Hallucis Longus Tendon

To ensure the best length of tendon is achieved, the foot and the great toe can be held in plantarflexion. A suture passer can be used to pass a suture through it (**Fig. 5**A). This process can be used to retract the tendon further and also to secure it to bring it out of the skin. Arthroscopic scissors are used going as far down into the FHL groove as possible and the tendon is cut under direct vision.

Next, the tendon is brought out through the medial portal using the stay suture and it is whip-stitched with a Fiberwire suture (Arthrex, Naples, FL; **Fig. 5**B).

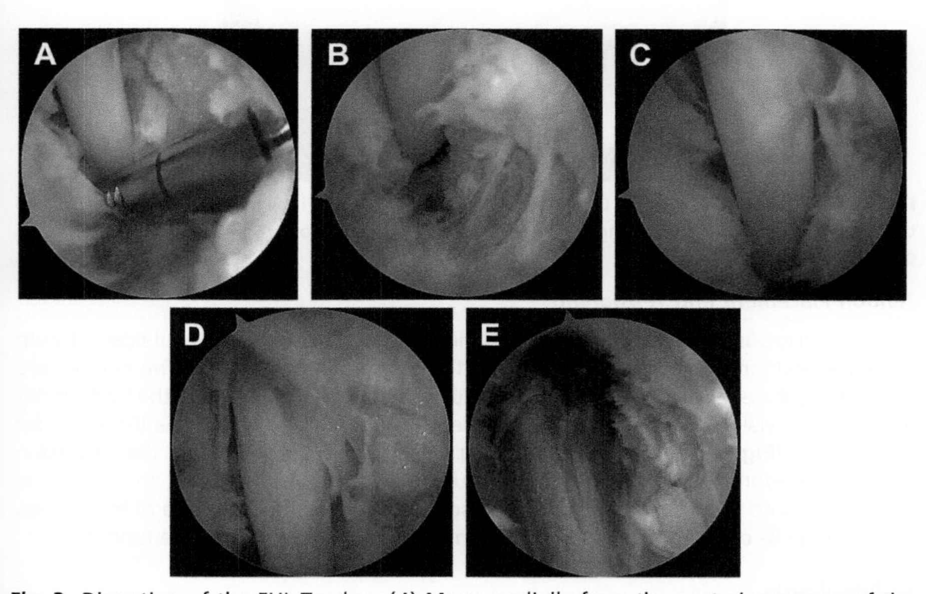

Fig. 3. Dissection of the FHL Tendon. (*A*) Move medially from the posterior process of the talus shaving toward the camera and identify the FHL tendon. (*B*) Next, clear the tunnel as much as possible to achieve the longest length of tendon. (*C*) The dissected tendon must be undamaged. (*D*) The FHL muscle can be tethered by fascia and tissue but, (*E*) this can be released to allow a direct line of pull.

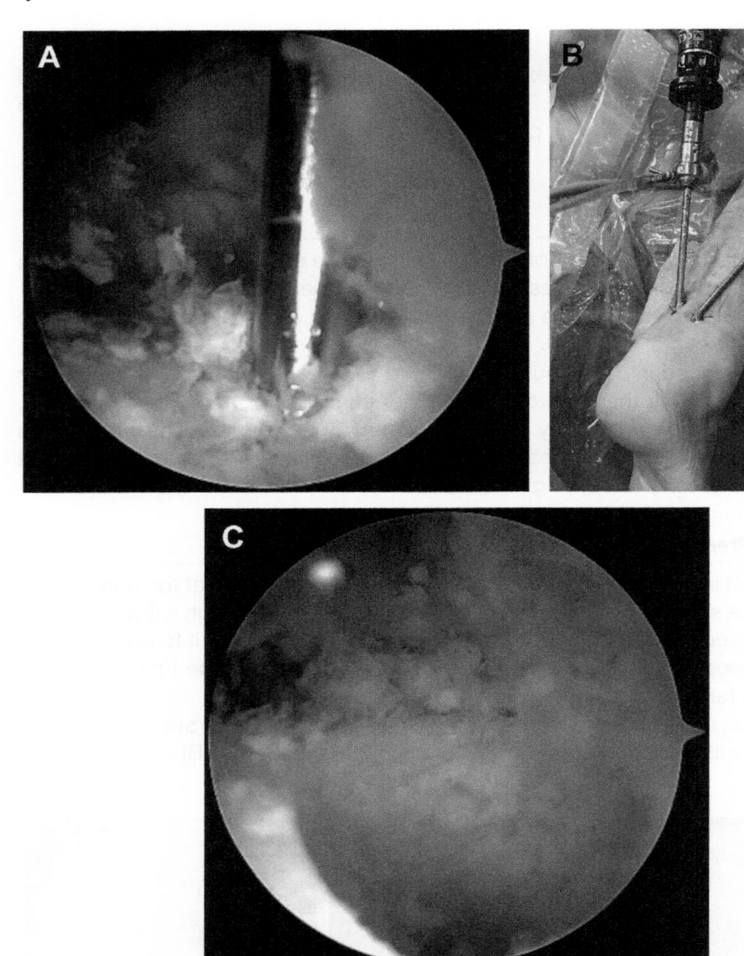

Fig. 4. Tunnel preparation. (*A*) Guide wire placement. (*B*) A drill is placed over this wire and the tunnel prepared. (*C*) Looking into the prepared tunnel through endoscope at the mouth of the tunnel.

Tendon Placement and Tensioning

The tendon is pushed back into the ankle while leaving the suture ends outside. A Beath pin is passed through the medial portal and into the calcaneal tunnel. The sutures are passed into the eyelet and the pin is pulled out from the inferior aspect of the foot. Under arthroscopic vision, the sutures can be pulled, taking the tendon into the tunnel under direct vision (**Fig. 6**). The tendon tensioning is by holding the foot in 20° plantarflexion while the tendon is pulled as far into the tunnel as possible. Typically, the tendon is out of sight into the tunnel leaving the muscle exposed at the entrance of the tunnel. A 20-mm by 6- or 7-mm diameter interference screw is inserted into the tunnel.

Technical note

Although dissection of the ankle needs to be kept to a minimum, it is important that the tendon has a direct passage to the tunnel and that it is not snagged on any tissue. It may be necessary to divide the deep crural fascia overlying the FHL muscle in a longitudinal fashion as proximally as necessary. This step can be done with a shaver or a blade.

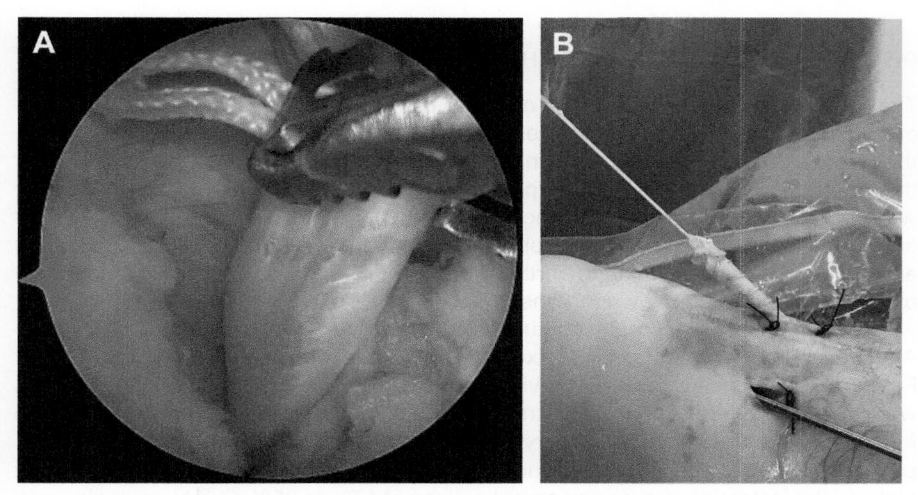

Fig. 5. (*A*) FHL Tendon visible with Suture going through it before harvesting it. (*B*) Tendon harvested and locking suture applied to tendon; out through the endoscopic portal, prior to placement in the tunnel already created in calcaneum.

Postoperative Management

If the patient is high risk, then it may be necessary to use a below-the-knee cast in equinus to let the soft tissues settle. However, generally the patient can be placed into a walker boot with 3 wedges and allowed to start immediate weight bearing to comfort. Thromboprohylaxis is used in line with current guidelines. Regular analgesia including antiinflammatories are used.

Rehabilitation

At 2 weeks, the patient is encouraged to start full weight bearing in a boot if they are not already doing so. The wedges are decreased over the next 3 weeks until the patient is full weight bearing in neutral at 6 weeks. Early plantarflexion exercises are commenced immediately, but no loaded dorsiflexion and no weight bearing exercises are undertaken until 6 weeks. At 6 weeks, the patient can go into a running shoe and commence on physiotherapy.

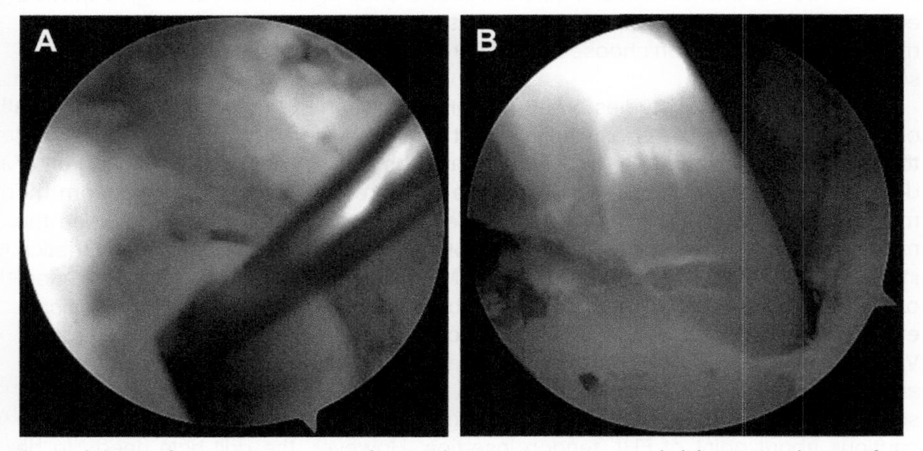

Fig. 6. (*A*) Interference Screw over the Guide Wire Being Inserted. (*B*) FHL Tendon Graft in Place after secured with Interference Screw.

DISCUSSION: ENDOSCOPIC FLEXOR HALLUCIS LONGUS TRANSFER

The FHL is a useful tendon transfer owing to its proximity and because its action occurs in the same phase as the Achilles tendon. However, there are power differences; the Achilles tendon has been shown to generate a peak tendon force much greater than the FHL.[28,29] Nonetheless, the power generated by the FHL is sufficient for quiet walking on the flat and even walking on stairs, which requires approximately 27° of ankle motion[30] and mean ankle flexion–extension moments of 137.2 NM for ascending and 107.5 NM for descending.[30] Furthermore, the FHL has been shown to be capable of significant hypertrophy when transferred.[31]

Open FHL transfer for chronic rupture has been shown to be a successful procedure. Abubeih and colleagues[32] showed excellent outcomes with the American Orthopaedic Foot and Ankle Society score improving from 57.4 to 95.3. They showed that the risks were low and that there was minimal morbidity including good preservation of great toe function. The average time for surgery was 52.9 minutes. There was 1 infection in the 21 patients in the study group. Other studies on open transfer have shown a considerably higher risk of infection and wound complications of 17% to 25%.[25,33] Neurologic complications have also been described. In Hahn's series,[33] there were issues in 2 out of 16 procedures, although other reports have not shown any neurologic injuries.

An endoscopic approach has been used successfully by a number of authors.[34] This technique does not seem to increase the operative time with tourniquet times of 42 to 56 minutes reported.[19,35,36] Although the series have been, small there seems to be a low risk of infection.[36] Neurologic injuries are a concern, but again their risk seemed to be low. In a series reported on by Husebye and associates,[36] there were 2 patients out of 6 who had a temporary dysfunction in the medical calcaneal nerve.

A study by Liu and colleagues[37] using matched pairs of cadaveric specimens showed that interference screw fixation for FHL provides similar biomechanical properties to the use of a bone tunnel (ultimate strength, peak stress, Young's modulus, failure strain and strain energy). They proposed that an interference screw was a practical option for FHL fixation to calcaneus. Also, they proposed the use of FiberLoop (Arthrex) suture onto the FHL tendon stump that, because of its braided pattern, likely provided a buttress against the threads of interference screws, increasing the pull out strength.[26] A cadaveric study by Wu and colleagues,[38] where 9 matched pairs of frozen cadavers had graft fixation done with interference screw insertion angles of 60° and 120°. Graft insertion at 2 different interference screw insertion angles showed equivalent biomechanical properties in terms of failure load and stiffness. They recommended that the surgeon choose the interference screw insertion angle based on personal preference.

There are no clinical studies on the preferred location of the calcaneal tunnel. The only evidence available is a finite element analysis using 2 computer programs[29] that suggest that although a more anterior attachment was associated with a greater degree of plantarflexion (37% more), there was greater power generated from the most posterior placement (39% more). There is a balance, therefore, between the maximum range of plantarflexion and the power generated, with a significant variation in the results, depending on the placement. Medial or lateral placement has little effect on the function of the ankle sagittal motion, but it would theoretically have a significant effect on the moment arm of the subtalar joint, as shown by Zifchock and Piazza.[39] Variations of only 6 mm in the medial–lateral insertion caused subtalar joint moment arms to change by approximately 5 mm.[30] A slightly medial placement does, however, seem to have a small advantage in power generation.[29] Hence, it is important to be cautious about point of FHL tendon insertion. However, the drill hole needs to be not too posterior, because there would be a risk of posterior wall blow out either during drilling or inserting the interference screw.[40]

A recent Brazilian study by Baumfeld and colleagues[41] performed an FHL transfer using an endoscopic technique in 6 patients (5 chronic and 1 rerupture). They also used an additional procedure to repair the preexisting gap in 3 tendoachilles. Using the Achilles tendon Total Rupture Score, they showed a major increase in the score from 17.8 (preoperatively) to 83.3 (postoperatively). In a study by Oksanen and coworkers,[42] 7 patients with an isolated FHL tendon transfer for chronic Achilles tendon rupture at an average of 27 months after the procedure, were able to return to their preactivity level, even though there was a decrease in isokinetic plantarflexion strength of the operative leg over the contralateral leg by an average of 16.1% at 30°/s and 26.7% at 90°/s. They also included preoperative and postoperative MRIs and showed that the cross-sectional area of FHL muscle was on average 51.5% larger on the operative side than the control side.

A study by Bruggeman and colleagues[43] evaluated wound complications after open Achilles repair showed a wound complication rate of 10% (17 of 164 patients). Of these 17 patients, 5 developed deep infections, and others sustained superficial infections. They found female sex and the use of tobacco or steroids showed a stronger correlation with the development of wound complications postoperatively.

The use of endoscopic FHL harvest and reconstruction of chronic Achilles tendon rupture using this technique would allow less soft tissue dissection, avoid violation of the plantar surface of the foot, decrease the chance of fracture through the osseous tunnel, and reduce complications associated with open FHL reconstruction with good clinical outcomes and return to preinjury activity levels, even in chronic Achilles tendon ruptures.

Pearls	Pitfalls
Foot positioning is crucial for relaxing the FHL; this allows a very distal harvest – place the big toe in maximum flexion and the ankle in equinus by getting an assistant to hold it during harvest.	The tibial verve is close to the FHL and the lateral plantar nerve is most commonly affected. Be gentle with the scope.
Gentle traction on the stay suture improves exposure of the FHL.	Too posterior of a tunnel is prone to wall blow out. Maintain at least 10 mm from the Achilles insertion to prevent this from happening.
Use a 1.6-mm K-wire as a guide for tunnel placement, entering from the medial portal.	If the tunnel is drilled all the way to the inferior calcaneus, still use a smaller screw. A prominent inferior screw can be problematic when weight bearing.
Adequate tension should be maintained on the FHL traction suture while advancing the screw; use an artery clip horizontally across the heel onto sutures if no assistant is available.	Check the position of ankle when inserting a Beath pin. The ankle should be in a dorsiflexed position so that bone tunnel is parallel to the Achilles tendon.
The screw diameter should at least be the same size as the tunnel size.	Poor interference fit in the tunnel: Check by pulling onto the tendon after its insertion. If loose, change for a larger diameter screw.
Consider using a FiberLoop on the FHL stump to improve the pull out strength of the interference screw.	Inadequate tension compared with the other side when the FHL is secured.

REFERENCES

1. Gabel S, Manoli A. Neglected rupture of the Achilles tendon. Foot Ankle Int 1994; 15(9):512–7.
2. Wapner KL, Pavlock GS, Hecht PJ, et al. Repair of chronic Achilles tendon rupture with flexor hallucis longus tendon transfer. Foot Ankle 1993;14(8):443–9.
3. Wilcox DK, Bohay DR, Anderson JG. Treatment of chronic Achilles tendon disorders with flexor hallucis longus tendon transfer/augmentation. Foot Ankle Int 2000;21(12):1004–10.
4. Mulier T, Pienaar H, Dereymaeker G, et al. The management of chronic Achilles tendon ruptures: gastrocnemius turn down flap with or without flexor hallucis longus transfer. Foot Ankle Surg 2003;9(3):151–6.
5. El Shewy MT, El Barbary HM, Abdel-Ghani H. Repair of chronic rupture of the Achilles tendon using 2 intratendinous flaps from the proximal gastrocnemius-soleus complex. Am J Sports Med 2009;37(8):1570–7.
6. Gerdes MH, Brown TD, Bell AL, et al. A flap augmentation technique for Achilles tendon repair. Postoperative strength and functional outcome. Clin Orthop Relat Res 1992;(280):241–6.
7. Abraham E, Pankovich AM. Neglected rupture of the Achilles tendon. Treatment by V-Y tendinous flap. J Bone Joint Surg Am 1975;57(2):253–5.
8. Panchbhavi VK, Trevino S. Clinical tip: a new clinical sign associated with metatarsophalangeal joint synovitis of the lesser toes. Foot Ankle Int 2007;28(5):640–1.
9. Maffulli N, Leadbetter WB. Free gracilis tendon graft in neglected tears of the Achilles tendon. Clin J Sport Med 2005;15(2):56–61.
10. Sarzaeem MM, Lemraski MM, Safdari F. Chronic Achilles tendon rupture reconstruction using a free semitendinosus tendon graft transfer. Knee Surg Sports Traumatol Arthrosc 2012;20(7):1386–91.
11. Maffulli N, Ajis A. Management of chronic ruptures of the Achilles tendon. J Bone Joint Surg Am 2008;90(6):1348–60.
12. Dalton GP, Wapner KL, Hecht PJ. Complications of Achilles and posterior tibial tendon surgeries. Clin Orthop Relat Res 2001;(391):133–9.
13. Mann RA, Holmes GB, Seale KS, et al. Chronic rupture of the Achilles tendon: a new technique of repair. J Bone Joint Surg Am 1991;73(2):214–9.
14. Myerson MS. Achilles tendon ruptures. Instr Course Lect 1999;48:219–30.
15. Silver RL, de la Garza J, Rang M. The myth of muscle balance. A study of relative strengths and excursions of normal muscles about the foot and ankle. J Bone Joint Surg Br 1985;67(3):432–7.
16. Coull R, Flavin R, Stephens MM. Flexor hallucis longus tendon transfer: evaluation of postoperative morbidity. Foot Ankle Int 2003;24(12):931–4.
17. Den Hartog BD. Flexor hallucis longus transfer for chronic Achilles tendonosis. Foot Ankle Int 2003;24(3):233–7.
18. Wapner KL, Hecht PJ, Mills RH. Reconstruction of neglected Achilles tendon injury. Orthop Clin North Am 1995;26(2):249–63.
19. Gossage W, Kohls-Gatzoulis J, Solan M. Endoscopic assisted repair of chronic Achilles tendon rupture with flexor hallucis longus augmentation. Foot Ankle Int 2010;31(4):343–7.
20. Lui TH. Endoscopic-assisted flexor hallucis longus transfer: harvest of the tendon at zone 2 or zone 3. Arthrosc Tech 2015;4(6):e811–4.
21. Lui TH. Lateral plantar nerve neuropraxia after FHL tendoscopy: case report and anatomic evaluation. Foot Ankle Int 2010;31(9):828–31.

22. Lui TH. Endoscopic assisted flexor hallucis tendon transfer in the management of chronic rupture of Achilles tendon. Knee Surg Sports Traumatol Arthrosc 2007; 15(9):1163–6.
23. van Dijk CN, Scholten PE, Krips R. A 2-portal endoscopic approach for diagnosis and treatment of posterior ankle pathology. Arthroscopy 2000;16(8):871–6.
24. DeCarbo WT, Hyer CF. Interference screw fixation for flexor hallucis longus tendon transfer for chronic Achilles tendonopathy. J Foot Ankle Surg 2008; 47(1):69–72.
25. Rahm S, Spross C, Gerber F, et al. Operative treatment of chronic irreparable Achilles tendon ruptures with large flexor hallucis longus tendon transfers. Foot Ankle Int 2013;34(8):1100–10.
26. Cohn JM, Sabonghy EP, Godlewski CA, et al. Tendon fixation in flexor hallucis longus transfer: a biomechanical study comparing a traditional technique versus biobasorbable interference screw fixation. Tech Foot Ankle Surg 2005;4(4): 214–21.
27. van Dijk CN, van Sterkenburg MN, Wiegerinck JI, et al. Terminology for Achilles tendon related disorders. Knee Surg Sports Traumatol Arthrosc 2011;19(5): 835–41.
28. Komi PV, Fukashiro S, Järvinen M. Biomechanical loading of Achilles tendon during normal locomotion. Clin Sports Med 1992;11(3):521–31.
29. Arastu MH, Partridge R, Crocombe A, et al. Determination of optimal screw positioning in flexor hallucis longus tendon transfer for chronic tendoachilles rupture. Foot Ankle Surg 2011;17(2):74–8.
30. Andriacchi TP, Andersson GB, Fermier RW, et al. A study of lower-limb mechanics during stair-climbing. J Bone Joint Surg Am 1980;62(5):749–57.
31. Hahn F, Meyer P, Maiwald C, et al. Treatment of chronic Achilles tendinopathy and ruptures with flexor hallucis tendon transfer: clinical outcome and MRI findings. Foot Ankle Int 2008;29(8):794–802.
32. Abubeih H, Khaled M, Saleh WR, et al. Flexor hallucis longus transfer clinical outcome through a single incision for chronic Achilles tendon rupture. Int Orthop 2018;42(11):2699–704.
33. Hahn F, Maiwald C, Horstmann T, et al. Changes in plantar pressure distribution after Achilles tendon augmentation with flexor hallucis longus transfer. Clin Biomech (Bristol, Avon) 2008;23(1):109–16.
34. Lui TH. Minimally invasive flexor hallucis longus transfer in management of acute Achilles tendon rupture associated with tendinosis: a case report. Foot Ankle Spec 2012;5(2):111–4.
35. Gonçalves S, Caetano R, Corte-Real N. Salvage flexor hallucis longus transfer for a failed Achilles repair: endoscopic technique. Arthrosc Tech 2015;4(5):e411–6.
36. Husebye EE, Molund M, Hvaal KH, et al. Endoscopic transfer of flexor hallucis longus tendon for chronic Achilles tendon rupture: technical aspects and short-time experiences. Foot Ankle Spec 2018;11(5):461–6.
37. Liu GT, Balldin BC, Zide JR, et al. A biomechanical analysis of interference screw versus bone tunnel fixation of flexor hallucis longus tendon transfers to the calcaneus. J Foot Ankle Surg 2017;56(4):813–6.
38. Wu Z, Li H, Chen S, et al. Interference screw insertion angle has no effect on graft fixation strength for insertional Achilles tendon reconstruction. Knee Surg Sports Traumatol Arthrosc 2018;26(12):3606–10.
39. Zifchock RA, Piazza SJ. Investigation of the validity of modeling the Achilles tendon as having a single insertion site. Clin Biomech (Bristol, Avon) 2004; 19(3):303–7.

40. El Shazly O, Abou El Soud MM, El Mikkawy DM, et al. Endoscopic-assisted Achilles tendon reconstruction with free hamstring tendon autograft for chronic rupture of Achilles tendon: clinical and isokinetic evaluation. Arthroscopy 2014;30(5):622–8.
41. Baumfeld D, Baumfeld T, Figueiredo AR, et al. Endoscopic flexor halluces longus transfer for chronic Achilles Tendon rupture - technique description and early post-operative results. Muscles Ligaments Tendons J 2017;7(2):341–6.
42. Oksanen MM, Haapasalo HH, Elo PP, et al. Hypertrophy of the flexor hallucis longus muscle after tendon transfer in patients with chronic Achilles tendon rupture. Foot Ankle Surg 2014;20(4):253–7.
43. Bruggeman NB, Turner NS, Dahm DL, et al. Wound complications after open Achilles tendon repair: an analysis of risk factors. Clin Orthop Relat Res 2004;(427):63–6.

Biologics in the Treatment of Achilles Tendon Pathologies

Cristian Indino, MD[a,*], Riccardo D'Ambrosi, MD[a], Federico G. Usuelli, MD[b]

KEYWORDS

• Achilles • Biologics • Platelet-rich plasma • Stem cells • Imaging

KEY POINTS

- Biologics have a role in the management of midportion Achilles tendinopathy as a step between conservative and surgical treatment or as an augmentation.
- The level of treatment recommendation for biologics treatment of insertional tendinopathy is yet to be determined.
- The authors created an algorithm (FARG [Foot and Ankle Reconstruction Group] algorithm) for the use of biologics in midportion tendinopathy inspired by the MRI-based classification and for categorizing patients according to the sports activity.
- Combining imaging with patient's functional requests could be the way to reach a protocol for the use of biologics for the treatment of midportion tendinopathy.

INTRODUCTION

Among the human tendons, the Achilles tendon is one of the most prone to pathologic conditions.[1,2] Unfortunately, the ability of tendons to heal spontaneously is very inefficient and unreliable because of their hypocellularity and hypovascularity.[3] Unlike bone, tendon repair is incomplete and does not result in tissue homologous to its prepathologic state[4,5]: a fibrovascular scar is formed and it leads to a mechanically weaker tissue than the natural tendon.[6] The subsequent possible strength loss may increase risk for reinjury or other complications. Furthermore, surgical treatments are sometimes unsuccessful, in which case the main part of these patients develops a chronic condition that is susceptible to recur.[5] These considerations have stimulated the necessity to enhance the outcome of Achilles tendon tendinopathies treatment; in this perspective, biologics propose attractive solutions to be investigated.[5]

In the last decade, the use of biologics for improving repair and healing of Achilles tendon has gained growing interest.[4,5] At present, strategies using biological augmentation techniques are being investigated for potential benefits in tendon healing: they

Disclosure Statement: Dr F.G. Usuelli: consultant for Zimmer-Biomet, Geistlich. Dr C. Indino and Dr R. D'Ambrosi have no disclosures.
[a] IRCCS Istituto Ortopedico Galeazzi, Via Riccardo Galeazzi, 4, Milan 20161, Italy; [b] Humanitas San Pio X, via Francesco Nava, 31, 20159 Milano, Lombardia, Italy
* Corresponding author.
E-mail address: cristian.indino@gmail.com

Foot Ankle Clin N Am 24 (2019) 471–493
https://doi.org/10.1016/j.fcl.2019.04.009
1083-7515/19/

may enhance the healing process by improving the biomechanical quality of repairing tissue with the aim of simulating the native tissue.[7]

Among the several biological therapies that have been proposed and investigated, the use of growth factors, platelet-rich plasma (PRP), adipose-derived stem cells (ADSCs), bone marrow aspirate concentrate (BMAC), peripheral blood mononuclear cells (PBMNCs), and scaffolds is the focus of this article.

BIOLOGICS IN ACHILLES TENDON PATHOLOGIC CONDITIONS

Achilles tendon pathologic conditions embrace insertional Achilles tendinopathy and midportion Achilles tendinopathy. Insertional Achilles tendinopathy accounts for approximately 20% to 25% of Achilles tendon disorders, whereas midportion Achilles tendinopathy accounts for another 66%.[8,9]

Midportion Achilles Tendinopathy

Midportion Achilles tendinopathy refers to a tendon disorder located 2 to 7 cm from the posterior calcaneal tuberosity[9] (**Fig. 1**). The mainstay of initial management in midportion Achilles tendinopathy is conservative based on rest or modification of the activities and of the training regimens, eccentric exercises, and use of orthosis.[9,10] This pathologic condition is characterized by good responses to conservative treatment, but it fails to resolve symptoms and to allow sports continuation in 24.0% to 45.5% of cases.[11] Surgical treatment is usually considered when conservative therapies fail: the most frequently performed procedures are open release of adhesions with or without resection of the peritenon, multiple tenotomies with or without augmentation with plantaris tendon or tendon transfers (peroneus brevis, flexor digitorum longus [FDL], flexor hallucis longus [FHL]), or transfer of a soleus pedicle graft, stripping of the peritenon, endoscopic tendon debridement.[9] The main concern about Achilles tendon surgery is the nonnegligible risk of wound-healing complications and nerve and soft tissues damage.[9,12,13]

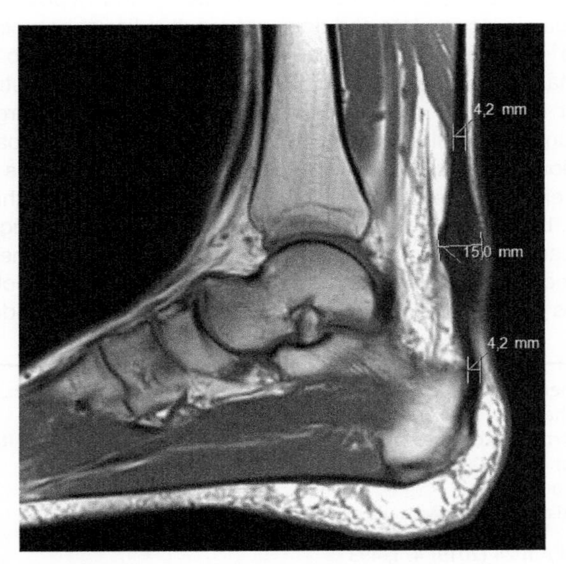

Fig. 1. MRI of midportion Achilles tendinopathy: T1 sagittal view shows midportion tendon thickening.

In this scenario, biologics therapies could have a role: they could support conservative strategies as biological augmentation; they could be considered a treatment option in patients recalcitrant to conservative strategies before considering surgery; and, finally, they can support surgery as biological augmentation, allowing a switch toward less invasive strategies with a lower rate of surgical complications.

Most studies focused on biological treatment of midportion Achilles tendinopathy and dealt with PRP injections, but many systematic reviews determined that high-level evidence does not support the use of PRP injections for a variety of clinical, sports, and instrumental outcomes in individuals with midportion Achilles tendinopathy[14–21] (**Fig. 2**). However, the variability of PRP formulations impedes the understanding of study data and the optimization of treatment protocols.[22]

Besides this, other biological therapies for midportion Achilles tendinopathy have been investigated. In randomized controlled clinical trials, PRP injections were prospectively compared with ADSCs injections (stromal vascular fraction) in a population of 44 patients affected by monolateral or bilateral midportion Achilles tendinopathy (28 tendons per group): both treatments were effective, but patients treated with ADSCs obtained faster results, and the investigators suggested that this treatment should be taken into consideration for those patients who require an earlier return to daily activities or sport.[23] Furthermore, in a review dealing with biologics in Achilles tendon healing, it appeared that ADSCs may be as effective as other mesenchymal stem cells (MSCs) as measured by their multipotency and proliferative efficiency and may have a higher concentration of the pluripotent stem cells compared with BMAC.[4]

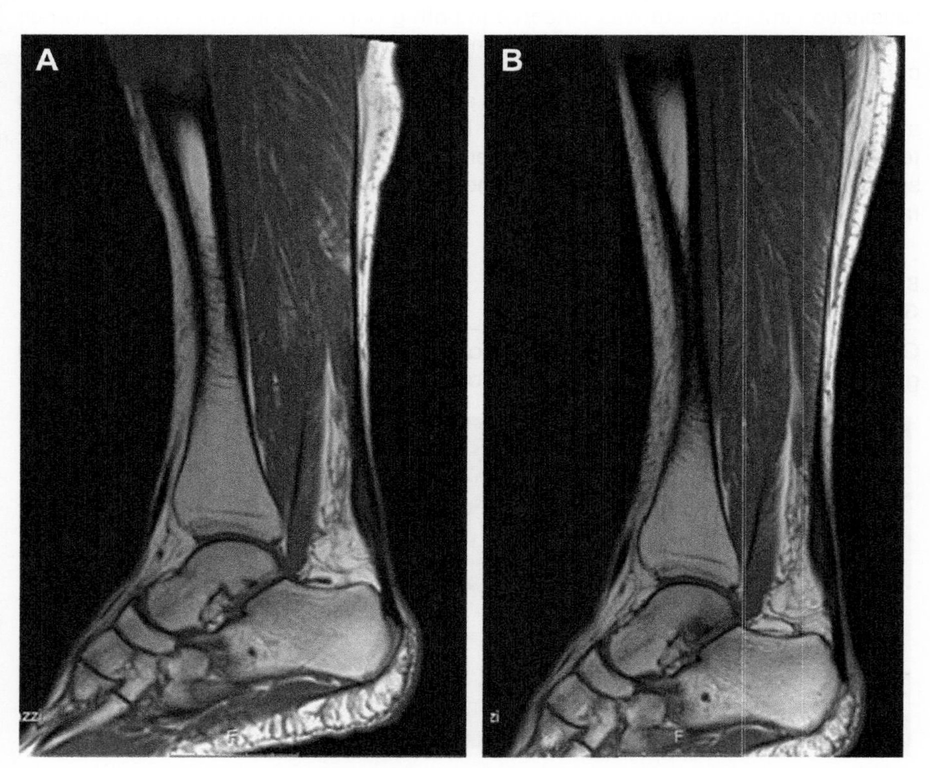

Fig. 2. (*A*) Pretreatment MRI appearance of midportion Achilles tendinopathy. (*B*) MRI appearance of the same patient 6 months after treatment with PRP injections.

Future investigation should focus on finding an ideal biological strategy for this pathologic condition, but it appears that biologics could play a role in the management of midportion Achilles tendinopathy as a step between conservative and surgical treatment or as an augmentation to optimize outcomes and lower complication rates of the treatment.

Insertional Achilles Tendinopathy

Insertional Achilles tendinopathy is situated at the insertion site of the Achilles tendon to the posterior calcaneal tuberosity, likely with the development of calcifications and bone spurs in the tendon at the bone insertion[9,24] (**Fig. 3**). For this pathologic condition, the good results obtained by conservative treatment of noninsertional disorders were not replicated: the success rate accounts for 28% to 32%.[25–27]

Currently, most studies focusing on biologics treatment of insertional Achilles tendon pathologic conditions deal with PRP in mixed cohorts of patients with insertional and noninsertional Achilles tendinopathies, and its use in this field remains controversial.[28] A prospective case series showed that PRP led to satisfaction in 28/30 patients of a mixed cohort with a 2-year follow-up (8 patients were affected by insertional Achilles tendinopathy), but both failures occurred in patients with insertional Achilles tendinopathy.[29] A retrospective case series compared 24 patients with insertional Achilles tendinopathy treated with 3 sessions of extracorporeal shock-wave therapy and 21 patients affected by insertional Achilles tendinopathy treated with 2 autologous PRP injections with a 6-month follow-up: a significant clinical and satisfaction improvement was detected in both groups without differences between the 2 groups, resulting in no better outcomes for PRP injections compared with extracorporeal shock-wave therapy.[30]

Higher-level studies with randomization and blinding are needed before determining a level of treatment recommendation for biologics strategies for insertional Achilles tendinopathy, whereas surgical treatment (debridement, calcifications and bone spur removal, tendon augmentation) is indicated in symptomatic patients who have failed conservative therapies.[27]

BIOLOGICS OPTIONS

Growth Factors

Growth factors, such as transforming growth factor-β (TGF-β), vascular endothelial growth factor (VEGF), platelet-derived growth factor (PDGF), and insulin-like growth

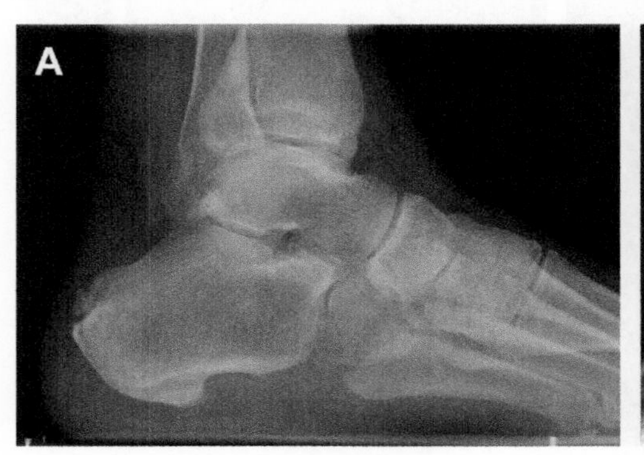

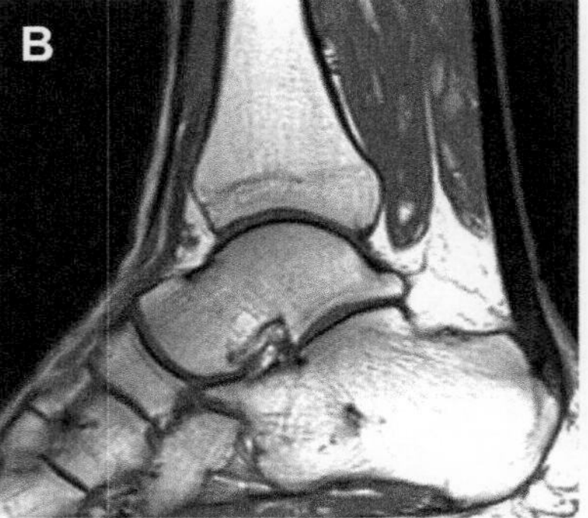

Fig. 3. Radiographs (*A*) and MRI (*B*) of a patient with insertional Achilles tendinopathy showing bone spurs and intratendinous calcifications at the bone insertion.

factor (IGF-I), are signal molecules involved in proliferation, differentiation cell chemotaxis, and synthesis of extracellular matrix. These molecules are produced by the tenocytes and white blood cells and are released from the platelets during the degranulation process. In the case of tendon injury, numerous growth factors are involved in activation and regulation of the cellular responses.[31]

Transforming growth factor–β

TGF-β is a family of proteins involved in many cellular processes and is present in 3 different isoforms (TGF-β1, -β2, and -β3) not always distinguishable regarding their effect on cell behavior. All 3 isoforms bind to cells via the same receptor, playing a key role in the healing process.[32]

TGF-β1 regulates cellular migration and proliferation and can increase the synthesis of collagen type I and III in tendon-derived cells; moreover, TGF-β1 is overexpressed in tendon in the early postinjury period but not in tendon sheath. Promising results have been reported using TGF-β1 complementary DNA-transduced BMSCs grafts, injections of TGF-β, and delivery of TGF-β by adenovirus-modified muscle grafts in rat Achilles tendon models.[33–35]

Maeda and colleagues[36] demonstrated that in acute injury the interruption to tendon continuity can cause a loss of tensile loading, resulting in the destabilization of the extracellular matrix and releasing too high levels of active TGF-β leading to tenocyte death. Furthermore, several in vivo and in vitro studies have shown that if the production of TGF-β1 is stopped, this can lead to a reduction in adhesion formation and increased range of motion in injured tendons. In an Achilles tendon model, mannose-6-phosphate has been shown to reduce activation of latent TGF-β, resulting in an increase in elastin production and increased strain and peak stress failure.[37,38] Recently, Potter and colleagues[39] evaluated the role of TGF-β1 in regulating tendon extracellular matrix after acute exercise in rats, showing that TGF-β1 signaling is necessary for the regulation of tendon cross-link formation as well as collagen and lysyl-oxidase gene transcription in an exercise-dependent manner. TGF-β therapy can increase mechanical strength of the healing Achilles tendon by the regulation of collagen synthesis, upregulation of cross-link formation, and enhanced matrix remodeling.[39]

Vascular endothelial growth factor

The VEGF family consists of several isoforms (VEGF-A, -B, -C, -D, and -E, and placenta growth factor) due to different messenger RNA (mRNA) splicing. VEGF isoforms exert their biological activity through 3 tyrosine kinase receptors, but the bioavailability depends on the isoform binding to the receptor.[40]

VEGF-A is known to be a regulator of neovascularization that is a prerequisite for tissue healing; however, it has been shown that excessive production of VEGF also can result in excessive scar formation.[41] In vitro studies showed that during tendon repair VEGF mRNA is increased, peaking at days 7 to 10, but returned to baseline by day 14, which suggests its function in neovascularization around the repair site.[42] In an Achilles tendon model, VEGF gene therapy increased TGF-β gene expression, and exogenous VEGF appears to increase tensile strength.[43] In a recent study, Tempfer and colleagues[44] blocked VEGF-A signaling using local injection of Bevacizumab, a monoclonal antibody, in a rat model with complete Achilles tendon rupture. After the treatment, angiogenesis was found to be significantly reduced in the Bevacizumab-treated repair tissue, accompanied by significantly reduced cross-sectional area, improved matrix organization, increased stiffness and Young's modulus, and maximum load and stress.[44]

Platelet-Derived Growth Factor

PDGF is a basic protein composed of 2 subunits, an A and a B chain, that exists in 3 different isoforms (PDGF-AA, PDGF-BB, and PDGF-AB). These isoforms act as chemotactic agents for inflammatory cells and help to increase type I collagen synthesis and induce TGF-β1 expression and IGF-I.[45]

Tenocytes can increase the expression of type I collagen with the addition of exogenous PDGF.[46] In vivo, a sustained delivery of PDGF-BB via a fibrin matrix led to an increase in cell density, cell proliferation, and type I collagen mRNA expression, and a fibrin/heparin delivery system demonstrated that PDGF-BB improved tendon function but not tendon structure.[47,48]

Insulin-like growth factor

IGF-I is one of the 3 single-chain polypeptides belonging to the IGF family (IGF-I, IGF-II, and insulin). Its expression increases during wound healing, and its absence is thought to impair dermal repair.[49] IGF-I has been successfully used by Kurtz and colleagues[50] to increase the rate of healing in the transacted rat Achilles tendon. Following transection, each tendon was treated with 25 μg of a recombinant variant form of IGF-I and showed a positive effect on healing within 24 hours after the transection and addition of IGF-I; this effect continued up until the tenth and last measurement, on day 15. Lyras and colleagues[51] have shown in an Achilles tendon rupture model treated with PRP that IGF-I increased expression in both epitenon and endotenon throughout the healing phases.

Platelet-Rich Plasma

PRP is the plasma fraction of the blood containing concentrated platelets and, in most cases, white blood cells. Because of the autologous nature, PRP is inherently safe, providing a natural conductive scaffold and containing many growth factors (eg, PDGF, TGF-β, VEGF, and hepatocyte growth factor), supposing to enhance tendon healing in this way.[52]

In 2009, a new classification was proposed to avoid the debates regarding the contents and the role of different preparations.[53] The classification separates the products following the presence of a cell's content (mostly leukocytes) and the fibrin architecture. Four main families of PRP have been proposed:

- Pure platelet-rich plasma, or leukocyte-poor platelet-rich plasma, is a preparation without leukocytes and with a low-density fibrin network after activation. It can be used as a liquid solution or in an activated gel form. Gel form is often used during surgery and can be injected. Many methods of preparation exist, particularly using cell separators (continuous flow plasmapheresis), even if this method is too heavy to be used easily in daily practice.
- Leukocyte- and platelet-rich plasma is a preparation with leukocytes and with a low-density fibrin network after activation. It can be used as a liquid solution or in an activated gel form. Most commercial systems belong to this family, and several protocols have been developed in the last few years, requiring the use of specific kits that allow minimum handling of the blood samples and maximum standardization of the preparations.
- Pure platelet-rich fibrin, or leukocyte-poor platelet-rich fibrin, is a preparation without leukocytes and with a high-density fibrin network. This product only exists in a strongly activated gel form and cannot be injected or used like traditional fibrin glues. However, because of its strong fibrin matrix, it can be handled like a

real solid material for other applications. Its main inconvenience remains its cost and relative complexity in comparison to the other forms of platelet-rich fibrin.

- Leukocyte- and platelet-rich fibrin products are preparations with leukocytes and with a high-density fibrin network, and these products only exist in a strongly activated gel form and cannot be injected or used like traditional fibrin glues. However, because of their strong fibrin matrix, they can be handled like a real solid material for other applications.

The use of PRP in Achilles tendon pathologic condition is still debated. A recent review aimed to compare the effectiveness of autologous blood-derived products (ABP) injection with that of placebo (sham injection or no injection or physiotherapy alone) in patients with Achilles tendinopathy.[54] Seven articles were included in the meta-analysis. The ABP injection and placebo revealed equal effectiveness in Victorian Institute of Sports Assessment - Achilles questionnaire (VISA-A) score improvement at 4 to 6 weeks, 12 weeks, 24 weeks, and 48 weeks. In meta-regression, there was no association between change in VISA-A score and duration of symptoms at 4 to 6 weeks (short term), 12 weeks (medium term), and 24 weeks (long term). The investigators concluded that ABP injection was not more effective than placebo (sham injection, no injection, or physiotherapy alone) in Achilles tendinopathy and that no association was found between therapeutic effects and duration of symptoms.[54]

A recent review identified 4 papers dealing with the use of PRP for Achilles tendon rupture[17]: no beneficial effects of PRP administration during and/or immediately after tendon suturing were reported and, in particular, Schepull and colleagues[55] hypothesized that PRP addition could even be detrimental in tissue healing because no biomechanical advantages and lower performance were reported in PRP patients with respect to the "suture-alone" group.

Adipose-Derived Stem Cells

In last several years, ADSCs have been the focus of numerous in vitro and in vivo studies for tendon regeneration. All this interest is mainly due to their high numbers in the human body (ADSCs are 5% of nucleated cells in adipose tissue), the simplicity of harvesting, and their rapid expansion and high proliferative potential[56,57] (**Fig. 4**). They can differentiate into different cellular lines, such as adipocytes, chondrocytes, osteoblasts, hepatocytes, pancreatic cells, muscle cells, and neuron-like cells both in vitro and in vivo.[56,57]

In tendon tissue, ADSCs can enhance the gene expression profile of cartilage oligomeric matrix protein (COMP), an extracellular matrix protein primarily present in cartilage. COMP is crucial to bind and organize collagen fibrils.[56,58] The use of ADSCs for the treatment of tendon pathologic conditions has been widely investigated in experimental animal models, with encouraging mechanical and histologic results.[57] ADSCs can induce tenocytes differentiation overexpressing the bone morphogenetic protein 12 gene.[57,59,60] Usuelli and colleagues[23] described the use of ADSCs to treat human noninsertional Achilles tendinopathy compared with PRP injection (28 patients in ADSCs group and 28 in PRP group). At final follow-up, there were no clinical (Visual Analog Scale pain, the VISA-A, the American Orthopaedic Foot and Ankle Society Ankle-Hindfoot Score, and the Short Form-36 [SF-36]) or imaging (MRI and ultrasonography [US]) differences between the 2 groups, and neither serious side effects nor adverse events were observed during the follow-up period: both treatments were effective, but patients treated with ADSCs obtained faster results and they should be taken into consideration for patients who require an earlier return to daily activities (**Fig. 5**).

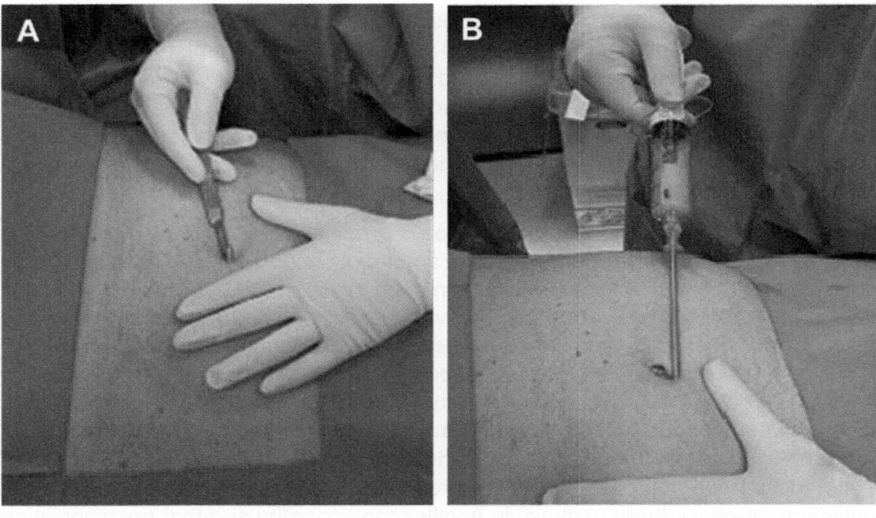

Fig. 4. Two phases of adipose tissue harvest to collect ADSCs. (*A*) Periumbilical incision. (*B*) Vacuum-syringe aspiration of abdominal adipose tissue.

Peripheral Blood Mononuclear Cells

Recently, several studies indicated PBMNCs (monocytes/macrophages and lymphocytes) as a new generation of regenerative autologous cell concentrate[61,62]: monocytes and macrophages promote tissue repair and guide regeneration.[62,63]

In fact, monocytes and macrophages have a plasticity comparable to marrow stem cells (they are able to differentiate and interact into the tissues depending on the surrounding microenvironment) and have multiple action mechanisms[64]: an angiogenic action thanks to the release of VEGF[65–67]; a regenerative action through the release of growth factors, cytokines, and messenger molecules[68–70]; and, furthermore, a recent study affirmed that osteo-inductive action is characteristic of monocyte population rather than stem cells population[71]; they are able to active resident MSCs through a paracrine effect and the release of exosomes[70,72–74]; they have an anti-inflammatory and immune-modulatory action through the polarization of macrophages M1 in M2[75–80]: in injured tissues with a healing delay, there is a majority of macrophages activated in M1 state (degenerative inflammatory), whereas polarization in M2 (macrophages activated in anti-inflammatory regenerative state) allows the regeneration of the injured or inflamed tissues.

Immunohistochemical studies have confirmed that inflammatory cells, such as mast cells, T cells, and macrophages, are present in the early stages of tendinopathies in humans.[81,82] Inflammation in the injured tendons is characterized by the infiltration of immune cells, such as neutrophils and macrophages. Initially, proinflammatory macrophages release cytokines at the repair site and promote degradation of the extracellular tendon matrix, inflammation, and apoptosis. In the later stages of tendon healing, macrophages repair tissues and release anti-inflammatory cytokines to alleviate inflammation and promote tendon remodeling.[83–85] Therefore, the balance between proinflammatory and anti-inflammatory cells (M1/M2) and soluble factors in the tendon-healing process has a major impact on the successful resolution of inflammation.

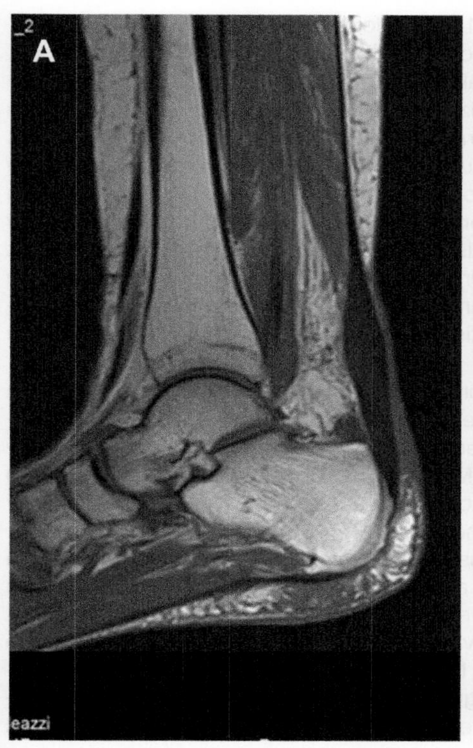

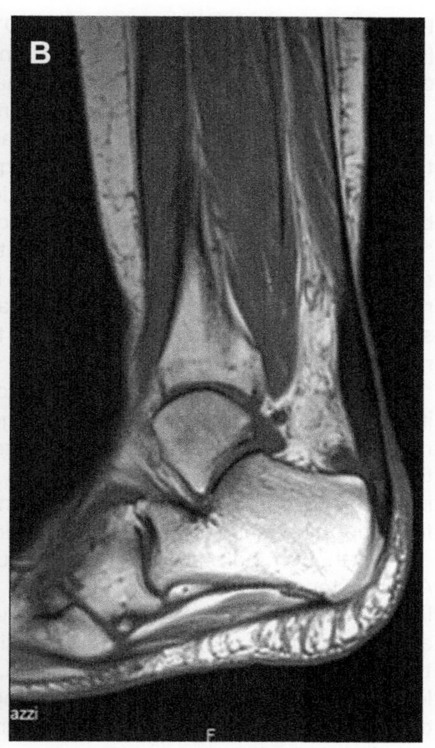

Fig. 5. (*A*) Pretreatment MRI appearance of midportion Achilles tendinopathy. (*B*) MRI appearance of the same patient 6 months after treatment with ADSCs injections.

Most tendons are surrounded by a layer of epithelial cells that could provide a source of fibroblasts to repair injured tendons. Epithelial cells can transdifferentiate into fibroblasts, which can then regenerate the damaged extracellular matrix. This process is triggered by the activation of a signal pathway called epithelial-mesenchymal transition. Sugg and colleagues[86] performed a tenotomy and a repair of the Achilles tendons of adult rats and studied and monitored changes in the macrophage phenotype (M1/M2) and related genes of both the extracellular matrix and the epithelial-mesenchymal transition pathways for a period of 4 weeks. The results suggest that changes in the phenotype of macrophages and the activation of epithelial-mesenchymal transition-related programs probably contribute first to the degradation of the injured tissue and then to the subsequent repair of the tendon tissue. The results also confirmed that the sequential transition between the M1 and M2 phenotypes supports the dual function of macrophages in the degradation and repair of damaged tendon tissue.

Moreover, Stolk and colleagues[87] stimulated tenocytes isolated from injured supraspinatus tendons with PBMNC. They demonstrated that tenocytes respond to an inflammatory microenvironment by altering surface receptors and release of cytokines, influencing the state polarization of macrophages and regulating the expression of collagen.[87] Furthermore, all these changes occurred both by direct cell-cell contact (macrophage-tenocytes) and by the release of endogenous factors (paracrine effect).

The role of monocytes-derived macrophages in tissue remodeling and repair is known for many tissues and pathologic conditions, and it is probably important in tendinopathy because infiltration of $CD14^+$ myeloid cells (monocytes) and $CD68^+$ (macrophages) has been extensively demonstrated, mainly by immunohistochemistry, cytofluorimetry, or mRNA expression analysis.[87–93]

Macrophages are activated and polarized under the influence of the surrounding matrix and the environment.[94] The balancing of the M1/M2 polarization influences the outcome of the repair, and an inadequate or unregulated resolution of the inflammation would lead to chronic inflammation and fibrosis.[95] Despite stem cells having been considered a promising solution for the treatment of degenerative disease by "disseminating" them inside damaged tissues, recently it has been observed that regenerative capacity of stem cells is influenced and regulated by local immune response to tissue damage and particularly, by monocytes/macrophages that represent a central component of response to tissue damage and are coordinators of tissue repairing and regeneration.[63,96]

It has recently been affirmed that monocytes from peripheral blood are able to induce the polarization of M1 macrophages in M2 in muscle tissue.[97] Given the fundamental inflammatory component of the tendon lesions and the imbalance in the relationship between macrophages M1 and M2 in both acute and chronic tendinitis, the injections of autologous circulating monocytes could represent a valid cell therapy for supporting injured or degenerated tendons.[82]

Even though there are no studies focusing exclusively on the treatment of human Achilles tendinopathies with PBMNCs, autologous cell therapy with the injection into the tissues of monocytes simply harvested from peripheral blood could represent a new therapeutic option with low invasiveness and a solid scientific rationale in the treatment of these pathologic conditions. Moreover, it could be associated with Achilles tendon surgical procedures as biological augmentation to enhance healing process, improve surgical outcomes, and reduce complication rates, allowing for less invasive strategies.

Bone Marrow Aspirate Concentrate

BMAC is the result of different density gradient centrifugations of bone marrow aspirated from the iliac crest.[98,99] This aspirate has a concentration of nucleated cells less than 0.01%, and its role is to deliver MSCs to the injured tendon.[100] This procedure concentrates the mononucleated cells, hematopoietic stem cells, and platelets in 1 layer and the red blood cells in another. The efficacy of cells contained in BMAC is to modulate the healing response of pathologic tendon by controlling inflammation, reducing fibrosis, and recruiting other cells, including tenocytes and MSCs.[101] An in vitro study demonstrated an increase in cell proliferation in Achilles tendon scaffolds seeded with bone marrow aspirate.[102] In the only in vivo study reporting outcomes in patients with sport-related Achilles tendon ruptures treated via open repair augmented with BMAC injection, a total of 27 patients treated with open repair and BMAC injection were reevaluated at a mean follow-up of 29.7 ± 6.1 months and no reruptures were noted. Of the patients, 92% returned to their sport at 5.9 ± 1.8 months. No soft tissue masses, bone formation, or tumors were observed in the operative extremity.[103]

Scaffolds

In recent years, several natural and synthetic materials, such as collagen, silk, or synthetic polymers, have been examined, and in some cases also hybrid materials with the aim to promote cellular growth and provide mechanical support for tendon repair.[104]

The ideal scaffold for Achilles tendon should allow a natural and fast bridging of tendinous defect as well as organized collagen-rich tissue with complete incorporation of the material within 8 weeks. Moreover, the scaffold should release chemotactic factors to promote the recruitment of progenitor cells.[105]

Polyhydroxyalkanoates is a material that possesses several of the above qualities. It is part of a family of biopolymers consisting of polyesters produced in nature by microorganisms to store energy and carbon. These materials, in particular, poly-3-hydroxybutyrate-*co*-3-hydroxyhexanoate (PHBHHx), are known to be compatible with many mesenchyme-derived cell types and have adaptable mechanical properties along with delayed biodegradability.[104] A study by Webb and colleagues[104] reported how tendons repair using PHBHHx scaffold was mechanically and histologically superior in comparison to controls.

Another treatment regards the use of decellularized tendon tissue as a scaffold, which maintains the native characteristics (ultrastructure, biochemical composition, and tensile strength of the tendon extracellular matrix) and preserves more than 90% of the proteoglycans and growth factors.[106] In vitro, the decellularized tendon slices were able to facilitate repopulation and attachment of fibroblasts. Farnebo and colleagues,[107] analyzing the use of decellularized grafts in rats, demonstrated an enhancement of mechanical properties and reduced immune response. Decellularized porcine tendon can also be recellularized with human tenocytes.[108]

An acellular human dermal allograft (GraftJacket; Wright Medical Technology, Inc, Arlington, TN, USA) reported significant improvement in mechanical strength and stiffness in biomechanical test. In in vivo studies, patients treated with GraftJacket showed a desirable return-to-activity time without complications.[109,110] Recently, interest has also increased about scaffolds of animal origin; in fact, the use of xenograft, in addition to suture repair, seems to improve tendon strength compared with isolated repair. The most used tissue is porcine small intestinal submucosa (SIS).[111] Preclinical studies demonstrated the ability of SIS to remodel tendon: SIS retains several biologically active growth factors, including VEGF, TGF-β, and fibroblast growth factor, which likely contribute to the behavior and migration of cells into the scaffold.[112,113] Moreover, SIS is subject to a rapid degradation, with 60% of the mass lost after 30 days and complete degradation within 90 days. After complete degradation, the extracellular matrix looks very similar to native tissue for vascularity and organization. A strength of SIS is its ability to recruit marrow-derived cells involved in the remodeling and repair process.[112,113]

IMAGING IN BIOLOGICS TREATMENT OF ACHILLES TENDON PATHOLOGIC CONDITIONS

Ultrasonography

Because of its easy accessibility, large tissue volume, and straight course, US is an ideal technique to evaluate the Achilles tendon. Moreover, the contralateral assessment results in a very easy and dynamic evaluation, which is easily accomplished with active and passive ankle movement. Color/power Doppler imaging can theoretically demonstrate hyperemia, increased vascularity, and varicosities.[114]

A recent systematic review confirms and recommends US's diagnostic role in patients with Achilles tendon pain. US can determine the type (full, partial, or even plantaris tendon) and level of rupture, define the extent of tissue damage and prognosis as well as aid in providing an indication for treatment selection (surgery or conservative treatment). Literature regarding US after regenerative treatment is scarce.[115] Recently, Albano and colleagues[116] assessed the correlation between US findings and clinical outcome after intratendinous injection of leucocyte-rich PRP or ADSCs in patients with noninsertional Achilles tendinopathy. Significant increase of tendon thickness measured using US (P = .012) and power Doppler signal (P = .027) was seen. There was no significant difference between pretreatment and posttreatment cross-sectional area, signal intensity, and echotexture (P>.217). None of the pretreatment parameters was a predictor of treatment outcome (P>.104).

MRI

MRI is an excellent technique for imaging the internal morphology of the Achilles tendon. It can easily distinguish between paratenonitis and tendinosis. MRI is not user-dependent and can provide multiplanar images of the Achilles. It is also useful in determining the extent of degeneration in the tendon, which is useful for preoperative planning. In last several years, dynamic MRI has been developed, and this procedure provides relevant images, particularly at the myotendinous junction level of the Achilles tendon.[114,115]

Few studies analyzed MRI changing after regenerative treatment. The study of Albano and colleagues[116] highlighted how, after ADSCs or PRP treatment, Achilles tendon increased its thickness, as measured using MRI (P = .013).

Oloff and colleagues[117] evaluated 13 individuals who underwent Achilles tendon surgery and PRP treatment and 13 individuals who underwent PRP treatment alone, correlating clinical outcomes pretreatment and posttreatment with MRI. At final follow-up, the MRI score did not correlate with the VISA-A questionnaire score (P = .13), whereas the Pearson's correlation test suggested a linear trend between the difference in MRI score and VISA-A questionnaire.

MRI is useful not only for assessing effects of biologic treatment of Achilles tendon pathologic conditions but also for creating an imaging-based classification. The classification of Achilles tendinopathy proposed by Oloff and colleagues[117] was based on MRI appearance and distinguished 5 grades of Achilles tendinopathy depending on the thickness of the tendon (ranging from hypertrophy to severe thickness) and on the signal changes of the tendon (ranging from homogeneous signal to greater than 50% of tendon with abnormal signal or partial tendon tear).

Sonoelastography

Sonoelastography (SE) is an image method based on US that analyzes the viscoelastic behavior of a tissue subjected to a deformation applied by the examiner during the execution of the diagnostic examination.[118] The SE uses the real-time Doppler US technique to render in images the vibration resulting from the propagation of a low-frequency wave (<1 kHz) through the examined tissue. This low frequency is generated by an external source, such as the pressure of the operator and propagated by means of a probe. The SE allows a conventional-type evaluation (B-mode) contextually to the evaluation of the elasticity of the investigated structures. The software returns the elastogram as a scale of colors that turn from blue, an indicator of maximum stiffness, to green and yellow, which indicate intermediate stiffness, up to red, indicating the greater elasticity.[118]

There is still a lack of consensus in the application of SE to detect tendon pathologic condition. In normal Achilles tendon, tissue can be classified into 3 grades: grade 1, blue (hardest tissue) to green (hard tissue); grade 2, yellow (intermediate tissue); or grade 3, red (soft tissue). During aging, Achilles tendon exhibited an increased stiffness when compared with young adults.[119]

In those patients with symptomatic Achilles tendons but normal US appearance, SE was able to highlight very early changes in tissue elasticity, due to initial edema and inflammation, usually missed at conventional US. SE demonstrated high to excellent sensitivity, specificity, and accuracy, and also a high agreement with US (k = 0.81) and clinical examination (k = 0.91).[119]

THE AUTHORS' ALGORITHM FOR USE OF BIOLOGICS IN MIDPORTION ACHILLES TENDINOPATHY (FOOT AND ANKLE RECONSTRUCTION GROUP ALGORITHM)

Over the years, numerous types of treatment have been proposed for chronic Achilles tendinopathies, but with the advent of regenerative medicine, the therapeutic possibilities have multiplied without a precise treatment algorithm. The authors created an algorithm for the use of biologics in midportion Achilles tendinopathy based on their clinical experience. Developing the FARG (Foot and Ankle Reconstruction Group) algorithm for midportion Achilles tendinopathy, the authors have been inspired by the MRI-based classification of tendinopathy described by Oloff and colleagues,[117] and they have categorized symptomatic patients according to their level of sporting activity:

- Sport-active patients (sports activity at least 2 times a week)
- Nonathletic patients (sports activity <2 times a week)

The treatment scheme is shown in **Table 1**. It is noteworthy that the major differences concern grades 1 and 2 of tendinopathy in which, considering the lower functional request, the nonathletic patient can more probably benefit from less invasive treatments.

BIOLOGICS IN ACUTE AND CHRONIC ACHILLES RUPTURES

In recent years, the use of regenerative medicine for the treatment of acute Achilles tendon rupture has been widely described. Zou and colleagues[120] hypothesized that PRP can be used as biological augmentation for surgical treatment of acute Achilles tendon rupture. Patients with acute Achilles tendon rupture were randomly assigned to either control group (isolated end-to-end Krackow suture) or PRP group (suture plus PRP). At 3 months, the PRP group had better isokinetic muscle. The PRP group also achieved higher SF-36 and Leppilahti scores at 6 and 12 months.

Table 1
Foot and Ankle Reconstruction Group algorithm for midportion Achilles tendinopathy

Sport-Active Patients	Achilles Tendinopathy Grade	Nonathletic Patients
Conservative treatment	Grade 0: Hypertrophy, with homogeneous signal	Conservative treatment
Biologic treatment[b]	Grade 1: Hypertrophy, with isolated signal changes in <25% of tendon	Conservative treatment
Stripping[a] + biologic treatment[b]	Grade 2: Hypertrophy, with signal changes in >1 area, or diffuse changes in >25% of tendon	Biologic[a] treatment[b]
Stripping[a] + biologic treatment[b]	Grade 3: Severe hypertrophy, <50% tendon signal changes, with interstitial tear	Stripping[a] + biologic treatment[b]
FHL transfer ± biologic treatment[b]	Grade 4: Severe thickening, >50% of tendon with abnormal signal, partial tendon tear	FHL transfer ± biologic treatment[b]

[a] Stripping technique as described by Maffulli and colleagues.[121]
[b] Authors' preferred biologic treatments are ADSCs and PBMNCs injections.

At 24 months, the PRP group had an improved ankle range of motion compared with the control group.[120]

In contrast, Schepull and colleagues[55] evaluated 30 patients with acute Achilles tendon rupture, 16 of whom were injected with 10 mL PRP at time of surgery. No significant group differences in elasticity modulus could be shown. There was no significant difference in heel raise index. The Achilles Tendon Total Rupture Score was lower in the PRP group, suggesting a detrimental effect. There was a correlation between the elasticity modulus at 7 and 19 weeks and the heel raise index at 52 weeks.

The use of PRP was analyzed also in an athlete population. Sánchez and colleagues[122] evaluated 12 athletes who underwent open suture repair after complete Achilles tendon tear.[122] Open suture repair in conjunction with a preparation rich in growth factors (PRGF) was performed in 6 athletes. Athletes receiving PRGF recovered their range of motion earlier, showed no wound complication, and took less time to take up gentle running and to resume training activities.

An immunohistochemistry study, moreover, showed that local application of PRP, in acute Achilles tendon rupture, can enhance the healing capacity by promoting better collagen I deposition, decreasing cellularity and vascularity, and increasing glycosaminoglycan content when compared with control samples.[123]

Concerning BMAC, only 1 study evaluated clinical effects in primary Achilles tendon repair. Stein and colleagues[103] reviewed patients with sport-related Achilles tendon ruptures treated via open repair augmented with BMAC injection. A total of 28 tendons were identified with a mean age of 38.3. At mean follow-up of 29.7 months, there were no reruptures. Walking without a boot was achieved at 1.8 months' participation, in light activity at 3.4 months, and 92% of patients returned to their sport at 5.9 months.

A recent meta-analysis aimed to determine if augmented surgical repair with gastrocnemius (3 studies) or plantaris tendon (1 study) of an acute Achilles tendon rupture improved subjective patient satisfaction without an increase in rerupture rates.[124] In 4 studies, 169 patients were analyzed, of which 83 participants were treated with augmented repair and 86 were treated with nonaugmented repair. Augmented repair led to similar responses when compared with nonaugmented repair for acute Achilles tendon rupture. The rerupture rates showed no significant difference for augmented versus nonaugmented repair. No differences in superficial and deep infections occurred in augmented (7 infections) and nonaugmented (8 infections) repair groups during postoperative follow-up. No significant differences in other complications were found between augmented (7.2%) and nonaugmented (8.1%) repair.[124]

The treatment of chronic Achilles tendon ruptures is still a challenge for foot and ankle surgeons, and given the lack of prospective randomized trials and the small number of the studies, a gold standard treatment has not been described. The key role in this pathologic condition is the size of tendon defects. Most of surgical repair involves tendon transfer or the use of an allograft or scaffold to cover the defect.[125] Several tendon transfer techniques have been described, including the peroneus brevis, FDL, and FHL.[125] Each of these techniques has its own pertinent anatomy, advantages, and disadvantages that should be taken into consideration before surgery. By using the peroneus brevis, it is possible to report a loss of eversion strength.[126] Concerning FDL, the risk is linked with a weakened toe flexion and development of lesser toe deformities. Moreover, the possibility of damaging the adjacent neurovascular bundle has been reported in the literature.[125]

One transfer technique described for chronic Achilles tendon rupture is the use FHL tendon: in addition to the mechanical function, comes into play also a biological mechanism due to the muscular proximity with the consequent contribution of blood and growth factors[127] (**Fig. 6**). Literature reports no functional deficits related to the FHL tendon harvest, but doubts remain regarding the potential to develop hallux claw deformity, decreased great toe push-off strength, and transfer metatarsalgia following FHL tendon harvest.[128,129]

Another strategy to fill the tendon defect involves the use of autograft or allograft tendon for augmentation. The use of fascia lata or hamstrings tendon has been widely described with excellent clinical results and with a high return to preinjury sport activity.[130–134]

Otherwise synthetic materials avoid the risks and the comorbidities related to tendon harvesting. In contrast, the literature reported a higher risk of wound complications, infection, and inflammatory reactions. Several published articles reported the use of different scaffolds, such as polymer-carbon fiber, Marlex mesh, or polyester tape, reporting a complication rate ranging from 17.3% to 31.3%.[135–139]

Another alternative for the treatment of neglected Achilles tendon rupture regards the use of acellular dermal human matrix. This patch can be used in the "burrito" technique or to augment a direct end-to-end repair in which the goal is early mobilization. There are similar xenograft options commercially available. These grafts have acellular collagen matrix derived from sources, such as equine pericardium or porcine urinary bladder matrix.[109,140,141]

SUMMARY AND FUTURE PERSPECTIVES

Achilles tendinopathies are challenging pathologic conditions considering the scarce tendency to healing and the average high-functional requests of the patients that are often young and active in sports activities. Conservative treatments for insertional Achilles tendinopathies have shown low success rate and biologics, and presently, have not shown better outcomes: surgery remains the main indication in patients resistant to conservative treatment.

In contrast, several studies have focused on biologics for the treatment of midportion Achilles tendinopathy with good outcomes. Despite this, because of the variability of the treatments evaluated and the wide spectrum of techniques and technologies available, standardized protocols have still not been created. Combining imaging appearance with patients' functional requests could be the way to reach a protocol for the use of biologics for the treatment of midportion Achilles tendinopathy and, for this perspective, the authors have described their actual protocol in this field.

Regenerative medicine has demonstrated the in vitro and in vivo ability to enhance tendon-healing processes, and biologics will gain more and more space as

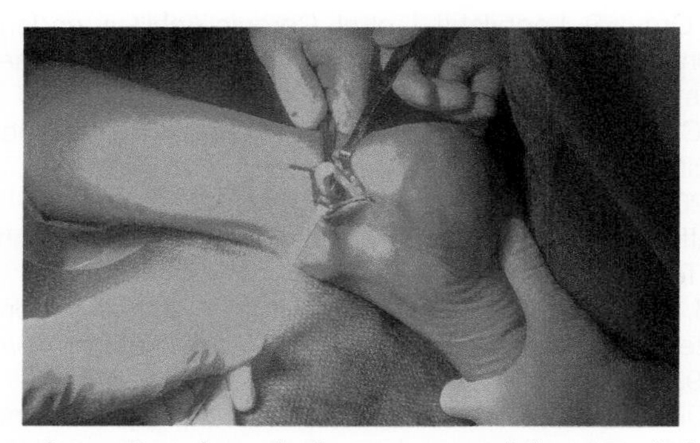

Fig. 6. FHL tendon harvesting through the posteromedial approach in a patient with chronic Achilles tendon rupture.

augmentation or support in surgical procedures for Achilles pathologic conditions and acute or chronic Achilles tears. Despite this, further scientific evaluation is needed to reach 3 goals that will widen the general use of biologics for Achilles tendon pathologic conditions:

1. To identify the most appropriate biologic tools to address these pathologic conditions
2. To achieve a strong level of treatment recommendation
3. To create evidence-based and personalized protocols of treatment.

REFERENCES

1. Maffulli N, Khan KM, Puddu G. Overuse tendon conditions: time to change a confusing terminology. Arthroscopy 1998;14:840–3.
2. Scott A, Ashe MC. Common tendinopathies in the upper and lower extremities. Curr Sports Med Rep 2006;5:233–41.
3. Benjamin M, Ralphs JR. Tendons and ligaments—an overview. Histol Histopathol 1997;12:1135–44.
4. Shapiro E, Grande D, Drakos M. Biologics in Achilles tendon healing and repair: a review. Curr Rev Musculoskelet Med 2015;8:9–17.
5. Docheva D, Müller SA, Majewski M, et al. Biologics for tendon repair. Adv Drug Deliv Rev 2015;84:222–39.
6. Gott M, Ast M, Lane LB, et al. Tendon phenotype should dictate tissue engineering modality in tendon repair: a review. Discov Med 2011;12:75–84.
7. LaPrade RF, Geeslin AG, Murray IR, et al. Biologic treatments for sports injuries II think tank-current concepts, future research, and barriers to advancement, part 1: biologics overview, ligament injury, tendinopathy. Am J Sports Med 2016;44:3270–83.
8. Kvist M. Achilles tendon injuries in athletes. Sports Med 1994;18:173–201.
9. Benazzo F, Marullo M, Indino C, et al. Achilles tendinopathy. In: Volpi P, editor. Arthroscopy and sport injuries: applications in high-level athletes. Cham (Switzerland): Springer International Publishing; 2016. p. 69–76.
10. Pearce CJ, Tan A. Non-insertional Achilles tendinopathy. EFORT Open Rev 2017;1:383–90.
11. Maffulli N, Kader D. Tendinopathy of tendo achillis. J Bone Joint Surg Br 2002;84:1–8.
12. Tallon C, Coleman BD, Khan KM, et al. Outcome of surgery for chronic Achilles tendinopathy. A critical review. Am J Sports Med 2001;29:315–20.
13. Paavola M, Orava S, Leppilahti J, et al. Chronic Achilles tendon overuse injury: complications after surgical treatment. An analysis of 432 consecutive patients. Am J Sports Med 2000;28:77–82.
14. Martin RL, Chimenti R, Cuddeford T, et al. Achilles pain, stiffness, and muscle power deficits: midportion Achilles tendinopathy revision 2018. J Orthop Sports Phys Ther 2018;48:A1–38.
15. Andia I, Maffulli N. Clinical outcomes of biologic treatment for chronic tendinopathy. Oper Tech Orthop 2016;26:98–109.
16. Di Matteo B, Filardo G, Kon E, et al. Platelet-rich plasma: evidence for the treatment of patellar and Achilles tendinopathy–a systematic review. Musculoskelet Surg 2015;99:1–9.
17. Filardo G, Di Matteo B, Kon E, et al. Platelet-rich plasma in tendon-related disorders: results and indications. Knee Surg Sports Traumatol Arthrosc 2016. https://doi.org/10.1007/s00167-016-4261-4.

18. Krogh TP, Ellingsen T, Christensen R, et al. Ultrasound-guided injection therapy of Achilles tendinopathy with platelet-rich plasma or saline: a randomized, blinded, placebo-controlled trial. Am J Sports Med 2016;44:1990–7.
19. Redler LH, Thompson SA, Hsu SH, et al. Platelet-rich plasma therapy: a systematic literature review and evidence for clinical use. Phys Sportsmed 2011;39: 42–51.
20. Sadoghi P, Rosso C, Valderrabano V, et al. The role of platelets in the treatment of Achilles tendon injuries. J Orthop Res 2013;31:111–8.
21. Unlu MC, Kivrak A, Kayaalp ME, et al. Peritendinous injection of platelet-rich plasma to treat tendinopathy: a retrospective review. Acta Orthop Traumatol Turc 2017;51:482–7.
22. Andia I, Martin JI, Maffulli N. Advances with platelet rich plasma therapies for tendon regeneration. Expert Opin Biol Ther 2018;18:389–98.
23. Usuelli FG, Grassi M, Maccario C, et al. Intratendinous adipose-derived stromal vascular fraction (SVF) injection provides a safe, efficacious treatment for Achilles tendinopathy: results of a randomized controlled clinical trial at a 6-month follow-up. Knee Surg Sports Traumatol Arthrosc 2017. https://doi.org/10.1007/s00167-017-4479-9.
24. van Dijk CN, van Sterkenburg MN, Wiegerinck JI, et al. Terminology for Achilles tendon related disorders. Knee Surg Sports Traumatol Arthrosc 2011;19: 835–41.
25. Wiegerinck JI, Kerkhoffs GM, van Sterkenburg MN, et al. Treatment for insertional Achilles tendinopathy: a systematic review. Knee Surg Sports Traumatol Arthrosc 2013;21:1345–55.
26. Fahlström M, Jonsson P, Lorentzon R, et al. Chronic Achilles tendon pain treated with eccentric calf-muscle training. Knee Surg Sports Traumatol Arthrosc 2003; 11:327–33.
27. Shakked RJ, Raikin SM. Insertional tendinopathy of the Achilles: debridement, primary repair, and when to augment. Foot Ankle Clin 2017;22:761–80.
28. Chimenti RL, Cychosz CC, Hall MM, et al. Current concepts review update: insertional Achilles tendinopathy. Foot Ankle Int 2017;38:1160–9.
29. Monto RR. Platelet rich plasma treatment for chronic Achilles tendinosis. Foot Ankle Int 2012;33:379–85.
30. Erroi D, Sigona M, Suarez T, et al. Conservative treatment for insertional Achilles tendinopathy: platelet-rich plasma and focused shock waves. A retrospective study. Muscles Ligaments Tendons J 2017;7:98–106.
31. Sharma P, Maffulli N. Tendon injury and tendinopathy: healing and repair. J Bone Jt Surg Am 2005;87:187–202.
32. Leksa V, Godar S, Schiller HB, et al. TGF-beta-induced apoptosis in endothelial cells mediated by M6P/IGFII-R and mini-plasminogen. J Cell Sci 2005;118: 4577–86.
33. Hou Y, Mao Z, Wei X, et al. Effects of transforming growth factor-beta1 and vascular endothelial growth factor 165 gene transfer on Achilles tendon healing. Matrix Biol 2009;28:324–35.
34. Kashiwagi K, Mochizuki Y, Yasunaga Y, et al. Effects of transforming growth factor-beta 1 on the early stages of healing of the Achilles tendon in a rat model. Scand J Plast Reconstr Surg Hand Surg 2004;38:193–7.
35. Majewski M, Porter RM, Betz OB, et al. Improvement of tendon repair using muscle grafts transduced with TGF-beta1 cDNA. Eur Cell Mater 2012;23: 94–101.

36. Maeda T, Sakabe T, Sunaga A, et al. Conversion of mechanical force into TGF-beta-mediated biochemical signals. Curr Biol 2011;21:933–41.
37. Jorgensen HG, McLellan SD, Crossan JF, et al. Neutralisation of TGF beta or binding of VLA-4 to fibronectin prevents rat tendon adhesion following transection. Cytokine 2005;30:195–202.
38. Katzel EB, Wolenski M, Loiselle AE, et al. Impact of Smad3 loss of function on scarring and adhesion formation during tendon healing. J Orthop Res 2011; 29:684–93.
39. Potter RM, Huynh RT, Volper BD, et al. Impact of TGF-β inhibition during acute exercise on Achilles tendon extracellular matrix. Am J Physiol Regul Integr Comp Physiol 2017;312:R157–64.
40. Stojadinovic O, Lee B, Vouthounis C, et al. Novel genomic effects of glucocorticoids in epidermal keratinocytes: inhibition of apoptosis, interferon-gamma pathway, and wound healing along with promotion of terminal differentiation. J Biol Chem 2007;282:4021–34.
41. Wilgus TA, Ferreira AM, Oberyszyn TM, et al. Regulation of scar formation by vascular endothelial growth factor. Lab Invest 2008;88:579–90.
42. Boyer MI, Watson JT, Lou J, et al. Quantitative variation in vascular endothelial growth factor mRNA expression during early flexor tendon healing: an investigation in a canine model. J Orthop Res 2001;19:869–72.
43. Zhang F, Liu H, Stile F, et al. Effect of vascular endothelial growth factor on rat Achilles tendon healing. Plast Reconstr Surg 2003;112:1613–9.
44. Tempfer H, Kaser-Eichberger A, Lehner C, et al. Bevacizumab improves Achilles tendon repair in a rat model. Cell Physiol Biochem 2018;46:1148–58.
45. Wurgler-Hauri CC, Dourte LM, Baradet TC, et al. Temporal expression of 8 growth factors in tendon-to-bone healing in a rat supraspinatus model. J Shoulder Elb Surg 2007;16:S198–203.
46. Wang XT, Liu PY, Tang JB. Tendon healing in vitro: genetic modification of tenocytes with exogenous PDGF gene and promotion of collagen gene expression. J Hand Surg Am 2004;29:884–90.
47. Thomopoulos S, Zaegel M, Das R, et al. PDGF-BB released in tendon repair using a novel delivery system promotes cell proliferation and collagen remodeling. J Orthop Res 2007;25:1358–68.
48. Thomopoulos S, Das R, Silva MJ, et al. Enhanced flexor tendon healing through controlled delivery of PDGF-BB. J Orthop Res 2009;27:1209–15.
49. Chetty A, Cao GJ, Nielsen HC. Insulin-like growth factor-I signaling mechanisms, type I collagen and alpha smooth muscle actin in human fetal lung fibroblasts. Pediatr Res 2006;60:389–94.
50. Kurtz CA, Loebig TG, Anderson DD, et al. Insulin-like growth factor I accelerates functional recovery from Achilles tendon injury in a rat model. Am J Sports Med 1999;27:363–9.
51. Lyras DN, Kazakos K, Georgiadis G, et al. Does a single application of PRP alter the expression of IGF-I in the early phase of tendon healing? J Foot Ankle Surg 2011;50:276–82.
52. Randelli P, Randelli F, Ragone V, et al. Regenerative medicine in rotator cuff injuries. Biomed Res Int 2014;2014:129515.
53. Dohan Ehrenfest DM, Rasmusson L, Albrektsson T. Classification of platelet concentrates: from pure platelet-rich plasma (P-PRP) to leucocyte- and platelet-rich fibrin (L-PRF). Trends Biotechnol 2009;27:158–67.

54. Lin MT, Chiang CF, Wu CH, et al. Meta-analysis comparing autologous blood-derived products (including platelet-rich plasma) injection versus placebo in patients with achilles tendinopathy. Arthroscopy 2018;34:1966–75.
55. Schepull T, Kvist J, Norrman H, et al. Autologous platelets have no effect on the healing of human Achilles tendon ruptures: a randomized single-blind study. Am J Sports Med 2011;39:38–47.
56. Longo UG, Lamberti A, Petrillo S, et al. Scaffolds in tendon tissue engineering. Stem Cells Int 2012;2012:517165.
57. Usuelli FG, D'Ambrosi R, Maccario C, et al. Adipose-derived stem cells in orthopaedic pathologies. Br Med Bull 2017;124:31–54.
58. Fuoco C, Petrilli LL, Cannata S, et al. Matrix scaffolding for stem cell guidance toward skeletal muscle tissue engineering. J Orthop Surg Res 2016;11:86.
59. Yan Z, Yin H, Nerlich M, et al. Boosting tendon repair: interplay of cells, growth factors and scaffold-free and gel-based carriers. J Exp Orthop 2018;5:1.
60. Akpancar S, Tatar O, Turgut H, et al. The current perspectives of stem cell therapy in orthopedic surgery. Arch Trauma Res 2016;5:e37976.
61. Zhang M, Huang B. The multi-differentiation potential of peripheral blood mononuclear cells. Stem Cell Res Ther 2012;3:48.
62. Ogle ME, Segar CE, Sridhar S, et al. Monocytes and macrophages in tissue repair: implications for immunoregenerative biomaterial design. Exp Biol Med (Maywood) 2016;241:1084–97.
63. Forbes SJ, Rosenthal N. Preparing the ground for tissue regeneration: from mechanism to therapy. Nat Med 2014;20:857–69.
64. Kuwana M, Okazaki Y, Kodama H, et al. Human circulating CD14+ monocytes as a source of progenitors that exhibit mesenchymal cell differentiation. J Leukoc Biol 2003;74:833–45.
65. Barnett FH, Rosenfeld M, Wood M, et al. Macrophages form functional vascular mimicry channels in vivo. Sci Rep 2016;6:36659.
66. Barbeck M, Unger RE, Booms P, et al. Monocyte preseeding leads to an increased implant bed vascularization of biphasic calcium phosphate bone substitutes via vessel maturation. J Biomed Mater Res A 2016;104:2928–35.
67. Hu K, Olsen BR. The roles of vascular endothelial growth factor in bone repair and regeneration. Bone 2016;91:30–8.
68. Caplan AI. New era of cell-based orthopedic therapies. Tissue Eng Part B Rev 2009;15:195–200.
69. Dong L, Wang C. Harnessing the power of macrophages/monocytes for enhanced bone tissue engineering. Trends Biotechnol 2013;31:342–6.
70. Champagne CM, Takebe J, Offenbacher S, et al. Macrophage cell lines produce osteoinductive signals that include bone morphogenetic protein-2. Bone 2002;30:26–31.
71. Henrich D, Seebach C, Verboket R, et al. The osteo-inductive activity of bone-marrow-derived mononuclear cells resides within the CD14+ population and is independent of the CD34+ population. Eur Cell Mater 2018;35:165–77.
72. Pajarinen J, Lin T, Gibon E, et al. Mesenchymal stem cell-macrophage crosstalk and bone healing. Biomaterials 2018. https://doi.org/10.1016/j.biomaterials.2017.12.025.
73. Pirraco RP, Reis RL, Marques AP. Effect of monocytes/macrophages on the early osteogenic differentiation of hBMSCs. J Tissue Eng Regen Med 2013;7:392–400.
74. Ekström K, Omar O, Granéli C, et al. Monocyte exosomes stimulate the osteogenic gene expression of mesenchymal stem cells. PLoS One 2013;8:e75227.

75. Schlundt C, Schell H, Goodman SB, et al. Immune modulation as a therapeutic strategy in bone regeneration. J Exp Orthop 2015;2:1.
76. Schlundt C, El Khassawna T, Serra A, et al. Macrophages in bone fracture healing: their essential role in endochondral ossification. Bone 2018;106:78–89.
77. Thomopoulos S, Parks WC, Rifkin DB, et al. Mechanisms of tendon injury and repair. J Orthop Res 2015;33:832–9.
78. Misharin AV, Cuda CM, Saber R, et al. Nonclassical Ly6C(-) monocytes drive the development of inflammatory arthritis in mice. Cell Rep 2014;9:591–604.
79. Utomo L, van Osch GJ, Bayon Y, et al. Guiding synovial inflammation by macrophage phenotype modulation: an in vitro study towards a therapy for osteoarthritis. Osteoarthritis Cartilage 2016;24:1629–38.
80. Mountziaris PM, Mikos AG. Modulation of the inflammatory response for enhanced bone tissue regeneration. Tissue Eng Part B Rev 2008;14:179–86.
81. Millar NL, Hueber AJ, Reilly JH, et al. Inflammation is present in early human tendinopathy. Am J Sports Med 2010;38:2085–91.
82. Dean BJ, Gettings P, Dakin SG, et al. Are inflammatory cells increased in painful human tendinopathy? A systematic review. Br J Sports Med 2016;50:216–20.
83. John T, Lodka D, Kohl B, et al. Effect of pro-inflammatory and immunoregulatory cytokines on human tenocytes. J Orthop Res 2010;28:1071–7.
84. Marsolais D, Côté CH, Frenette J. Neutrophils and macrophages accumulate sequentially following Achilles tendon injury. J Orthop Res 2001;19:1203–9.
85. Manning CN, Havlioglu N, Knutsen E, et al. The early inflammatory response after flexor tendon healing: a gene expression and histological analysis. J Orthop Res 2014;32:645–52.
86. Sugg KB, Lubardic J, Gumucio JP, et al. Changes in macrophage phenotype and induction of epithelial-to-mesenchymal transition genes following acute Achilles tenotomy and repair. J Orthop Res 2014;32:944–51.
87. Stolk M, Klatte-Schulz F, Schmock A, et al. New insights into tenocyte-immune cell interplay in an in vitro model of inflammation. Sci Rep 2017;7:9801.
88. Murray PJ, Allen JE, Biswas SK, et al. Macrophage activation and polarization: nomenclature and experimental guidelines. Immunity 2014;4:14–20.
89. Michalski MN, McCauley LK. Macrophages and skeletal health. Pharmacol Ther 2017;174:43–54.
90. Guiteras R, Flaquer M, Cruzado JM. Macrophage in chronic kidney disease. Clin Kidney J 2016;9:765–71.
91. Millar NL, Akbar M, Campbell AL, et al. IL-17A mediates inflammatory and tissue remodelling events in early human tendinopathy. Sci Rep 2016;6:27149.
92. Blomgran P, Blomgran R, Ernerudh J, et al. A possible link between loading, inflammation and healing: immune cell populations during tendon healing in the rat. Sci Rep 2016;6:29824.
93. Mauro A, Russo V, Di Marcantonio L, et al. M1 and M2 macrophage recruitment during tendon regeneration induced by amniotic epithelial cell allotransplantation in ovine. Res Vet Sci 2016;105:92–102.
94. Dakin SG, Werling D, Hibbert A, et al. Macrophage sub-populations and the lipoxin A4 receptor implicate active inflammation during equine tendon repair. PLoS One 2012;7:e32333.
95. Douglas MR, Morrison KE, Salmon M, et al. Why does inflammation persist: a dominant role for the stromal microenvironment? Expert Rev Mol Med 2002;4:1–18.
96. Julier Z, Park AJ, Briquez PS, et al. Promoting tissue regeneration by modulating the immune system. Acta Biomater 2017;53:13–28.

97. Arnold L, Henry A, Poron F, et al. Inflammatory monocytes recruited after skeletal muscle injury switch into antiinflammatory macrophages to support myogenesis. J Exp Med 2007;204:1057–69.
98. Cottom JM, Plemmons BS. Bone marrow aspirate concentrate and its uses in the foot and ankle. Clin Podiatr Med Surg 2018;35:19–26.
99. Salamanna F, Contartese D, Nicoli Aldini N, et al. Bone marrow aspirate clot: a technical complication or a smart approach for musculoskeletal tissue regeneration? J Cell Physiol 2018;233:2723–32.
100. Hegde V, Shonuga O, Ellis S, et al. A prospective comparison of 3 approved systems for autologous bone marrow concentration demonstrated nonequivalency in progenitor cell number and concentration. J Orthop Trauma 2014;28:591–8.
101. Imam MA, Holton J, Horriat S, et al. A systematic review of the concept and clinical applications of bone marrow aspirate concentrate in tendon pathology. SICOT J 2017;3:58.
102. Broese M, Toma I, Haasper C, et al. Seeding a human tendon matrix with bone marrow aspirates compared to previously isolated hBMSCs—an in vitro study. Technol Health Care 2011;19:469–79.
103. Stein BE, Stroh DA, Schon LC. Outcomes of acute Achilles tendon rupture repair with bone marrow aspirate concentrate augmentation. Int Orthop 2015;39:901–5.
104. Webb WR, Dale TP, Lomas AJ, et al. The application of poly(3-hydroxybutyrate-co-3-hydroxyhexanoate) scaffolds for tendon repair in the rat model. Biomaterials 2013;34:6683–94.
105. Suckow MA, Hodde JP, Wolter WR, et al. Repair of experimental Achilles tenotomy with porcine renal capsule material in a rat model. J Mater Sci Mater Med 2007;18:1105–10.
106. Ning LJ, Zhang Y, Chen XH, et al. Preparation and characterization of decellularized tendon slices for tendon tissue engineering. J Biomed Mater Res A 2012;100:1448–56.
107. Farnebo S, Woon CY, Bronstein JA, et al. Decellularized tendon-bone composite grafts for extremity reconstruction: an experimental study. Plast Reconstr Surg 2014;133:79–89.
108. Lohan A, Stoll C, Albrecht M, et al. Human hamstring tenocytes survive when seeded into a decellularized porcine Achilles tendon extracellular matrix. Connect Tissue Res 2013;54:305–12.
109. Lee DK. Achilles tendon repair with acellular tissue graft augmentation in neglected ruptures. J Foot Ankle Surg 2007;46:451–5.
110. Lee DK. A preliminary study on the effects of acellular tissue graft augmentation in acute Achilles tendon ruptures. J Foot Ankle Surg 2008;47:8–12.
111. Wisbeck JM, Parks BG, Schon LC. Xenograft scaffold full-wrap reinforcement of Krackow Achilles tendon repair. Orthopedics 2012;35:e331–4.
112. Gilbert TW, Stewart-Akers AM, Simmons-Byrd A, et al. Degradation and remodeling of small intestinal submucosa in canine Achilles tendon repair. J Bone Joint Surg Am 2007;89:621–30.
113. Zantop T, Gilbert TW, Yoder MC, et al. Extracellular matrix scaffolds are repopulated by bone marrow-derived cells in a mouse model of Achilles tendon reconstruction. J Orthop Res 2006;24:1299–309.
114. Mahoney JM. Imaging techniques and indications. Clin Podiatr Med Surg 2017;34:115–28.

115. Dams OC, Reininga IHF, Gielen JL, et al. Imaging modalities in the diagnosis and monitoring of Achilles tendon ruptures: a systematic review. Injury 2017;48:2383–99.
116. Albano D, Messina C, Usuelli FG, et al. Magnetic resonance and ultrasound in Achilles tendinopathy: predictive role and response assessment to platelet-rich plasma and adipose-derived stromal vascular fraction injection. Eur J Radiol 2017;95:130–5.
117. Oloff L, Elmi E, Nelson J, et al. Retrospective analysis of the effectiveness of platelet-rich plasma in the treatment of Achilles tendinopathy: pretreatment and posttreatment correlation of magnetic resonance imaging and clinical assessment. Foot Ankle Spec 2015;8:490–7.
118. Klauser AS, Miyamoto H, Bellmann-Weiler R, et al. Sonoelastography: musculoskeletal applications. Radiology 2014;272:622–33.
119. Fusini F, Langella F, Busilacchi A, et al. Real-time sonoelastography: principles and clinical applications in tendon disorders. A systematic review. Muscles Ligaments Tendons J 2018;7:467–77.
120. Zou J, Mo X, Shi Z, et al. A prospective study of platelet-rich plasma as biological augmentation for acute Achilles tendon rupture repair. Biomed Res Int 2016;2016:9364170.
121. Longo UG, Ramamurthy C, Denaro V, et al. Minimally invasive stripping for chronic Achilles tendinopathy. Disabil Rehabil 2008;30:1709–13.
122. Sánchez M, Anitua E, Azofra J, et al. Comparison of surgically repaired Achilles tendon tears using platelet-rich fibrin matrices. Am J Sports Med 2007;35:245–51.
123. Alsousou J, Thompson M, Harrison P, et al. Effect of platelet-rich plasma on healing tissues in acute ruptured Achilles tendon: a human immunohistochemistry study. Lancet 2015;385:S19.
124. Zhang YJ, Zhang C, Wang Q, et al. Augmented versus nonaugmented repair of acute Achilles tendon rupture: a systematic review and meta-analysis. Am J Sports Med 2018;46:1767–72.
125. Steginsky BD, Van Dyke B, Berlet GC. The missed Achilles tear: now what? Foot Ankle Clin 2017;22:715–34.
126. Gallant GG, Massie C, Turco VJ. Assessment of eversion and plantar flexion strength after repair of Achilles tendon rupture using peroneus brevis tendon transfer. Am J Orthop (Belle Mead NJ) 1995;24:257–61.
127. Den Hartog BD. Flexor hallucis longus transfer for chronic Achilles tendonosis. Foot Ankle Int 2003;24:233–7.
128. Richardson DR, Willers J, Cohen BE, et al. Evaluation of the hallux morbidity of single-incision flexor hallucis longus tendon transfer. Foot Ankle Int 2009;30:627–30.
129. Coull R, Flavin R, Stephens MM. Flexor hallucis longus tendon transfer: evaluation of postoperative morbidity. Foot Ankle Int 2003;24:931–4.
130. Duhamel P, Mathieu L, Brachet M, et al. Reconstruction of the Achilles tendon with a composite anterolateral thigh free flap with vascularized fascia lata: a case report. J Bone Joint Surg Am 2010;92:2598–603.
131. Lee JW, Yu JC, Shieh SJ, et al. Reconstruction of the Achilles tendon and overlying soft tissue using antero-lateral thigh free flap. Br J Plast Surg 2000;53:574–7.
132. Maffulli N, Leadbetter WB. Free gracilis tendon graft in neglected tears of the Achilles tendon. Clin J Sport Med 2005;15:56–61.

133. Maffulli N, Longo UG, Spiezia F, et al. Free hamstrings tendon transfer and interference screw fixation for less invasive reconstruction of chronic avulsions of the Achilles tendon. Knee Surg Sports Traumatol Arthrosc 2010;18:269–73.
134. Usuelli FG, D'Ambrosi R, Manzi L, et al. Clinical outcomes and return to sports in patients with chronic Achilles tendon rupture after minimally invasive reconstruction with semitendinosus tendon graft transfer. Joints 2017;5:212–6.
135. Howard CB, Winston I, Bell W, et al. Late repair of the calcaneal tendon with carbon fibre. J Bone Joint Surg Br 1984;66:206–8.
136. Ozaki J, Fujiki J, Sugimoto K, et al. Reconstruction of neglected Achilles tendon rupture with Marlex mesh. Clin Orthop Relat Res 1989;(238):204–8.
137. Choksey A, Soonawalla D, Murray J. Repair of neglected Achilles tendon ruptures with Marlex mesh. Injury 1996;27:215–7.
138. Jennings AG, Sefton GK. Chronic rupture of tendo Achillis. Long-term results of operative management using polyester tape. J Bone Joint Surg Br 2002;84:361–3.
139. Jennings AG, Sefton GK, Newman RJ. Repair of acute rupture of the Achilles tendon: a new technique using polyester tape without external splintage. Ann R Coll Surg Engl 2004;86:445–8.
140. Barber FA, McGarry JE, Herbert MA, et al. A biomechanical study of Achilles tendon repair augmentation using GraftJacket matrix. Foot Ankle Int 2008;29:329–33.
141. Grove JR, Hardy MA. Autograft, allograft and xenograft options in the treatment of neglected Achilles tendon ruptures: a historical review with illustration of surgical repair. Foot Ankle J 2008;1:1.

Minimally Invasive and Endoscopic Approach for the Treatment of Noninsertional Achilles Tendinopathy

Craig C. Akoh, MD[a,*], Phinit Phisitkul, MD[b]

KEYWORDS

• Sclerotherapy • Prolotherapy • Achilles tendinopathy • Endoscopy
• Achilles stripping • Longitudinal tenotomy • Minimally invasive

KEY POINTS

- The goals of minimally invasive surgery are to debride degenerative tendon, stimulate healing, and, when appropriate, repair damaged tendon with minimal soft tissue trauma.
- Sclerosing agents have been described to aid in the reduction of neovascularization that occurs in Achilles tendinopathy.
- Percutaneous longitudinal tenotomy is a minimally invasive technique that uses multiple longitudinal incisions into the Achilles tendon to promote neovascularization and healing.
- Endoscopy allows for the treatment of diffuse Achilles tendinopathy and concomitant paratenon involvement.
- Minimally invasive techniques offer a safe surgical options with earlier recovery and less pain and scarring compared with traditional open surgeries.

INDICATION FOR SURGERY

Surgical intervention can be indicated for noninsertional Achilles tendinopathy after 6 months of conservative management.[1,2] Retrospective studies have shown than up to 29% of individuals treated nonoperatively will go on to require surgery.[3,4] In addition, 41% of patients will develop symptoms on the contralateral side.[3] Classic

Disclosure Statement: The authors report the following potential conflicts of interest or sources of funding: P.P. is a paid consultant for Arthrex and Restor 3D, receives royalties from Arthrex; and has stock/stock options in First Ray and Mortise Medical. Full ICMJE author disclosure forms are available for this article online, as supplementary material.

[a] Department of Orthopedics and Rehabilitation, University of Wisconsin School of Medicine and Public Health Madison, 600 Highland Avenue, Room 6220, Madison, WI 53705-2281, USA;
[b] Tri-State Specialists, LLP, 2730 Pierce Street Suite 300, Sioux City, IA 51104, USA
* Corresponding author.
E-mail address: ccakoh@gmail.com

Foot Ankle Clin N Am 24 (2019) 495–504
https://doi.org/10.1016/j.fcl.2019.04.007
foot.theclinics.com
1083-7515/19/

contraindications to open surgery include vascular insufficiency, active infection, poor skin integrity, and severe medical comorbidities.[1,5] Paavlov reported up to an 11% complication rate following open surgery, with 54% of the complications relating to wound issues.[6] Minimally invasive techniques have been shown to offer similar satisfaction rates as open procedures with less morbidity and complications.[7] Thus, minimally invasive techniques offer a safe surgical options in patients who may otherwise be contraindicated to undergoing open procedures. In addition, it can offer an earlier recovery with less pain and scarring compared with traditional open surgeries.

SCLEROTHERAPY AND PROLOTHERAPY

The goals of minimally invasive surgery are to debride degenerative tendon, stimulate healing, and, when appropriate, repair damaged tendon with minimal soft tissue trauma.[8] Sclerosing agents have been described to aid in the reduction of neovascularization that occurs in Achilles tendinopathy, as seen in **Fig. 1**. Polidocanol was first used as a local anesthetic but has been also found to have sclerosing properties. Sclerosing agents are typically injected under ultrasound guidance at the ventral aspect of the diseased tendon.[9] Alfredson published a double-blinded randomized pilot study comparing 20 consecutive healthy patients (mean age 59.3 years old) who were treated with either polidocanol (5 μg/mL) or lidocaine hydrochloride (5 mg/mL) for recalcitrant midportion Achilles tendinopathy.[9] At a mean follow-up of 3 months, the visual analog scores (VAS) for pain significantly improved from 77 to 41 for the polidocanol group compared with only 66 to 64 for the lidocaine group. In addition, 50% of the individuals in the polidocanol group were satisfied with their treatment compared with 0% of the lidocaine group. Interestingly, of the individuals who were pain free, 100% had absent neovascularization of the Achilles tendon on ultrasonographic follow-up. For the crossover group, individuals who initially received lidocaine were subsequently given polidacanol, and they were found to have improved VAS pain scores from 64 to 16. Lind and colleagues[10] published a 2-year prospective study on 42 patients with midportion Achilles tendinopathy. Patients were treated with ultrasound-guided percutaneous polidocanol (5 mg/mL) injections. At a mean follow-up of 23 months, 37 out of the 42 patients (88.1%) were satisfied their treatment outcomes. The mean VAS pain scores improved significantly from 75 to 7. Ultrasonographic evaluation showed a decrease in tendon thickness from 10 to 8 mm, and 71% of the cohort had a complete reversal of neovascularization.

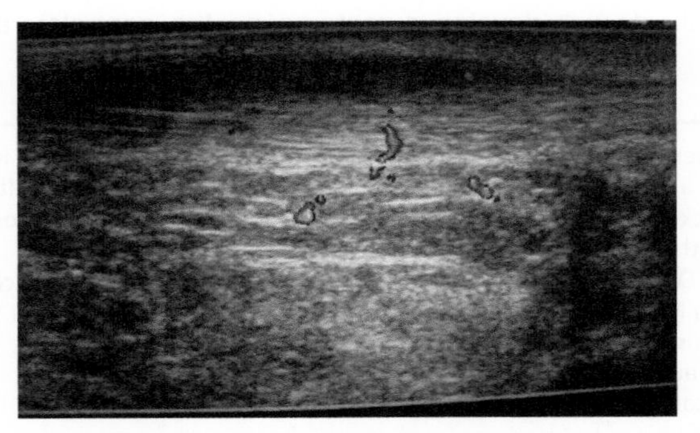

Fig. 1. Achilles tendinopathy with neovascularization. The color Doppler ultrasonographic image illustrates neovascularization along the ventral aspect of the Achilles tendon highlighted in red.

Willberg and colleagues[11] published a double-blinded randomized study to assess the dose effect of polidocanol. Fifty-two consecutive patients with chronic midportion Achilles tendinopathy received up to 3 treatments of either 5 or 10 mg/mL of polidocanol. At a mean follow-up of 14 months, there was no difference in patient-reported satisfaction between the low- and high-dosage groups (69.2% and 73.1%, respectively). The low-dosage group had a significant improvement of the mean VAS pain scores during activity from 66 to 25. The high-dosage group improved similarly from a pretreatment VAS of 66 to 24 posttreatment. The authors concluded that there was no difference between dosage groups for patient-reported satisfaction and mean VAS pain scores. Clementson and colleagues[12] published their retrospective study on 25 patients (mean age 51.5 years) with midportion tendinopathy receiving 10 mg/mL of polidocanol. Patients without ultrasonographic evidence of neovascularization were excluded. The results showed that 19 out of 25 patients (76%) had good or excellent results and were able to resume their previous activity level.

Prolotherapy is another minimally invasive technique that uses the injection of an irritant solution around the diseased tendon to reduce neovascularization.[13,14] Maxwell and colleagues[15] published a prospective study of 36 consecutive patients (mean age 52.6 years) with recalcitrant midportion and insertional chronic tendinosis. In Maxwell's study, the cohort was given an ultrasound-guided injection of 25% hyperosmolar dextrose solution (1 mL 50% dextrose, 1 mL of 2% lignocaine) for a mean of 4 sessions. The VAS pain scores significantly improved at rest and with exertion by 88.2% and 78.1%, respectively. Yelland and colleagues[16] performed an Australian multicenter single-blinded randomized control trial that compared eccentric loading exercises with hyperosmolar prolotherapy (20% glucose/0.1% lignocaine/0.1% ropivacaine) and combined treatment. Patients were treated weekly for 4 to 12 treatments. From their cohort of 43 patients, they measured the Victorian Institute of Sport Assessment-Achilles (VISA-A), VAS pain scores, stiffness, and limitation of activities scores. At 12 months follow-up, 67% of patients were asymptomatic and 87% were very satisfied with their outcomes. In addition, the mean improvement of VISA-A scores at 12 months follow-up were 23.7, 27.5, and 41.1 for eccentric training, prolotherapy only, and combined treatment, respectively. The midsubstance tendinopathy patients experienced an 88.7% and 83.2% improvement in VAS pain scores at rest and pain with sporting activity, respectively. In addition, 55% of the patients with tendinopathy had decreased neovascularization on ultrasonographic evaluation. A meta-analysis of all randomized control trials for prolotherapy and sclerotherapy showed an overall weighted mean improvement in outcome scores to be 36 points.[14] This meta-analysis reported a complication rate of 0.5% (3 out of 600 cases).[14]

Although there have been reported good results with sclerotherapy, some authors have questioned its efficacy.[14,17–19] van Sterkenburg and colleagues published a retrospective single-institution study on 48 patients (53 Achilles tendon) with midportion Achilles tendinopathy. Their cohort (mean age 45 years) was treated with 3 sessions of polidocanol injections and were followed for a mean of 3.9 years. At the short-term 6-week follow-up, only 44% of patients experienced pain relief and only 47% of patients had decreased neovascularization on ultrasonographic evaluation. At 3.9 years follow-up (75% follow-up rate), 15 out of 36 patients (41.7%) underwent operative intervention. Although Yelland's study showed significant clinical improvement in VISA-A scores, the percentage of individuals meeting minimal clinical important change (20 points) were similar between the eccentric exercise group (73%) and prolotherapy group (79%). Although complication rates are low,[14] reported complications including sural nerve pain,[12] partial Achilles tear,[15] and venous thrombosis[20,21] have been reported for sclerotherapy and prolotherapy.

PERCUTANEOUS LONGITUDINAL TENOTOMIES AND MINIMALLY INVASIVE TENDON STRIPPING

Percutaneous longitudinal tenotomy is a minimally invasive technique that uses multiple longitudinal incisions into the Achilles tendon to promote neovascularization and healing.[22,23] This technique is best used for patients with focal tendinopathy less than 3 cm and without peritendinitis.[22,23] The technique described by Maffulli and colleagues[23] places the patient in the prone position and uses a knife blade to make several longitudinal stab incisions over the diseased tendon under ultrasound guidance. With the cutting edge of the knife pointing cranially, the foot is maximally dorsiflexed. The knife is then turned so that the cutting edge is facing caudally, and the foot is maximally plantarflexed. Four more stab incision are made (proximal-lateral, proximal-medial, distal-lateral, and distal-medial) and the previous steps are repeated.

Testa and colleagues[22] reported their retrospective study on 75 athletes who underwent ultrasound-guided percutaneous longitudinal tenotomies for recalcitrant Achilles tendinopathy with less than 3 cm of tendon involvement. Short-term follow-up showed that 83% of the cohort return to sports at a mean time of 6.5 months. At long-term follow-up (mean 4.25 years, 84% follow-up), they found that 87.3% of the cohort continued to have symptomatic relief and 74.6% continued to play sports. The authors concluded that although patients with focal tendinopathy did well with percutaneous tenotomies, patients with diffuse tendinopathy took longer to return to sports. Maffulli and colleagues[23] published a retrospective study on 39 runners (mean age 45 years) who underwent ultrasound-guided percutaneous longitudinal tenotomies for midportion tendinopathy without peritendinitis. At a mean follow-up of 17 years, although calf circumference was smaller than the unaffected side, 77% reported good or excellent outcomes and 60% returned to their baseline activities.

The percutaneous ultrasonic tenotomy (Tenex Health, Lake Forest, CA) is a newer technology to perform percutaneous longitudinal tenotomy procedures for chronic noninsertional Achilles tendinopathy.[24] This technique uses ultrasound guidance to place a probe percutaneously at the site of the diseased tendon. The device uses a microtip that pistons within the diseased tendon to stimulate a healing response. Although there is some promising animal data on the ability of percutaneous ultrasonic tenotomy to reorganize collagen, there is a paucity of human clinical data.[25] Sanchez and colleagues[24] reported complications in 6 patients who presented to his institution after undergoing this procedure at outside facilities and recommended against its use. Complications after the percutaneous tenotomy procedures include postoperative hematoma, superficial infection, Achilles rupture, deep vein thrombosis, and complex regional pain syndrome.[22] Percutaneous longitudinal tenotomy is not recommended for diffuse tendinopathy or for patients with peritendinitis.

Minimally invasive tendon stripping is another option that focuses on releasing ventral adhesions and disrupting the ventral neovascularization seen in Achilles tendinopathy. Options for minimally invasive stripping include mini-open, percutaneous needling,[26] or sliding sutures.[27] Alfredson[26] performed a randomized control trial comparing percutaneous ventral tendon stripping with mini-open tendon stripping. In his study, 31 patients (37 tendons) (mean age 47 years) were randomized into the mini-open group (15 patients) and percutaneous group (16 patients). The mini-open group used a small lateral incision and stripped the ventral Achilles with a scalpel. The percutaneous group used a 14 gauge needle to ventrally strip the Achilles tendon. The results showed that, at a mean follow-up of 18 months, 83% and 74% of the respective mini-open and percutaneous groups were satisfied. The VAS improved from 69 to 6 and 75 to 2 for the mini-open and percutaneous groups, respectively. They concluded that there was no difference between percutaneous and mini-open stripping.

Naidu and colleagues[28] performed a modified stripping technique using a near-circumferential blunt hook around the diseased Achilles tendon ventrally. Mini-open paratenon releases were performed with corticosteroid infusion for 26 patients (mean age 53 years, 29 tendons) with noninsertional Achilles tendinopathy. At a mean follow-up of 13 months, VAS scores significantly decreased from 8.7 to 2.4. Seventy-three percent of the tendons had significant pain improvement and 86% of the cohort was satisfied with their outcome. There were 2 patients with delayed wound healing treated conservatively and no Achilles ruptures.

ENDOSCOPIC PARATENON DEBRIDEMENT

Endoscopy has been described as a safe treatment of diffuse noninsertional Achilles tendinopathy.[29–31] Endoscopy allows for the treatment of diffuse Achilles tendinopathy and concomitant paratenon involvement. First described by Maquirriain in 1998,[32] Achilles endoscopy technique has been evolved to modern techniques.[30] As described by Steenstra and van Dijk,[30] the patient is placed in the prone position and local anesthetic is placed at the site of tendinopathy. Landmarks including the sural nerve, posterior tibial bundle, and Achilles tendon are drawn onto the skin. Then, distal-lateral and proximal-medial portals are made along the Achilles tendon. The 30° arthroscopic camera is then introduced into the distal portal and the shaver proximally to break up paratenon adhesions (**Fig. 2**). Care should be taken during debridement not to damage the posterior tibial bundle distally or the sural nerve proximally at the myotendinous junction.

Maquirriain and colleagues[33] published a preliminary prospective study on 7 patients (mean age 41.7 years) with chronic Achilles tendinopathy who underwent endoscopic debridement. These patients participated in recreational sports and included 2 patients with peritendinitis, 4 with combined peritendinitis and tendinosis, and 1 with a chronic partial Achilles tear. All patients with peritendinitis underwent paratenon debridement, whereas patients with tendinosis underwent longitudinal

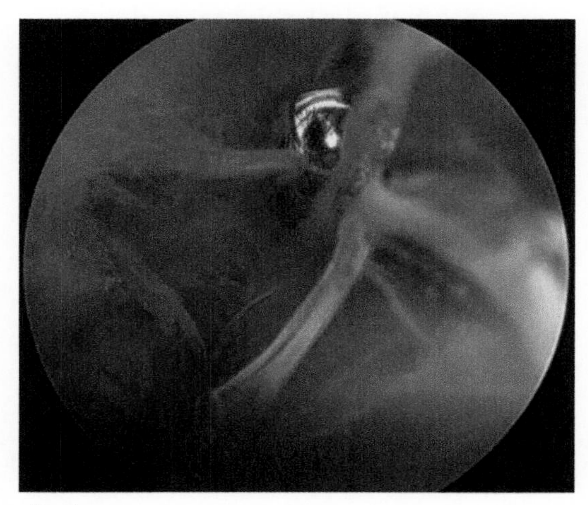

Fig. 2. Paratenon adhesions.

tenotomies using a retrograde knife blade. At a mean follow-up of 16 months, the mean Achilles Tendinopathy Scoring System (ATSS) improved from 39 to 89. However, the patient with a partial tear only improved from 27 to 53. Vega and colleagues[34] retrospectively studied 8 recreational athletes (mean age 43.2 years) who underwent endoscopic paratenon debridement and longitudinal tenotomies. At a mean follow-up of 27 months, all patients were pain free and had excellent Nelen clinical outcome scores. Clinically, the nodular swelling improved in all patients. All patients were able to return to normal daily activities at 3 months and return to sports at 6 months postoperatively. No complications were noted. Thermann and colleagues[35] published a short-term clinical study on endoscopy treatment of recalcitrant midportion Achilles tendinopathy. The authors followed 8 patients (mean age 52 years) who underwent endoscopy paratenon debridement. At 6 months follow-up, the median VAS pain score improved from 40 preoperatively to 97.5 postoperatively. The median VAS global satisfaction at follow-up was 85. There were no postoperative short-term complications noted.

Maquirriain[29] reported on the long-term outcomes of endoscopic treatment of noninsertional Achilles tendinopathy. He evaluated 24 patients (mean age 45.5 years) who underwent 24 unilateral procedures and 3 bilateral. At a mean follow-up of 7.7 years, 85.1% and 14.9% of the cohort reported excellent or good outcomes, respectively. The VISA-A score improved from 37.1 preoperatively to 97.55 postoperatively. The ATSS score improved from 32.7 to 97.3 and the mean postoperative VAS pain score (0–10 scale) was 0.22. Two complications (7.4%) occurred in the cohort, including 1 delayed keloid formation and a fistula formation treated conservatively. Steenstra and van Dijk[30] published their results of 20 patients who underwent endoscopic debridement for noninsertional Achilles tendinopathy. At a mean follow-up of 6 years, their cohort had SF-6 and Foot and Ankle Outcome Scores comparable with normal patients.

PLANTARIS TENDON RELEASE

Plantaris tendon release is other minimally invasive option for Achilles tendinopathy (**Fig. 3**). The plantaris tendon has been described as a potential cause of midportion Achilles tendinopathy. One cadaveric study showed that the plantaris tendon is stiffer

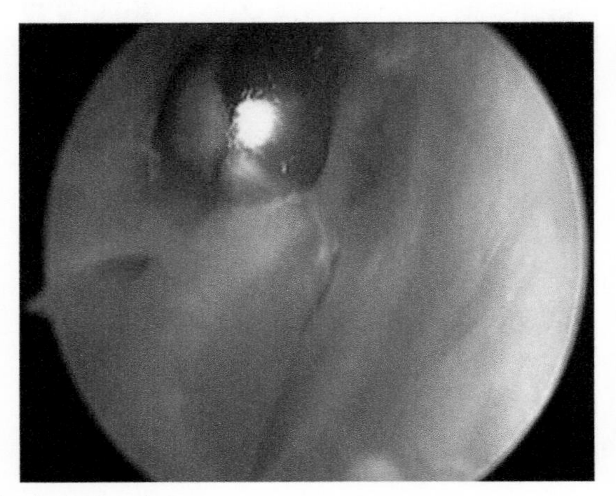

Fig. 3. Endoscopic plantaris release.

than the Achilles tendon, potentially leading to compression of the Achilles tendon and inflammation.[36] Plantaris involvement may explain continued medial-sided symptoms and may lead to continued symptoms if not addressed at the time of percutaneous stripping.[37–39]

Masci and colleagues[40] studied 9 tendons in 8 patients (mean age 39 years) treated with percutaneous stripping and plantaris excision. At 6 months follow-up, there was increased Achilles tissue organization on ultrasonography, and VISA-A scores improved from 56.8 preoperatively to 93.3 postoperatively. van Sterkenburg and colleagues[41] described 3 cases of medial-sided midportion Achilles tendinopathy who underwent a mini-open plantaris release. The authors used a posteromedial incision and released the plantaris distally with a tendon stripper. The authors noted good pain relief and function 6 weeks and 1 year postoperatively. Of note, one of the cases had a larger incision due to significant adhesions, and another case was aborted because of the tightness of the Achilles tendon. Calder and colleagues[42] studied 32 elite athletes (mean age 27.2 years) who underwent combined mini-open longitudinal tendon stripping and plantaris release for noninsertional Achilles tendinopathy. At a mean follow-up of 22.4 months, there was a 91% satisfaction rate with a mean time to return to elite-level sports at 10.3 weeks. The mean VAS pain score improved from 5.8 preoperatively to 0.8 postoperatively. The mean Foot and Ankle Outcome Score improved in all domains, especially for athletes with peritendinitis without intrinsic tendinosis. Complications included 4 athletes with stiffness and 1 with a superficial wound infection.

Bedi and colleagues[43] performed a prospective consecutive study on 15 elite athletes (mean age 32 years) who underwent open ventral paratenon scraping and plantaris release for noninsertional Achilles tendinopathy. Thirteen out of 15 patients returned to full competition at 12 weeks postoperatively. At 6 months, the mean VISA-A scores improved from 51 preoperatively to 95 postoperatively. One patient had a superficial wound infection treated with oral antibiotics. The other patient had a revision paratenon stripping procedure for continued pain. At follow-up of 25 months, there was a 93.3% satisfaction rate.

Pearce and colleagues[44] performed a retrospective study on 11 patients (mean age 36.5 years) who underwent endoscopic paratenon stripping and plantaris division for recalcitrant noninsertional Achilles tendinopathy. At a mean follow-up of 30 months, 8 out of 11 patients (72.7%) were satisfied with their treatment. The mean American Orthopedic Foot and Ankle Society score improved from 68 to 92. The Ankle Osteoarthritis Scale for pain and disability also improved from 28% to 8% and 38% to 10%, respectively. There were no complications and no patient required further surgery.

Overall, combined plantaris release and longitudinal symptoms may improve symptoms for patients with medial-sided Achilles pain with diffuse tendinopathy. However, future randomized control trials are needed to determine whether an isolated plantaris release can improve symptoms.

AUGMENTATION

Tendon transfers are traditionally performed for severe Achilles tendinopathy and allow for additional mechanical support and offloading.[45] Lui[46] published a technique guide on endoscopic flexor hallucis longus (FHL) transfer for noninsertional Achilles tendinopathy.[46] In his technique, Lui arthroscopically releases the FHL just proximal to the knot of Henry and reroutes it proximally through the calcaneal bone tunnel and onto the Achilles tendon. Lui[46] reported on 5 patients (mean age 46 years) who underwent endoscopic FHL transfer for recalcitrant midportion Achilles tendinopathy. At a follow-up of 19.8 months, the mean ATSS improved from 29.4 preoperatively to 89 postoperatively.

SUMMARY

Minimally invasive techniques for noninsertional Achilles tendinopathy can be used for recalcitrant cases. Sclerotherapy and prolotherapy have shown to be effective, but some authors have questioned the generalizability of these results. Percutaneous longitudinal tenotomies have been reported to have good outcomes for focal disease but may not improve results when compared with eccentric Achilles training. Percutaneous stripping and endoscopic debridement are better options for diffuse lesions with associated peritendinitis. Plantaris releases can be performed via mini-open or endoscopic approaches and can be useful in diffuse disease in patients with primarily medial-sided Achilles pain. Overall, minimally invasive surgery provides similar benefits as open procedures with reduced complications and morbidity.

REFERENCES

1. Clanton TO, Waldrop NE. Athletic injuries of the soft tissues of the foot and ankle. In: Coughlin MJ, Saltzman CL, Anderson RB, editors. Mann's surgery of the foot and ankle. Philadelphia: Elsevier Inc.; 2014. p. 1531–687.
2. Johnston E, Scranton P Jr, Pfeffer GB. Chronic disorders of the Achilles tendon: results of conservative and surgical treatments. Foot Ankle Int 1997;18(9):570–4.
3. Paavola M, Kannus P, Paakkala T, et al. Long-term prognosis of patients with Achilles tendinopathy. An observational 8-year follow-up study. Am J Sports Med 2000;28(5):634–42.
4. Kvist M. Achilles tendon injuries in athletes. Sports Med 1994;18(3):173–201.
5. Singh A, Calafi A, Diefenbach C, et al. Noninsertional tendinopathy of the Achilles. Foot Ankle Clin 2017;22(4):745–60.
6. Paavola M, Orava S, Leppilahti J, et al. Chronic Achilles tendon overuse injury: complications after surgical treatment. An analysis of 432 consecutive patients. Am J Sports Med 2000;28(1):77–82.
7. Lohrer H, David S, Nauck T. Surgical treatment for Achilles tendinopathy - a systematic review. BMC Musculoskelet Disord 2016;17:207.
8. Scott AT, Le IL, Easley ME. Surgical strategies: noninsertional Achilles tendinopathy. Foot Ankle Int 2008;29(7):759–71.
9. Alfredson H, Ohberg L. Sclerosing injections to areas of neo-vascularisation reduce pain in chronic Achilles tendinopathy: a double-blind randomised controlled trial. Knee Surg Sports Traumatol Arthrosc 2005;13(4):338–44.
10. Lind B, Ohberg L, Alfredson H. Sclerosing polidocanol injections in mid-portion Achilles tendinosis: remaining good clinical results and decreased tendon thickness at 2-year follow-up. Knee Surg Sports Traumatol Arthrosc 2006;14(12):1327–32.
11. Willberg L, Sunding K, Ohberg L, et al. Sclerosing injections to treat midportion Achilles tendinosis: a randomised controlled study evaluating two different concentrations of Polidocanol. Knee Surg Sports Traumatol Arthrosc 2008;16(9):859–64.
12. Clementson M, Lorén I, Dahlberg L, et al. Sclerosing injections in midportion Achilles tendinopathy: a retrospective study of 25 patients. Knee Surg Sports Traumatol Arthrosc 2008;16(9):887–90.

13. Reeves K. Prolotherapy: basic science, clinical studies, and technique. In: TA L, editor. Pain procedures in clinical practice. Philadelphia: Hanley and Belfus; 2000. p. 172–90.
14. Morath O, Kubosch EJ, Taeymans J, et al. The effect of sclerotherapy and prolotherapy on chronic painful Achilles tendinopathy - a systematic review including meta-analysis. Scand J Med Sci Sports 2018;28(1):4–15.
15. Maxwell NJ, Ryan MB, Taunton JE, et al. Sonographically guided intratendinous injection of hyperosmolar dextrose to treat chronic tendinosis of the Achilles tendon: a pilot study. AJR Am J Roentgenol 2007;189(4):W215–20.
16. Yelland MJ, Sweeting KR, Lyftogt JA, et al. Prolotherapy injections and eccentric loading exercises for painful Achilles tendinosis: a randomised trial. Br J Sports Med 2011;45(5):421–8.
17. van Sterkenburg MN, de Jonge MC, Sierevelt IN, et al. Less promising results with sclerosing ethoxysclerol injections for midportion achilles tendinopathy: a retrospective study. Am J Sports Med 2010;38(11):2226–32.
18. Kearney RS, Parsons N, Metcalfe D, et al. Injection therapies for Achilles tendinopathy. Cochrane Database Syst Rev 2015;(5):CD010960.
19. Coombes BK, Bisset L, Vicenzino B. Efficacy and safety of corticosteroid injections and other injections for management of tendinopathy: a systematic review of randomised controlled trials. Lancet 2010;376(9754):1751–67.
20. Geukens J, Rabe E, Bieber T. Embolia cutis medicamentosa of the foot after sclerotherapy. Eur J Dermatol 1999;9(2):132–3.
21. Natali J. Lesion of the triceps surae after sclerosing injection in the territory of the external saphenous vein. Phlebologie 1987;40(2):315–24 [in French].
22. Testa V, Capasso G, Benazzo F, et al. Management of Achilles tendinopathy by ultrasound-guided percutaneous tenotomy. Med Sci Sports Exerc 2002;34(4):573–80.
23. Maffulli N, Oliva F, Testa V, et al. Multiple percutaneous longitudinal tenotomies for chronic Achilles tendinopathy in runners: a long-term study. Am J Sports Med 2013;41(9):2151–7.
24. Sanchez PJ, Grady JF, Saxena A. Percutaneous ultrasonic tenotomy for Achilles tendinopathy is a surgical procedure with similar complications. J Foot Ankle Surg 2017;56(5):982–4.
25. Kamineni S, Butterfield T, Sinai A. Percutaneous ultrasonic debridement of tendinopathy - a pilot Achilles rabbit model. J Orthop Surg Res 2015;10:70.
26. Alfredson H. Ultrasound and Doppler-guided mini-surgery to treat midportion Achilles tendinosis: results of a large material and a randomised study comparing two scraping techniques. Br J Sports Med 2011;45(5):407–10.
27. Longo UG, Ramamurthy C, Denaro V, et al. Minimally invasive stripping for chronic Achilles tendinopathy. Disabil Rehabil 2008;30(20–22):1709–13.
28. Naidu V, Abbassian A, Nielsen D, et al. Minimally invasive paratenon release for non-insertional Achilles tendinopathy. Foot Ankle Int 2009;30(7):680–5.
29. Maquirriain J. Surgical treatment of chronic Achilles tendinopathy: long-term results of the endoscopic technique. J Foot Ankle Surg 2013;52(4):451–5.
30. Steenstra F, van Dijk CN. Achilles tendoscopy. Foot Ankle Clin 2006;11(2):429–38, viii.
31. Phisitkul P. Endoscopic surgery of the Achilles tendon. Curr Rev Musculoskelet Med 2012;5(2):156–63.
32. Maquirriain J. Endoscopic release of Achilles peritenon. Arthroscopy 1998;14(2):182–5.

33. Maquirriain J, Ayerza M, Costa-Paz M, et al. Endoscopic surgery in chronic Achilles tendinopathies: a preliminary report. Arthroscopy 2002;18(3):298–303.
34. Vega J, Cabestany JM, Golanó P, et al. Endoscopic treatment for chronic Achilles tendinopathy. Foot Ankle Surg 2008;14(4):204–10.
35. Thermann H, Benetos IS, Panelli C, et al. Endoscopic treatment of chronic midportion Achilles tendinopathy: novel technique with short-term results. Knee Surg Sports Traumatol Arthrosc 2009;17(10):1264–9.
36. Lintz F, Higgs A, Millett M, et al. The role of Plantaris Longus in Achilles tendinopathy: a biomechanical study. Foot Ankle Surg 2011;17(4):252–5.
37. Spang C, Alfredson H, Docking SI, et al. The plantaris tendon: a narrative review focusing on anatomical features and clinical importance. Bone Joint J 2016; 98-b(10):1312–9.
38. Masci L, Spang C, van Schie HT, et al. How to diagnose plantaris tendon involvement in midportion Achilles tendinopathy - clinical and imaging findings. BMC Musculoskelet Disord 2016;17:97.
39. Alfredson H. Midportion Achilles tendinosis and the plantaris tendon. Br J Sports Med 2011;45(13):1023–5.
40. Masci L, Spang C, van Schie HT, et al. Achilles tendinopathy - do plantaris tendon removal and Achilles tendon scraping improve tendon structure? A prospective study using ultrasound tissue characterisation. BMJ Open Sport Exerc Med 2015;1(1):e000005.
41. van Sterkenburg MN, Kerkhoffs GM, van Dijk CN. Good outcome after stripping the plantaris tendon in patients with chronic mid-portion Achilles tendinopathy. Knee Surg Sports Traumatol Arthrosc 2011;19(8):1362–6.
42. Calder JD, Freeman R, Pollock N. Plantaris excision in the treatment of non-insertional Achilles tendinopathy in elite athletes. Br J Sports Med 2015;49(23): 1532–4.
43. Bedi HS, Jowett C, Ristanis S, et al. Plantaris excision and ventral paratendinous scraping for Achilles tendinopathy in an athletic population. Foot Ankle Int 2016; 37(4):386–93.
44. Pearce CJ, Carmichael J, Calder JD. Achilles tendinoscopy and plantaris tendon release and division in the treatment of non-insertional Achilles tendinopathy. Foot Ankle Surg 2012;18(2):124–7.
45. Martin RL, Manning CM, Carcia CR, et al. An outcome study of chronic Achilles tendinosis after excision of the Achilles tendon and flexor hallucis longus tendon transfer. Foot Ankle Int 2005;26(9):691–7.
46. Lui TH. Treatment of chronic noninsertional Achilles tendinopathy with endoscopic Achilles tendon debridement and flexor hallucis longus transfer. Foot Ankle Spec 2012;5(3):195–200.

Nonsurgical Treatment Options for Insertional Achilles Tendinopathy

Connor P. Dilger, BS, Ruth L. Chimenti, DPT, PhD*

KEYWORDS

- Eccentric exercise • Rehabilitation • Physical therapy
- Extracorporeal shock wave therapy • Achilles tendonitis • Pain

KEY POINTS

- Exercise is a first-line treatment strategy for all patients with insertional Achilles tendinopathy (IAT) (grade A recommendation).
- When exercise is unsuccessful, extracorporeal shock wave therapy (ESWT) is the next best nonoperative treatment option to reduce IAT pain (grade B recommendation).
- There are a variety of other nonoperative treatment options that can be used either to enhance the effects of exercise and ESWT or to try before surgical intervention, but there is currently little evidence to support their efficacy.

INTRODUCTION

Nonoperative care is a first-line approach for treating insertional Achilles tendinopathy (IAT). Although surgical procedures for IAT have long differed from those done for midportion Achilles tendinopathy (AT), this disease-specific approach is fairly new in rehabilitation. For example, the eccentric exercise protocol published by Alfredson and colleagues[1] in 1998 was long considered the gold standard nonoperative treatment of AT. It was not until 2008 that a version of this exercise protocol was published with a modification to better target care for patients with IAT.[2] In the last decade there has been a greater emphasis on understanding the pain mechanisms and response to treatment in people with IAT rather than considering the midportion and insertional AT diagnoses as a single patient population. Although patients with chronic IAT have traditionally not done as well with nonoperative treatment compared with patients with midportion AT, there is the potential for this patient population to have better outcomes with nonoperative care now that disease-specific treatments are being designed and tested.

Department of Physical Therapy and Rehabilitation Science, University of Iowa, 500 Newton Road, 1-252 Medical Education Building, Iowa City, IA 52242, USA
* Corresponding author.
E-mail address: ruth-chimenti@uiowa.edu

Foot Ankle Clin N Am 24 (2019) 505–513
https://doi.org/10.1016/j.fcl.2019.04.004
foot.theclinics.com
1083-7515/19/

This article provides grades of recommendation for nonoperative treatments of IAT as well as estimates of the treatment effect size on IAT pain. Although other symptoms associated with IAT (eg, stiffness) and level of disability (eg, limitations in walking distance) are valuable in understanding the effect of an intervention on an individual, this article focuses on pain because it was assessed in nearly all of the reviewed studies and facilitated comparisons between treatments. The levels of evidence and grades of recommendation are consistent with standards set by other reviews on the treatment of AT (**Box 1**, **Table 1**).[3–5] The PEDro scores from the Physiotherapy Evidence Database were used when available to define a high-quality randomized controlled trial (RCT) (score $\geq$ 6 out of 10) when available.

Exercise: Grade A Treatment Recommendation

Exercise is the primary treatment strategy for all patients with IAT, but the ideal parameters (type, dose, combination with additional treatments) of exercise are still unknown. In this article the evidence for eccentric exercise has been grouped by 1 parameter related to the range of motion through which the exercise is performed, including (1) to end-range ankle dorsiflexion, and (2) with reduced range of ankle dorsiflexion. In addition to eccentric exercise, physical therapists also use heavy slow-resistance training and isometric exercise, which have been shown to provide pain relief for other types of tendinopathy.[6,7] Eccentric exercise has long been considered the gold standard for exercise interventions for tendinopathy, and testing of these other types of exercise has not yet been translated to the IAT population.

Eccentric, Full Range of Ankle Dorsiflexion

The standard eccentric exercise protocol using full range of ankle dorsiflexion motion does have some therapeutic benefit, with an average decrease of 1.8 to 2.8 in pain ratings on an 11-point scale at 3-month to 4-month follow-up (level I, II, and III evidence).[8–10] However, after completing this type of exercise program, on average pain persisted at a rating of 2 to 5.[8–10] Moreover, there is a high rate of nonresponse to eccentric exercise with end-range dorsiflexion with 70% of participants reporting poor results (level IV evidence).[11]

Box 1
Levels of evidence and grades of recommendation

Levels of evidence (given to individual studies)
- Level I: high-quality randomized controlled trial (RCT) or systematic review
- Level II: prospective comparative study, lesser-quality RCT, or systematic review
- Level III: retrospective or case-control study
- Level IV: case series or case study
- Level V: expert opinion

Grades of recommendation (given to treatment options)
- Grade A: treatment option is supported by strong evidence (consistent with a preponderance of level I and/or II studies)
- Grade B: treatment option is supported by moderate evidence (consistent with a single level I study or a preponderance of level II studies)
- Grade C: treatment option is supported by weak evidence (single level II study, or a preponderance of level III and IV studies)
- Grade I: insufficient evidence exists to make a treatment recommendation

Table 1
Summary of grades of recommendation for treatment options

Nonoperative	
Exercise	Grade A
Extracorporeal shock wave therapy	Grade B
Soft tissue treatment	Grade I
Nutritional supplement	Grade I
Iontophoresis	Grade I
Education	Grade I
Stretching	Grade I
Heel lifts	Grade I
Injections	Grade I

Eccentric, Reduced Range of Motion

Eccentric exercise can be modified for patients with IAT by reducing the range of motion during the exercise. By reducing the amount of ankle dorsiflexion, this modification reduces the amount of compression on the soft tissues at the tendon insertion[12] and, based on clinical experience, also reduces the level of pain reported during the exercise. With a modified eccentric exercise protocol, pain has been shown to decrease from 5.4 at baseline to 3.0 at 3 months and 1.0 by 1 year (level II evidence, n = 16).[13] Similarly, a case series of patients with IAT reported a high rate of patient satisfaction, with 67% able to resume their preinjury levels of activity.[2] In summary, all studies show a decrease in pain with eccentric exercise, but this effect may be greatest when the exercise is modified for the IAT population.

Extracorporeal Shock Wave Therapy: Grade B Treatment Recommendation

Extracorporeal shock wave therapy (ESWT) is commonly used after patients have not responded well to other nonoperative treatments, such as eccentric exercise or injections.[9,14–17] Use of ESWT is an emerging research with 4 level IV studies published since 2016 supporting the use of this treatment of IAT.[14–17] However, some studies exclude patients with enthesophytes or Haglund deformity, and so these positive findings may not be generalizable to all patients with IAT.[9,16]

Among nonresponders to other nonoperative treatments, including exercise, an RCT by Rompe and colleagues[9] found that ESWT was more effective at reducing pain than a full-range eccentric exercise program (eccentric group, 6.8–5.0; ESWT, 7.0–3.0; level I evidence). Even though the ESWT group had a 2-point greater decrease in pain compared with the eccentric exercise group, at 4 months the ESWT group still reported a load-induced pain level of 3.0.[9] Several other clinical trials (levels II and III) have shown similar results with greater than or equal to 2-point decrease in pain with ESWT but maintain a final pain level of 3 to 5 at short-term and long-term follow-up.[18–20]

Supplemental Nonoperative Treatments: Grade I Treatment Recommendation

There are a variety of other nonoperative treatment options that are used in combination with other treatments, and it is therefore difficult to assess their effectiveness individually. The addition of soft tissue treatment with Astym to an eccentric exercise program resulted in reduced pain at 3-month and 1-year follow-up, but the soft tissue treatment did not provide significantly more pain relief (**Table 2**).[13] Similarly, the

Table 2
Levels of evidence supporting grade A treatment recommendation of exercise for insertional Achilles tendinopathy

LoE, Study Design	IAT Sample	Intervention	Findings	Effect on Pain		Author, Year
Eccentric Exercise, End-range Dorsiflexion						
Level I, RCT PEDro = 8/10	N = 50	Eccentric exercise, end-range dorsiflexion (n = 25) vs ESWT (n = 25, also in **Table 3**)	• Both groups had decreased pain relative to baseline • ESWT had greater decrease in pain than eccentric exercise	Eccentric exercise	Baseline: 6.8 ± 1.0 4 mo: 5.0 ± 2.3	Rompe et al,[9] 2008
				ESWT	Baseline: 7.0 ± 0.8 4 mo: 3.0 ± 2.3	
Level I, RCT PEDro = 7/10	N = 36	Eccentric, end-range dorsiflexion, plus standard care (n = 16) vs standard care (stretching, ice, heel lifts, night splint) (n = 20)	• Both groups had decreased pain relative to baseline • No differences in pain between groups	Eccentric exercise	Baseline: 4.6 ± NR 3 mo: 2.4 ± 2.0	Kedia et al,[8] 2014
				Standard care	Baseline: 3.6 ± NR 3 mo: 1.5 ± 2.2	
Level IV, case series	N = 30	Eccentric exercise, end-range dorsiflexion	• One-third of participants (n = 10) had decrease in pain relative to baseline • Pain on 0–100 scale	Responders	Baseline: 68.3 ± 7.0 3 mo: 13.3 ± 13.2	Fahlstrom et al,[11] 2003
				Nonresponders	Baseline: 79.5 ± 11.2 3 mo: 75.4 ± 11.2	
Level IV, case series	N = 10	Eccentric exercise, end-range dorsiflexion	• Pain decreased relative to baseline	—	Baseline: 6 ± 2.5 3 mo: 3.2 ± 2.7	Knobloch,[10] 2007
Eccentric Exercise, Reduced-range Dorsiflexion						
Level I, RCT PEDro = 7/10	N = 16	Eccentric exercise, reduced-range dorsiflexion (n = 9) vs eccentric exercise plus Astym soft tissue treatment (n = 7)	• Both groups had decreased pain relative to baseline • No differences in pain between groups	Exercise	Baseline: 5.4 (3.6–7.2) 3 mo: 3.0 (1.5–4.4) 1 y: 1.0 (0.0–2.6)	McCormack et al,[13] 2016
				Astym + exercise	Baseline: 4.6 (2.8–6.4) 3 mo: 1.7 (0.8–2.8) 1 y: 0.7 (0.0–1.9)	
Level IV, case series	N = 27	Eccentric exercise, reduced range of ankle dorsiflexion	• Two-thirds of participants (n = 18) had decrease in pain relative to baseline • Pain on 0–100 scale	Responders	Baseline: 69.9 ± 18.9 3 mo: 21.0 ± 20.6	Jonsson et al,[2] 2008
				Nonresponders	Baseline: 77.5 ± 8.6 3 mo: 58.1 ± 14.8	

The effect on pain is reported on a 0 to 10 scale, unless otherwise noted, as mean ± standard deviation (SD) or mean (95% confidence interval [CI]).

Abbreviations: LoE, level of evidence; NR, not reported.

Table 3
Levels of evidence supporting grade B treatment recommendation of extracorporeal shock wave therapy for insertional Achilles tendinopathy

LoE, Study Design	IAT Sample	Intervention	Findings	Effect on Pain		Author, Year
Level I, RCT PEDro = 8/10	N = 50	ESWT (n = 25) vs eccentric exercise, full range of ankle dorsiflexion (n = 25, also in **Table 2**)	• Both groups had decreased pain relative to baseline • ESWT had greater decrease in pain than eccentric exercise	ESWT Eccentric	Baseline: 7.0 ± 0.8 4 mo: 3.0 ± 2.3 Baseline: 6.8 ± 1.0 4 mo: 5.0 ± 2.3	Rompe et al,[9] 2008
Level II, RCT PEDro = 5/10	N = 64	ESWT (n = 32) vs ESWT with nutraceuticals (n = 32, also see Table 5)	• Both groups had decreased pain relative to baseline • ESWT with nutraceuticals had greater decrease in pain than ESWT alone	ESWT ESWT + nutraceuticals	Baseline: 7.0 ± 1.3 2m: 4.5 ± 3.0 6m: 2.9 ± 2.3 Baseline: 7.1 ± 1.7 2 mo: 4.5 ± 3.0 6 mo: 2.0 ± 1.8	Notarnicola et al,[18] 2012
Level II, RCT PEDro = 4/10	N = 60	ESWT (n = 30) vs CHELT (n = 30)	• Both groups had decreased pain relative to baseline • CHELT had greater decrease in pain than ESWT	ESWT CHELT	Baseline: 7.0 ± 1.2 6 mo: 3.3 ± 1.0 Baseline: 7.0 ± 1.0 6 mo: 1.7 ± 1.0	Notarnicola et al[20], 2014
Level III, case-control study	N = 68	ESWT (n = 35) vs control: nonoperative management (n = 33)	• ESWT group had decrease in pain relative to baseline • Control group did not have decrease in pain relative to baseline	ESWT Control	Baseline: 7.9 ± 2.0 3 mo: 2.9 ± 2.1 12 mo: 2.8 ± 2.0 Baseline: 8.6 ± 1.1 3 mo: 7.2 ± 1.3 12 mo: 7.0 ± 1.4	Furia,[19] 2006

(*continued on next page*)

Table 3
(continued)

LoE, Study Design	IAT Sample	Intervention	Findings	Effect on Pain		Author, Year
Level IV, case series	N = 67	ESWT	• Decrease in pain relative to baseline	Baseline: 3.9/6 ± 0.8 15 mo (±7 mo): 2.1/6 ± 0.8		Wu,[17] 2016
Level IV, case series	N = 45	ESWT (n = 24) and PRP (n = 21, see Table 5)	• Decrease in pain relative to baseline	ESWT	Baseline: 6.4 ± 1.3 4 mo: 2.5 ± 2.3 6 mo: 1.5 ± 2.1	Erroi et al,[15] 2017
				PRP	Baseline: 5.9 ± 1.0 4 mo: 3.0 ± 1.9 6 mo: 2.6 ± 1.9	
Level IV, case series	N = 40	ESWT and eccentric exercise	• Decrease in pain relative to baseline	Baseline: 7.6 ± 0.6 6 mo: 2.8 ± 0.7 12 mo: 1.9 ± 1.2		Pavone et al,[14] 2016
Level IV, Case series	N = 12	ESWT	• Decrease in pain relative to baseline	Baseline: 6.7 (0–10) 4 mo: 4.4 (1–8) 2 y: 2.8 (0–10)		Taylor et al,[16] 2016

The effect on pain is reported on a 0 to 10 scale, unless otherwise noted, as mean ± SD or mean (95% CI).
Abbreviations: CHELT, cold air and high energy laser therapy; PRP, platelet-rich plasma.

addition of arginine supplementation with other nutraceuticals to ESWT made no difference to 2-month outcomes but did produce a slightly greater decrease in pain at 6-month follow-up (**Table 3**).[18] Particularly for patients with concomitant retrocalcaneal bursitis or paratendinitis, other common adjuncts to therapy include nonsteroidal antiinflammatory medications, iontophoresis,[21] and ice. Education on how to modify activities to increase activity level while minimizing aggravation of IAT symptoms may be beneficial.[22]

Weighing the need for stretching versus the need for heel lifts ultimately depends on the needs and preferences of the patient. On the one hand there is some biomechanical evidence to suggest that activities that require greater ankle dorsiflexion increase both tendon elongation (tensile strain) and compression (compressive strain) at the tendon insertion.[12,23] Therefore clinicians often recommend use of a heel lift, particularly during higher-level activities. Exercise treatments that require end-range dorsiflexion aggravate IAT symptoms for many patients and contribute to the lower rates of 30% to 50% patient satisfaction with, respectively, eccentric exercise into end-range dorsiflexion or use of stretching alone (level IV evidence).[11,24] In contrast, particularly for patients with limited ankle dorsiflexion, stretching may be a beneficial part of the intervention. Weight-bearing stretches and night splints have been used in combination with other treatments as standard of care and have resulted in decreased pain at long-term follow-up (see **Table 2**).[8]

Injections: Grade I Treatment Recommendation

There are a variety of injections offered for IAT, but none have sufficient levels of evidence to support a treatment recommendation. There is a consensus to avoid corticosteroid injections for treatment of tendinopathy because of concern about contributing to further tendon degeneration and potential tear.[25] However, particularly for patients with IAT who have concomitant retrocalcaneal bursitis, the use of a corticosteroid injection may be considered as a supplement to care for those who are initially nonresponders to an exercise intervention (level IV evidence).[26] Another option for patients who have failed other nonoperative treatment options is sclerosing therapy with polidocanol to target neovascularization (level IV evidence).[27] In addition platelet-rich plasma injections have been shown to reduce pain in some patients with chronic IAT following extensive use of other nonoperative treatments (level IV evidence).[15,28]

SUMMARY

Most nonoperative treatments for IAT have insufficient evidence to support treatment recommendations, with exercise and ESWT as notable exceptions (see **Table 1**). Exercise has the highest level of evidence supporting the ability of this treatment option to reduce IAT pain (grade A recommendation). The effects of exercise may be enhanced by the use of a wide variety of other treatments, including soft tissue treatment, nutritional supplements, iontophoresis, education, stretching, and heel lifts (grade I recommendation). When exercise is unsuccessful, ESWT seems to be the next best nonoperative treatment option to reduce IAT pain (grade B recommendation). After other nonoperative treatment options have been exhausted, injections may be considered, particularly as a means to facilitate participation in an exercise program (grade I recommendation).

The limitations of this review article are linked to limitations in reported outcome measures. This article focuses on pain, because it is often the primary outcome measure of research studies. However, certain treatments may be more effective for other symptoms, such as stiffness, or disability, which this article dos not capture. Also, the summary of results assumes that all studies had participants rate activity-related or load-related pain at the Achilles tendon insertion, but this was often not specified in research articles. In addition to intensity, the context (eg, during activity vs at rest), location, and duration are all components of the sensory-discriminative aspect of pain and are each needed to interpret the clinical significance of a change in pain. In addition, this article only provides a grade of recommendation for 2 nonoperative treatments; more research is needed to provide evidence-based recommendations for IAT.

ACKNOWLEDGMENT

This publication was supported by the National Institute of Arthritis and Musculoskeletal and Skin Diseases (NIAMS) of the National Institutes of Health under award number K99AR071517.

REFERENCES

1. Alfredson H, Pietila T, Jonsson P, et al. Heavy-load eccentric calf muscle training for the treatment of chronic Achilles tendinosis. Am J Sports Med 1998;26(3):360–6.
2. Jonsson P, Alfredson H, Sunding K, et al. New regimen for eccentric calf-muscle training in patients with chronic insertional Achilles tendinopathy: results of a pilot study. Br J Sports Med 2008;42(9):746–9.
3. Irwin TA. Current concepts review: insertional Achilles tendinopathy. Foot Ankle Int 2010;31(10):933–9.
4. Chimenti RL, Cychosz CC, Hall MM, et al. Current concepts review update: insertional Achilles tendinopathy. Foot Ankle Int 2017;38(10):1160–9.
5. Martin RL, Chimenti R, Cuddeford T, et al. Achilles pain, stiffness, and muscle power deficits: midportion Achilles tendinopathy revision 2018. J Orthop Sports Phys Ther 2018;48(5):A1–38.
6. Beyer R, Kongsgaard M, Hougs Kjaer B, et al. Heavy slow resistance versus eccentric training as treatment for Achilles tendinopathy: a randomized controlled trial. Am J Sports Med 2015;43(7):1704–11.
7. Rio E, Kidgell D, Purdam C, et al. Isometric exercise induces analgesia and reduces inhibition in patellar tendinopathy. Br J Sports Med 2015;49(19):1277–83.
8. Kedia M, Williams M, Jain L, et al. The effects of conventional physical therapy and eccentric strengthening for insertional Achilles tendinopathy. Int J Sports Phys Ther 2014;9(4):488–97.
9. Rompe JD, Furia J, Maffulli N. Eccentric loading compared with shock wave treatment for chronic insertional Achilles tendinopathy. A randomized, controlled trial. J Bone Joint Surg Am 2008;90(1):52–61.
10. Knobloch K. Eccentric training in Achilles tendinopathy: is it harmful to tendon microcirculation? Br J Sports Med 2007;41(6):e2 [discussion: e2].
11. Fahlstrom M, Jonsson P, Lorentzon R, et al. Chronic Achilles tendon pain treated with eccentric calf-muscle training. Knee Surg Sports Traumatol Arthrosc 2003;11(5):327–33.
12. Chimenti RL, Flemister AS, Ketz J, et al. Ultrasound strain mapping of Achilles tendon compressive strain patterns during dorsiflexion. J Biomech 2016;49(1):39–44.
13. McCormack JR, Underwood FB, Slaven EJ, et al. Eccentric exercise versus eccentric exercise and soft tissue treatment (Astym) in the management of

insertional Achilles tendinopathy: a randomized controlled trial. Sports Health 2016;8(3):230–7.
14. Pavone V, Cannavo L, Di Stefano A, et al. Low-energy extracorporeal shock-wave therapy in the treatment of chronic insertional Achilles tendinopathy: a case series. Biomed Res Int 2016;2016:7123769.
15. Erroi D, Sigona M, Suarez T, et al. Conservative treatment for Insertional Achilles Tendinopathy: platelet-rich plasma and focused shock waves. A retrospective study. Muscles Ligaments Tendons J 2017;7(1):98–106.
16. Taylor J, Dunkerley S, Silver D, et al. Extracorporeal shockwave therapy (ESWT) for refractory Achilles tendinopathy: a prospective audit with 2-year follow up. Foot (Edinb) 2016;26:23–9.
17. Wu Z, Yao W, Chen S, et al. Outcome of extracorporeal shock wave therapy for insertional Achilles tendinopathy with and without Haglund's deformity. Biomed Res Int 2016;2016:6315846.
18. Notarnicola A, Pesce V, Vicenti G, et al. SWAAT study: extracorporeal shock wave therapy and arginine supplementation and other nutraceuticals for insertional Achilles tendinopathy. Adv Ther 2012;29(9):799–814.
19. Furia JP. High-energy extracorporeal shock wave therapy as a treatment for insertional Achilles tendinopathy. Am J Sports Med 2006;34(5):733–40.
20. Notarnicola A, Maccagnano G, Tafuri S, et al. CHELT therapy in the treatment of chronic insertional Achilles tendinopathy. Lasers Med Sci 2014;29(3):1217–25.
21. Kilfoil RL Jr, Shtofmakher G, Taylor G, et al. Acetic acid iontophoresis for the treatment of insertional Achilles tendonitis. BMJ Case Rep 2014;2014 [pii: bcr2014206232].
22. Sartorio F, Zanetta A, Ferriero G, et al. The EdUReP approach plus manual therapy for the management of insertional Achilles tendinopathy. J Sports Med Phys Fitness 2018;58(5):664–8.
23. Chimenti RL, Bucklin M, Kelly M, et al. Insertional Achilles tendinopathy associated with altered transverse compressive and axial tensile strain during ankle dorsiflexion. J Orthop Res 2016;35(4):910–5.
24. Verrall G, Schofield S, Brustad T. Chronic Achilles tendinopathy treated with eccentric stretching program. Foot Ankle Int 2011;32(9):843–9.
25. Coombes BK, Bisset L, Vicenzino B. Efficacy and safety of corticosteroid injections and other injections for management of tendinopathy: a systematic review of randomised controlled trials. Lancet 2010;376(9754):1751–67.
26. Wetke E, Johannsen F, Langberg H. Achilles tendinopathy: a prospective study on the effect of active rehabilitation and steroid injections in a clinical setting. Scand J Med Sci Sports 2015;25(4):e392–9.
27. Ohberg L, Alfredson H. Sclerosing therapy in chronic Achilles tendon insertional pain-results of a pilot study. Knee Surg Sports Traumatol Arthrosc 2003;11(5):339–43.
28. Monto RR. Platelet rich plasma treatment for chronic Achilles tendinosis. Foot Ankle Int 2012;33(5):379–85.

Minimally Invasive and Endoscopic Treatment of Haglund Syndrome

Tun Hing Lui, MBBS (HK), FRCS (Edin), FHKAM, FHKCOS*,
Cho Yau Lo, MBChB (CUHK), FRCSEd, FHKAM, FHKCOS,
Yuk Chuen Siu, MBChB (CUHK), FRCSEd, FHKAM, FHKCOS

KEYWORDS

• Haglund syndrome • Minimally invasive • Tendoscopy • Endoscopy • Osteotomy
• Achilles tendon

KEY POINTS

- Haglund syndrome is a triad of posterosuperior calcaneal prominence (Haglund deformity), retrocalcaneal bursitis, and insertional Achilles tendinopathy.
- Insertional Achilles tendinopathy associated with Haglund syndrome is due to bony impingement and chemical attrition.
- The sources of pain in Haglund syndrome include the posterior calcaneal wall cartilage, retrocalcaneal and subcutaneous adventitial bursa, and the Achilles tendon.
- Most of the surgical treatment options for Haglund syndrome can be performed endoscopically or under minimally invasive approaches.

INTRODUCTION

Haglund syndrome is a triad of posterosuperior calcaneal prominence (Haglund deformity), retrocalcaneal bursitis, and insertional Achilles tendinopathy and presents with posterior heel pain at retrocalcaneal region and sometimes Achilles insertional pain.[1–3] It usually affects middle-aged people, women more than men, and it is often bilateral and presents with posterior heel pain, swelling, redness, and poststatic dyskinesia. Differential diagnoses include traumatic causes such as stress fracture of calcaneus or malunion of tongue-type calcaneal fracture,[4] infective causes such as tuberculosis of calcaneus,[5] neoplastic causes such as osteochondroma of calcaneum,[6] and inflammatory causes such as seronegative spondyloarthropathies.

There is no conflict of interest in preparation of this article.
No figure was borrowed from another source.
Department of Orthopaedics and Traumatology, North District Hospital, 9 Po Kin Road, Sheung Shui, NT, Hong Kong SAR 999077, China
* Corresponding author.
E-mail address: luithderek@yahoo.co.uk

Foot Ankle Clin N Am 24 (2019) 515–531
https://doi.org/10.1016/j.fcl.2019.04.006
foot.theclinics.com

It is general belief that Haglund deformity frequently associates with insertional Achilles tendinopathy[7–9] although recent studies[10–13] challenged this association. There is a 25% frequency of Haglund syndrome within the insertional Achilles tendinopathy population, but the insertional Achilles tendinopathy is more often found in the Haglund syndrome population.[14,15] The tendinopathy is caused by chemical attrition and bony mechanical abrasion. It is postulated that the anterior Achilles insertion rubs against the bony prominence, particularly when associated with a tight or contracted gastroc-soleus-Achilles myotendinous complex, resulting in local damage to the tendon and even intratendinous longitudinal tears.[13,16,17] In patients with cavovarus foot, the hindfoot varus can also cause the calcaneus to impinge against the Achilles tendon. An anatomic and radiological study confirmed the existence of communications between the retrocalcaneal bursa and the Achilles tendon, especially in the anteroinferior portion of the tendon.[18] This can serve as a route for chemical attrition of the tendon by the inflamed retrocalcaneal bursa. These explain why insertional Achilles tendinopathy associated with Haglund syndrome tends to involve the anterior part of the tendon, although the posterior fibers of the tendon have the highest strain on biomechanical testing.[17] Actually, "attritional Achilles tendinopathy" and "Achilles impingement tendinopathy" are better terms for the "insertional Achilles tendinopathy" associated with Haglund syndrome.[12,19] It results from frictional wear of the posterosuperior calcaneal eminence and is associated with marrow edema at the superior lateral calcaneal eminence rather than the Achilles tendon insertion.[19] Haglund deformity defined radiologically by the parallel pitch lines and the Fowler angle are found to have low predictive value for Haglund syndrome with a high false-negative rate.[12,14,20,21] The impinging osseous prominence shown in radiograph may not be as big as expected, partly because of the presence of the cartilaginous cap.[12,22] These radiological measurements could not be used as predictors for the preoperative symptoms or the postoperative outcome.[14,23,24]

In contrast to the common description of Haglund deformity as lateral prominence of the calcaneal tuberosity, impingement tendinopathy is the least common laterally and most common centrally.[12] Localization of a bone deformity and tendinopathy in the same sagittal section of an MRI scan can assist with the diagnosis in equivocal cases.[12] Impingement tendinopathy has a high association with distal insertional changes at the bony attachment (59.3%).[12] It is not known whether these insertional changes precede impingement tendinopathy. This could occur if insertional changes extend proximally, causing a thickening of the tendon, with secondary impingement and mechanical abrasion. In contrast, the impingement tendinopathy could occur first and extend distally or increase tension on the viable posterior fibers that extend to the distal insertion.[12] Moreover, Achilles tendinopathy with the appearance of Haglund syndrome can have proximal extension 5 cm from the insertion in 40% of patients.[12]

The posterior fibers of the Achilles tendon sustain more force owing to an increased lever arm, which results in more dystrophy of these fibers. This dystrophy results in degeneration of the tendon and deposition of calcification at the superficial fibers and posterior calcaneal step spur at the posterior insertion of the Achilles tendon.[25,26] On the other hand, calcification can also occur at the anterior part of the tendon, resulting from the prominent bursal projection, which tents the Achilles and hence results in degenerative tendon fibers.[25] The posterior calcaneal step spur and Achilles tendon calcification has predictive value for the Haglund syndrome and posterior heel pain.[14,21,25]

The retrocalcaneal bursa locates between the Achilles tendon and the upper third of the posterior calcaneal cortex. It serves as a spacer between axes of the ankle joint and Achilles tendon.[25] In primary case, a retrocalcaneal bursitis can be confirmed radiologically by less radiolucency of the retrocalcaneal recess of Kager triangle on a positive lateral radiograph of the ankle.[27] Haglund deformity should be reserved for defining a posterior prominence or hyperconvexity with loss of calcaneal recess because this corresponds with impingement.[12] However, in patients who already underwent endoscopic calcaneoplasty for the same pathology, the appearance of the retrocalcaneal recess on a conventional lateral standing radiograph cannot be used as a reliable diagnostic criterion because the scar tissue formation causes the persistent obliteration of the retrocalcaneal recess.[28]

Histologic evaluation of the posterior calcaneal wall cartilage in patients with insertional Achilles tendinopathy showed degenerative arthritic changes, and the severity of such changes is directly correlated to the degree of functional impairment.[29] This implies that the posterior calcaneal wall cartilaginous degeneration may also be a source of insertional pain.

Superficial adventitious Achilles tendon bursitis can also occur in Haglund syndrome.[30] Immunohistochemical examinations found that the subcutaneous bursa had the highest degree of innervation when compared with the retrocalcaneal bursa, the Achilles tendon, and the calcaneal bone[31]; this suggests that the subcutaneous bursa, which is traditionally not included in surgical treatment, may be a clinically important source of insertional pain.[31]

Impingement tendinopathy is less likely to respond to nonoperative treatment than noninsertional Achilles tendinopathy.[12] However, because of unpredictable surgical result, all possibilities of conservative treatment should still be performed before surgery.[23] The goal of treatment is to reduce the local inflammation and relieve the tension of Achilles tendon. Conservative first-line therapy includes reduction of activity levels, administration of nonsteroidal antiinflammatory drugs (NSAID), adaptation of footwear, heel wedges, and orthoses or immobilization.[32] Eccentric stretching exercises should be integral components of physiotherapy and can achieve a 40% reduction in pain.[32] Extracorporeal shock wave therapy (ESWT) is hypothesized to improve symptoms by promoting neovascularization and angiogenesis at the tendon-bone junction and inducing degeneration of epidermal nerve fibers with subsequent reinnervation.[33,34] It has been shown to reduce pain by 60% with a patient satisfaction of 80%.[32] However, the therapeutic effect of ESWT in patients with Haglund deformity is worse than that in those without deformity.[35] There is limited evidence to support the use of injections with platelet-rich plasma, dextrose (prolotherapy), or polidocanol (sclerotherapy).[35]

Operative therapy is indicated after 6 months of unsuccessful conservative therapy.[36] Patients with tenderness of the Achilles tendon insertion without obvious signs of inflammation who demonstrate confluent areas of intrasubstance signal changes on MRI are not likely to respond to nonoperative treatment. Early operative intervention is indicated in this group of patients in order to have earlier functional recovery.[37]

All potential sources of heel pain should be examined and treated during the operation.[38] The calcaneal bone, the superficial and retrocalcaneal bursa, and the Achilles tendon have all been considered the source of insertional pain, either alone or in combination.[38] These can be differentiated clinically by the locations of swelling and tenderness. Thompson's test should be performed in all cases to rule out associated Achilles tendon rupture. MRI scan is the investigation of choice for surgical planning, because this gives a much better understanding of the structures that are affected in Haglund syndrome.[25]

MINIMALLY INVASIVE AND ENDOSCOPIC APPROACHES

There are many surgical treatment options including retrocalcaneal bursa excision, calcaneal ostectomy, or osteotomy.[39–48] Open Achilles tendon detachment, calcaneoplasty, bursectomy, pathologic tendon-tissue debridement, and tendon reattachment of the Achilles tendon is a common surgical management of Haglund syndrome combined with insertional Achilles tendinopathy.[49] Surgical approaches include lateral,[16,39,50,51] central tendon splitting with or without tendon detachment,[8,50–56] and transverse incision.[57] Because in 95% of patients, calcification is located at the middle one-third of the Achilles insertion point, the tendon-splitting midline incision can expose the calcification site sufficiently.[58] A transverse incision allows a wide exposure and adequate debridement of the Achilles tendon insertion, less soft tissue injury from aggressive retraction, and a safe osteotomy of the posterosuperior corner of the calcaneus.[57] However, the open procedures are associated with high rate of complications including Achilles tendon avulsion, persistent posterior heel pain, wound breakdown, scar tenderness, altered heel sensation, nerve injuries (sural nerve), incisional neuroma, and ankle stiffness.[10,30,39,59] Recent development of endoscopic and minimally invasive approaches will have fewer complications and better outcome.[56,60–63] It is thought that endoscopic approach may not be possible to entirely remove the posterior calcaneal step spur or all diseased tissue in patients with full-thickness intratendinous calcifications, and it may be a more appropriate treatment for patients with disease characterized primarily by enlargement of the posterior superior calcaneal tuberosity.[56] However, recent advances in endoscopic and minimally invasive surgeries allow surgeons to deal with different pathologies of Haglund syndrome.

Treatment of Haglund Impingement

Endoscopic calcaneoplasty

van Dijk reported the first series of endoscopic calcaneoplasty in 2001 through medial and lateral portals with the patient in prone position.[64] This technique has been used successfully for the patients with pathologies limited to the retrocalcaneal bursitis and the posterosuperior border of the os calcis.[16,30,59–61,65–67] So far, there is no definite guideline on how much bone need to be removed during calcaneoplasty.[20,23,68,69] However, it is important not to leave any sharp bony prominence on either side of the posterosuperior calcaneal tubercle during endoscopic calcaneoplasty. The adequacy of bone excision is confirmed by the absence of impingement with the ankle in full dorsiflexion.[2] Besides simple mechanical decompression of the retrocalcaneal space, endoscopic calcaneoplasty can remove the degenerated posterior calcaneal wall cartilage that may also be a source of insertional pain. The exposed subchondral bone and bone marrow progenitor cells can form new fibrocartilage within a few weeks to restore the posterior coverage of the calcaneus.[29]

Open calcaneoplasty demonstrated a significant weakness of the Achilles tendon insertion especially in osteoporotic bone that might lead to Achilles tendon avulsion if aggressive rehabilitation is adopted.[70] Compared with open calcaneoplasty, endoscopic calcaneoplasty tends to resect less bone and the medial and lateral flares of the Achilles insertion are preserved and risk of Achilles tendon avulsion will be minimized.[25,71,72] However, Ortmann reported a case of Achilles tendon rupture 3 weeks after an endoscopic calcaneoplasty.[73]

Besides prone position, some investigators advocated endoscopic calcaneoplasty in supine position with more logical view on the monitor and a more ergonomic hand position.[22,25,74,75] A triangular support can be placed under the knee to flex the hip, knee, and ankle and stabilize the foot on the operating table. The plantarflexed ankle and flexed knee will relax the gastrosoleus and facilitate exposure of the retrocalcaneal recess and the Achilles insertion (**Fig. 1**).[74]

Percutaneous dorsal closing wedge calcaneal osteotomy

Dorsal closing wedge calcaneal osteotomy is a technique for the treatment of Haglund triad by reorientating bursal projection and avoiding bone resection adjacent to the Achilles tendon. It provides an increase in the blood supply to the region by way of an osteotomy.[25] It tilts the heel prominence anteriorly to reduce the posterior prominence of the heel and the lever arm. Moreover, the osteotomy slightly elevates the insertion of the Achilles tendon and would address slight equinus, which creates an effect similar to an Achilles tendon lengthening. The orientation of Achilles tendon fibers at the calcaneal insertion are also effectively altered, thereby reducing stress, which decompresses the enthesis and provides relief from pain associated with related insertional Achilles tendinopathy and retrocalcaneal bursitis.[2,25]

It is considered a safe procedure with good results.[2,76] However, it is technically demanding. The position of vertex of osteotomy is of paramount importance, because

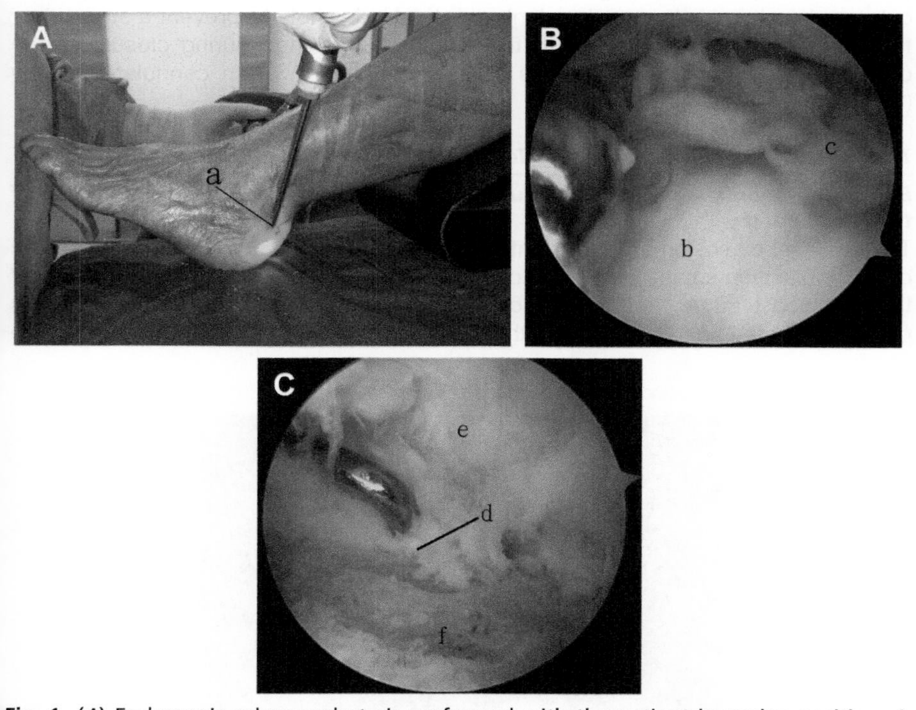

Fig. 1. (*A*) Endoscopic calcaneoplasty is performed with the patient in supine position. A triangular support is put under the knee to flex the knee and ankle. (*B*) Endoscopic view shows the inflamed retrocalcaneal bursa. (*C*) Endoscopic view after endoscopic calcaneoplasty shows the insertion point of the Achilles tendon. (a) Posterolateral portal; (b) posterosuperior calcaneal tubercle; (c) inflamed retrocalcaneal bursa; (d) insertional point of the Achilles tendon; (e) Achilles tendon; (f) exposed cancellous surface after endoscopic calcaneoplasty.

this determines whether or not the heel is placed horizontally. If the vertex is kept posterior, a forward rotation of the tuberosity is obtained. If the vertex is anterior, an elevation of the tuberosity is achieved, resulting in horizontalization of the heel in a cavus foot preoperatively.[25]

Complications of osteotomy include wound breakdown, nerve injury, nonunion, and widening of the heel and sharp plantar calcaneal cortex with proximal and posterior migration of the heel pad. Nonunion is a significant complication and is attributed to instability of the osteotomy site and proximal migration of the posterior calcaneal process due to breakage of plantar bone-bridge at the apex of the wedge osteotomy and the unopposed traction from the Achilles tendon.[2]

Minimally invasive calcaneal osteotomy has been developed to reduce some of the complications.[77,78] The safe zone of osteotomy extending 11.2 ± 2.7 mm anterior to the line joining the plantar aponeurosis origin to the posterosuperior apex of the calcaneus to avoid the sural nerve.[78] Two diagonal drill tracts at the planned osteotomy site of the posterior calcaneal tubercle. These results in 4 drill holes at the dorsomedial, dorsolateral, plantar-medial, and plantar-lateral corners of the planned osteotomy site.[77] Bone is cut with a Shannon straight flute burr (Vilex in Tennessee, Inc. McMinnville, TN, USA) from plantar dorsally through the drill holes (**Fig. 2**). This can avoid accidental cut of the plantar calcaneal cortex. Moreover, the plantar cortical holes help to prevent a stress riser to propagate all the way through the plantar bone hinge during closure of the osteotomy.[2] The osteotomy site is stabilized with a 7.3 mm cannulated screw (Synthes).

Treatment of Impingement Achilles Tendinopathy

Endoscopic debridement of ventral surface of Achilles tendon: proximal extension of the tendinopathy

The proximal extension of tendinopathy should be properly addressed. Endoscopic calcaneoplasty in supine position allows easy debridement of the ventral surface of the diseased tendon.[74] After endoscopic calcaneoplasty, the triangular support is placed under the heel. This will flex the hip and extend the knee. This allows a more

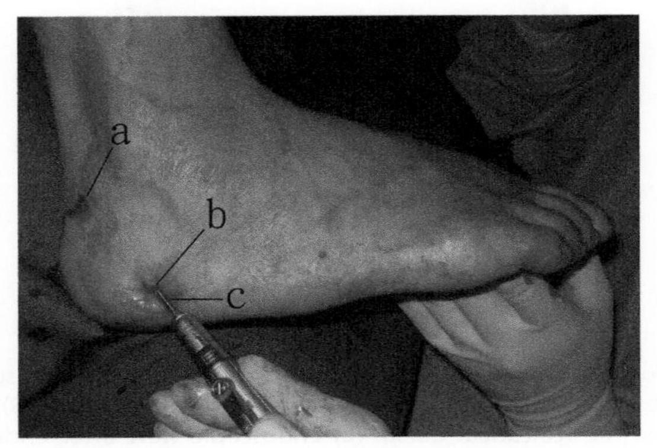

Fig. 2. Percutaneous dorsal closing wedge calcaneal osteotomy. A Shannon straight flute burr cutting the bone from plantar dorsally through the plantar lateral drill hole. (a) Stab incision for the dorsolateral drill hole; (b) stab incision for the plantar lateral drill hole; (c) Shannon straight flute burr.

ergonomic hand position for resection of the fibrous adhesions and neovasculature of the ventral surface of the diseased tendon (**Fig. 3**).[74]

Debridement of Achilles insertion: associated insertional tendinopathy

Open debridement of the Achilles insertion allows all pathologies of the associated insertional tendinopathy to be addressed, including osseous abnormalities and intratendinous necrosis. The success rate of greater than 70% is contrasted by complication rates of up to 40%.[32] Endoscopic debridement of the Achilles insertion may reduce the complication rates. After resection of the impinging bone, a superior-to-inferior resection of the Achilles insertion is performed with an arthroscopic shaver with preservation of the medial and lateral flares of the Achilles insertion. Cadaver study demonstrated that this direction of partial resection of the Achilles insertion offers the greatest margin of safety.[79] Sometimes, patient may have pain over the flares of the Achilles insertion, which may need detachment and debridement. In case of calcification located at the posterior part of the Achilles insertion, surgeon can consider debridement of the posterior part of the Achilles insertion from superficial surface of the tendon, especially if endoscopic resection of the subcutaneous adventitial bursa is also indicated. However, there is tendency of excessive resection and weakening of the Achilles insertion, and anchor suture augmentation may be needed.

The Achilles tendon should be reattached, if detached by more than 50%.[32,80] The tendon is usually reattached to its insertion by means of suture anchors via the portal incisions.[38,81,82] This allows anatomic repair but the point-to-point tendon healing may not restore the full strength and stability of the Achilles tendon.[83] Alternatively, the tendon can be reattached to the exposed cancellous surface after endoscopic calcaneoplasty. This provides larger contact area between tendon and bone surface and promotes the healing of the Achilles tendon.[83–85]

Sometimes, Achilles tendon tear can occur in Haglund syndrome. The fan-shaped Achilles insertion may make it more difficult to assess the extent of the lesion on only a few 2-dimensional MRI images.[86] An extensive endoscopic assessment after

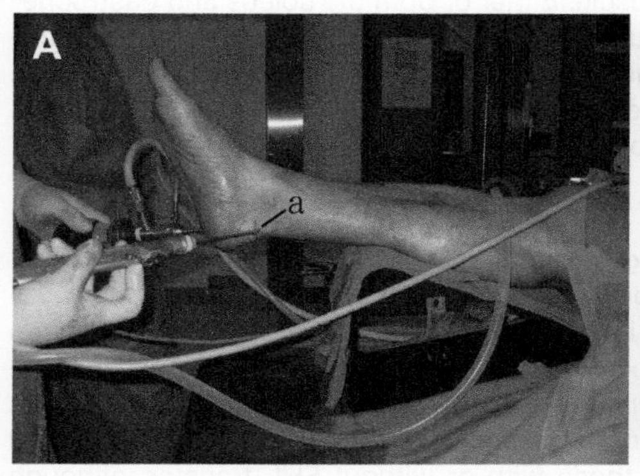

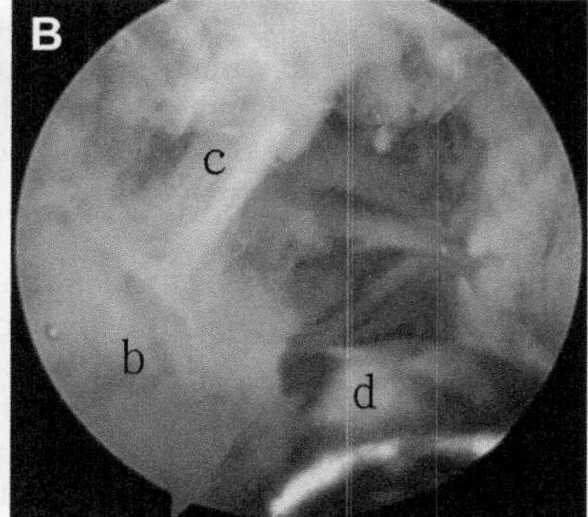

Fig. 3. (*A*) After endoscopic calcaneoplasty, the triangular support is placed under the heel. This will flex the hip and extend the knee. This allows a more ergonomic hand position for resection of the fibrous adhesions and neovasculature of the ventral surface of the diseased tendon. (*B*) Endoscopic view shows the fibrous adhesions at the ventral surface of the Achilles tendon. (a) Posteromedial portal; (b) Achilles tendon; (c) fibrous adhesions; (d) arthroscopic shaver.

endoscopic calcaneoplasty is recommended. Endoscopic repair can be considered if there is Achilles tendon tear.[86]

Endoscopic gastrocnemius ± soleus aponeurotic recession

Gastrocnemius recession may be indicated for the subset of patients with gastrocnemius contracture, failed previous reconstructions, or as an adjunct procedure combined with tendon debridement and/or flexor hallucis longus (FHL) transfer.[56] Patients without spurs tend to have greater improvement after gastrocnemius recession than patients with spurs.[56] This is commonly performed in adjunct with other procedures. Recently, Tallerico and colleagues[87] conducted a pilot study of isolated gastrocnemius recession for treatment of chronic insertional Achilles tendinopathy and concluded that it can provide high satisfaction, pain relief, and a faster recovery period with few or no complications. However, there is still insufficient evidence to provide a recommendation for isolated gastrocnemius recession as the sole treatment of insertional Achilles tendinopathy.[56]

Anatomically, the Achilles tendon rotates approximately 90° from its origin to insertion. The middle facet of the posterior calcaneal wall has the soleus attachment medially and laterally to the lateral head of gastrocnemius. The inferior facet has the attachment of the medial head of gastrocnemius.[25,30] In order to release the tension of the tendon fibers directly impinged by the posterosuperior bony prominence, it is logical to release the soleus aponeurosis together with the gastrocnemius aponeurosis because the medial tendon fibers are more commonly involved than the lateral fibers in impingement tendinopathy.[12] Most of the endoscopic gastrocnemius recession techniques are Strayer-type in which the extramuscular gastrocnemius aponeurosis is released. There is a risk of injury to the sural nerve. Villanueva and colleagues[88] reported a new ultra–minimally invasive surgical technique of ultrasound-guided gastrocnemius recession, which may reduce the risk of injury to the sural nerve. Moreover, patients who underwent a gastrocnemius recession did exhibit deficits in plantarflexion power and endurance and gastrocnemius recession may not be appropriate for athletic patients.[56] Recently, technique of endoscopic gastrocnemius intramuscular aponeurotic recession has been reported (**Fig 4**).[89,90] The working area is between the soleus and gastrocnemius aponeuroses and 3 cm proximal to the distal border of the medial gastrocnemius muscle. Either or both the soleus and gastrocnemius aponeurosis can be released through the same approach. The sural nerve is protected by the gastrocnemius muscle during the release. Because gastrosoleus muscle tendon unit remains intact during endoscopic intramuscular aponeurotic recession, the resultant deficit in plantarflexion power may be less than the Strayer-type endoscopic gastrocnemius recession.[90]

Endoscopic-assisted flexor hallucis longus transfer

Flexor hallucis longus (FHL) tendon augmentation is a safe adjunct to tendon debridement and partial ostectomy for chronic insertional Achilles tendinopathy and has been advocated in heavy patients older than age 50 years and those with extensive insertional Achilles tendon disease and/or when greater than 75% of the tendon is excised.[17,56,80,91,92] However, pain, functional outcome, or patient satisfaction may not be significantly different between those with or without FHL transfer, although ankle plantar flexor strength will be significantly improved with FHL transfer without functional weakness in the great toe.[56,91] It may not be necessary for primary cases and may be reserved for those with failed previous surgery or extensive tendon degeneration.[56,91] The addition of an FHL transfer may be associated with increased wound healing problems.[17] Endoscopic-assisted FHL transfer has been described to

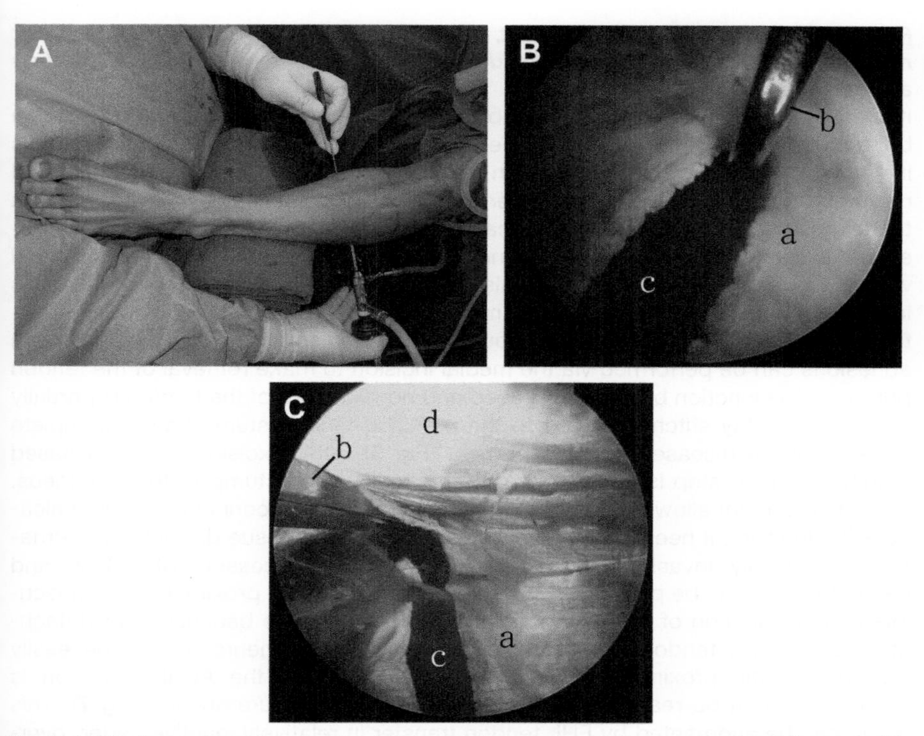

Fig. 4. (*A*) Endoscopic gastrocnemius intramuscular aponeurotic recession is performed with the patient in supine position. (*B*) The gastrocnemius aponeurosis is released with a retrograde knife. (*C*) Release of the soleus aponeurosis. (a) Gastrocnemius aponeurosis; (b) retrograde knife; (c) gastrocnemius muscle; (d) soleus aponeurosis.

minimize soft tissue dissection and wound problems.[93] The tendon can be harvested under sustentaculum tali or at its phalangeal insertion. The patient is in prone position and endoscopic calcaneoplasty and debridement of the Achilles tendon is performed via the posteromedial and posterolateral portals. The posteromedial portal is made a bit more proximal than usual and is in line with the plantar surface of first metatarsal and sustentaculum tali.[94] After debridement of the Achilles tendon and posterosuperior calcaneal tubercle, the FHL tendon at the posterior ankle (zone 1) is identified.[94] Zone 2 FHL tendoscopy is performed via the plantar and posteromedial portal if the tendon is planned to be harvested under sustentaculum tali. Alternatively, the tendon can be harvested at its phalangeal insertion (zone 3) by means of a tendon stripper via a plantar incision at the proximal phalanx of the hallux.[95]

Endoscopic subcutaneous adventitial Achilles bursa resection

Endoscopic resection of an inflamed subcutaneous adventitial Achilles bursa can be performed in prone or supine position. The portals for endoscopic calcaneoplasty should be made slightly more posterior than usual. The portal skin incision can be retracted posteriorly to allow endoscopic access to the subcutaneous bursa. If detachment of the Achilles insertion is planned, it is better performed after resection of the subcutaneous bursa. Intact Achilles tendon provides a stable platform for manipulation of the arthroscope and shaver during bursa resection.[96]

Resection of diseased tendon segment, minimally invasive gastrosoleus aponeurotic recession, reattachment of Achilles tendon: extensive tendinopathy with calcification and calcaneal step spur

It is general belief that endoscopic debridement should be avoided in patients with bone formation within the distal Achilles tendon insertion and open debridement is indicated.[22] Actually, this situation can be dealt with by combined endoscopic and minimally invasive approaches. After endoscopic calcaneoplasty, the Achilles tendon insertion together with the calcaneal step spur can be detached with arthroscopic shaver and burr. The medial and lateral flare of the tendon can be released with a Supercut scissors via the portals. After complete detachment of the Achilles insertion, the tendon is retrieved to a medial incision 4 to 6 cm from Achilles insertion. Sometimes, finger dissection around the tendon to breakdown peritendinous adhesions can be performed via the medial incision to make retrieval of the tendon possible. The junction between diseased and normal parts of the tendon is partially cut. Locking stay stitch is sewed to the proximal tendon stump before complete excision of the diseased tendon segment (**Fig 5**). After excision of the diseased tendon, the next step is to reattach the proximal tendon stump to the calcaneus. V-Y advancement allows the tendon to be extended and reconnected to the calcaneus.[92] However, it needs an extensive incision and soft tissue dissection. Alternatively, minimally invasive intramuscular aponeurotic recession of soleus and gastrocnemius can be performed via a medial incision 3 cm proximal to the musculotendinous junction of the gastrocnemius. This is possible because after detachment of Achilles tendon, its tension is lost and the aponeuroses can be easily retrieved to the proximal medial incision (**Fig 6**). After the Achilles tendon is extended, it can be reattached to the calcaneus with suture anchor (**Fig 7**). This repair can be augmented by FHL tendon transfer in relatively inactive, older, overweight patients to improve the Achilles tendon function.[97] In case of extensive tendinopathy requiring excision of a long tendon segment, the tendon gap can be reconstructed by double-thickness FHL tendon transfer (**Fig 8**).[95] The FHL tendon is harvested at its phalangeal insertion as described in previous session. The FHL tendon will pass through a bone tunnel of the posterior calcaneal tubercle before sewing to the proximal stump of the Achilles tendon. It is better to keep resection

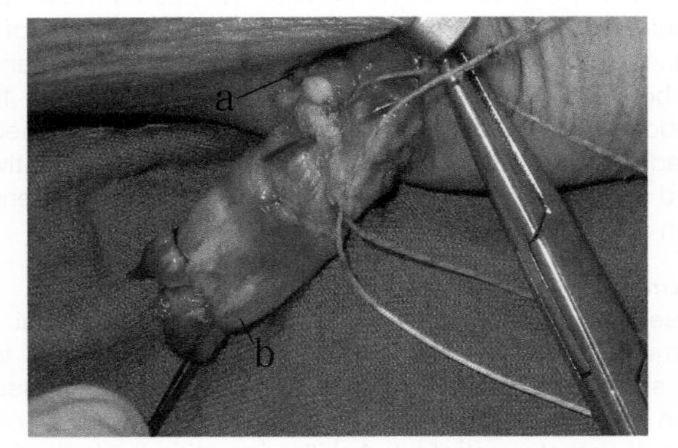

Fig. 5. The Achilles tendon is retrieved to the medial incision. It is partially cut at the junction between diseased and normal tendon tissue. Locking stay stitch is applied to the normal tendon stump before complete excision of the diseased tendon. (a) Medial incision; (b) Achilles tendon.

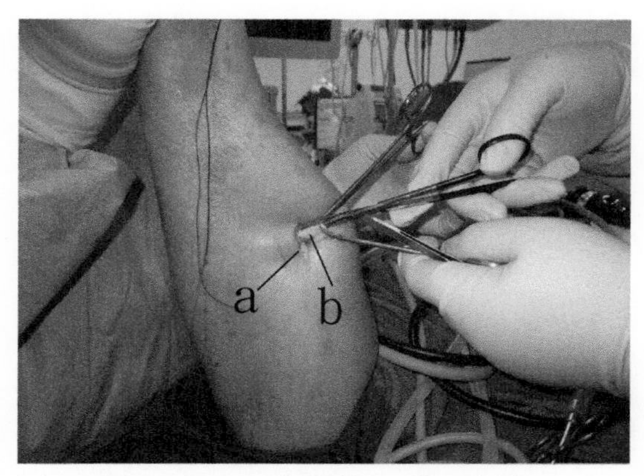

Fig. 6. The patient is in prone position with the knee flexed. The aponeuroses of gastrocnemius and soleus are retrieved to the proximal medial incision for release. (a) Proximal medial incision; (b) aponeuroses of gastrocnemius and soleus.

of the posterosuperior calcaneal tubercle to a minimum in order to reserve bone for anchorage of the FHL tendon.

RESULTS

The results after open Haglund resection and bursectomy are varying. In patients with posterior heel pain, resection of the posterosuperior part of the calcaneus and removal of the degenerative and calcified soft tissue lead to good clinical results of about 76%.[22] Endoscopic calcaneoplasty and tendoscopic treatment for insertional Achilles tendinopathy results in minimal complications when performed properly by experienced foot and ankle surgeons.[30,60] When compared with open approaches it was determined that the endoscopic approach to treatment of insertional Achilles tendinopathy is superior to open approaches.[65,98]

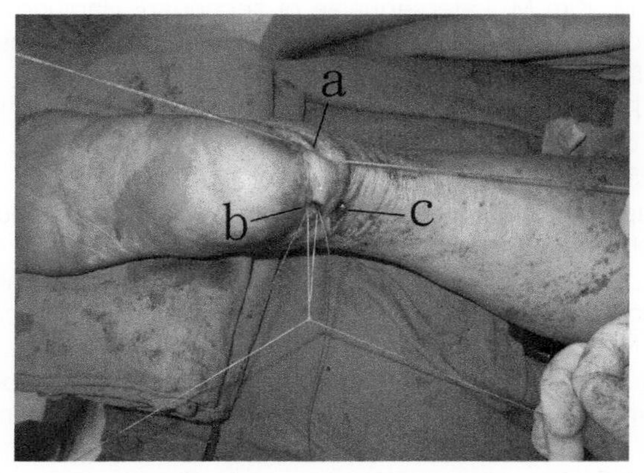

Fig. 7. The Achilles tendon is reattached to the calcaneus by means of suture anchors inserted via the posteromedial and posterolateral portals. (a) Posterolateral portal incision; (b) posteromedial portal incision; (c) medial incision.

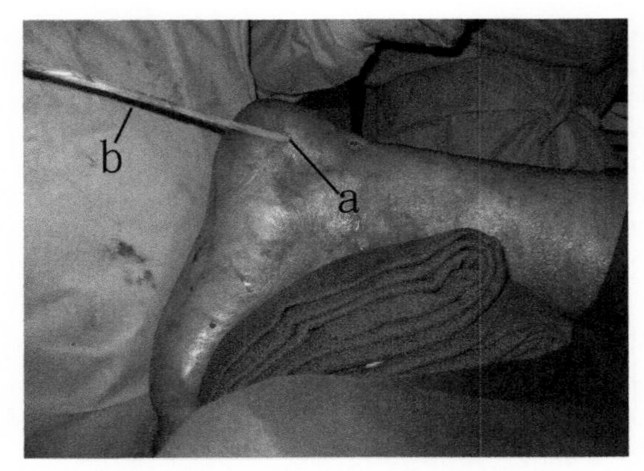

Fig. 8. FHL tendon is harvested from its phalangeal insertion and retrieved to the posteromedial portal incision. It is ready for double-thickness reconstruction of the Achilles tendon. (a) Posteromedial portal incision; (b) FHL tendon.

SUMMARY

With the advance in foot and ankle endoscopy and minimally invasive surgery, most of the pathologies of the Haglund syndrome can be managed by minimally invasive approaches. However, further large-scale prospective study is needed to evaluate their safety and efficacy.

REFERENCES

1. Haglund P. Beitrag zur Klinik der Achillessehne. Zeitschr Orthop Chir 1928;49:49–58.
2. Georgiannos D, Kitridis D, Bisbinas I. Dorsal closing wedge calcaneal osteotomy for the treatment of Insertional Achilles Tendinopathy: a technical tip to optimize its results and reduce complications. Foot Ankle Surg 2018;24:115–8.
3. Labib SA, Pendleton AM. Endoscopic calcaneoplasty: an improved technique. J Surg Orthop Adv 2012;21(3):176–80.
4. Jung H, Yoo M, Kim M. Late sequelae of secondary Haglund's deformity after malunion of tongue type calcaneal fracture: report of two cases. Foot Ankle Int 2002;23:1014–7.
5. Gillott E, Ray P. Tuberculosis of the calcaneum masquerading as Haglund's deformity: a rare case and brief literature review. BMJ Case Rep 2013;2013 [pii: bcr2013009252].
6. Jung H, Carag J, Park J, et al. Osteochondroma of the calcaneus presenting as Haglund's deformity. Foot Ankle Surg 2011;17:e20–2.
7. Yodlowski ML, Scheller AD Jr, Minos L. Surgical treatment of Achilles tendinitis by decompression of the retrocalcaneal bursa and the superior calcaneal tuberosity. Am J Sports Med 2002;30:318–21.
8. Nunley JA, Ruskin G, Horst F. Long-term clinical outcomes following the central incision technique for insertional Achilles tendinopathy. Foot Ankle Int 2011;32:850–5.
9. Johansson KJ, Sarimo JJ, Lempainen LL, et al. Calcific spurs at the insertion of the Achilles tendon: a clinical and histological study. Muscles Ligaments Tendons J 2013;2:273–7.

10. Clain MR, Baxter DE. Achilles tendinitis. Foot Ankle Int 1992;13:482–7.
11. Kang S, Thordarson DB, Charlton TP. Insertional Achilles tendinitis and Haglund's deformity. Foot Ankle Int 2012;33:487–91.
12. Bullock MJ, Mourelatos J, Mar A. Achilles impingement tendinopathy on magnetic resonance imaging. J Foot Ankle Surg 2017;56:555–63.
13. Shibuya N, Thorud JC, Agarwal MR, et al. Is calcaneal inclination higher in patients with insertional achilles tendinosis? A case-controlled, cross-sectional study. J Foot Ankle Surg 2012;51:757–61.
14. Lu CC, Cheng YM, Fu YC, et al. Angle analysis of Haglund syndrome and its relationship with osseous variations and Achilles tendon calcification. Foot Ankle Int 2007;28:181–5.
15. Sundararajan PP, Wilde TS. Radiographic, clinical, and magnetic resonance imaging analysis of insertional Achilles tendinopathy. J Foot Ankle Surg 2014;53(2): 147–51.
16. Oshri Y, Palmanovich E, Brin YS, et al. Chronic insertional Achilles tendinopathy: surgical outcomes. Muscles Ligaments Tendons J 2012;2:91–5.
17. Shakked RJ, Raikin SM. Insertionai tendinopathy of the achilles debridement, primary repair, and when to augment. Foot Ankle Clin 2017;22(4):761–80.
18. Pękala PA, Henry BM, Pękala JR, et al. The Achilles tendon and the retrocalcaneal bursa. An anatomical and radiological study. Bone Joint Res 2017;6(7): 446–51.
19. Schweitzer D, Karasick D. MR imaging of disorders of the Achilles tendon. AJR Am J Roentgenol 2000;175:613–25.
20. Fowler A, Philip JF. Abnormality of the calcaneus as a cause of painful heel. Its diagnosis and operative treatment. Br J Surg 1945;32:494–8.
21. Burhenne LJ, Connell DG. Xeroradiography in the diagnosis of the Haglund syndrome. Can Assoc Radiol J 1986;37(3):157–60.
22. Jerosch J, Schunck J, Sokkar SH. Endoscopic calcaneoplasty (ECP) as a surgical treatment of Haglund's syndrome. Knee Surg Sports Traumatol Arthrosc 2007; 15(7):927–34.
23. Schneider W, Niehus W, Knahr K. Haglund's syndrome: disappointing results following surgery – a clinical and radiographic analysis. Foot Ankle Int 2000;21: 26–30.
24. Kim KC, Shin HK, Kang DH. Clinical utility of radiographic measurements of insertional Achilles tendinitis with Haglund's deformity. J Korean Foot Ankle Soc 2005; 9:188–92.
25. Syed TA, Perera A. A proposed staging classification for minimally invasive management of Haglund's syndrome with percutaneous and endoscopic surgery. Foot Ankle Clin 2016;21(3):641–64.
26. Lyman J, Weinhold PS, Almekinders LC. Strain behavior of the distal Achilles tendon. Am J Sports Med 2004;32:457–61.
27. van Sterkenburg MN, Muller B, Maas M, et al. Appearance of the weight-bearing lateral radiograph in retrocalcaneal bursitis. Acta Orthop 2010;81:387–90.
28. Wiegerinck JI, Zwiers R, van Sterkenburg MN, et al. The appearance of the pre-Achilles fat pad after endoscopic calcaneoplasty. Knee Surg Sports Traumatol Arthrosc 2015;23:2400–5.
29. Palmanovich E, Oshri Y, Brin YS, et al. Insertional Achilles tendinopathy is associated with arthritic changes of the posterior calcaneal cartilage: a retrospective study. J Foot Ankle Res 2015;8:44.
30. Phisitkul P. Endoscopic surgery of the Achilles tendon. Curr Rev Musculoskelet Med 2012;5:156–63.

31. Andersson G, Backman LJ, Christensen J, et al. Nerve distributions in insertional Achilles tendinopathy - a comparison of bone, bursae and tendon. Histol Histopathol 2017;32(3):263–70.
32. Baumbach SF, Braunstein M, Mack MG, et al. Insertional Achilles tendinopathy: differentiated diagnostics and therapy. Unfallchirurg 2017;120(12):1044–53.
33. Ohtori S, Inoue G, Mannoji C, et al. Shock wave application to rat skin induces degeneration and reinnervation of sensory nerve fibres. Neurosci Lett 2001; 315:57–60.
34. Wang CJ, Wang FS, Yang KD, et al. Shock wave therapy induces neovascularization at the tendon–bone junction. A study in rabbits. J Orthop Res 2003;21: 984–9.
35. Wu Z, Yao W, Chen S, et al. Outcome of extracorporeal shock wave therapy for insertional achilles tendinopathy with and without Haglund's deformity. Biomed Res Int 2016;2016:6315846.
36. Irwin TA. Current concepts review: insertional Achilles tendiopathy. Foot Ankle Int 2010;31:933–9.
37. Nicholson CW, Berlet GC, Lee TH. Prediction of the success of nonoperative treatment of insertional Achilles tendinosis based on MRI. Foot Ankle Int 2007; 28(4):472–7.
38. Maquirriain J. Endoscopic Achilles tenodesis: a surgical alternative for chronic insertional tendinopathy. Knee Surg Sports Traumatol Arthrosc 2007;15:940–3.
39. Vaishya R, Agarwal AK, Azizi AT, et al. Haglund's syndrome: a commonly seen mysterious condition. Cureus 2016;8:e820.
40. Watson AD, Anderson RB, Davis WH. Comparison of results of retrocalcaneal decompression for retrocalcaneal bursitis and insertional Achilles tendinosis with calcific spur. Foot Ankle Int 2000;21:638–42.
41. Sammarco GJ, Taylor AL. Operative management of Haglund's deformity in the nonathlete: a retrospective study. Foot Ankle Int 1998;19:724–9.
42. Stephens MM. Haglund's deformity and retrocalcaneal bursitis. Orthop Clin North Am 1994;25:41–6.
43. Schunck J, Jerosch J. Operative treatment of Haglund's syndrome. Basics, indications, procedures, surgical techniques, results and problems. Foot Ankle Surg 2005;11:123–30.
44. Miller AE, Vogel TA. Haglund's deformity and the Keck and Kelly osteotomy: a retrospective analysis. J Foot Surg 1989;28:23–9.
45. Pauker M, Katz K, Yosipovitch Z. Calcaneal osteotomy for Haglund disease. J Foot Surg 1992;31:588–9.
46. Jones DC, James SL. Partial calcaneal osteotomy for retrocalcaneal bursitis. Am J Sports Med 1984;12:72–3.
47. Angermann P. Chronic retrocalcaneal bursitis treated by resection of the calcaneus. Foot Ankle 1990;10:285–7.
48. Boffeli TJ, Peterson MC. The keck and kelly wedge calcaneal osteotomy for Haglund's Deformity: a technique for reproducible results. J Foot Ankle Surg 2012; 51:398–401.
49. Vega J, Baduell A, Malagelada F, et al. Endoscopic Achilles tendon augmentation with suture anchors after calcaneal exostectomy in Haglund syndrome. Foot Ankle Int 2018;39(5):551–9.
50. Natarajan S, Narayanan VL. Haglund deformity – surgical resection by the lateral approach. Malays Orthop J 2015;9:1–3.

51. Anderson JA, Suero E, O'Loughlin PF, et al. Surgery for retrocalcaneal bursitis: a tendon-splitting versus a lateral approach. Clin Orthop Relat Res 2008;466: 1678–82.
52. Fridrich F. Tendon-splitting approach for the surgical treatment of Haglund's deformity and associated condition. Evaluation and results. Acta Chir Orthop Traumatol Cech 2009;76:212–7.
53. Ahn JH, Ahn CY, Byun CH, et al. Operative treatment of haglund syndrome with central achilles tendon-splitting approach. J Foot Ankle Surg 2015;54:1053–6.
54. McAlister JE, Hyer CF. Safety of Achilles detachment and reattachment using a standard midline approach to insertional enthesophytes. J Foot Ankle Surg 2015;54:214–9.
55. Gillis CT, Lin JS. Use of a central splitting approach and near complete detachment for insertional calcific achilles tendinopathy repaired with an achilles bridging suture. J Foot Ankle Surg 2016;55:235–9.
56. Chimenti RL, Cychosz CC, Hall MM, et al. Current concepts review update: insertional achilles tendinopathy. Foot Ankle Int 2017;38(10):1160–9.
57. Maffulli N, Del Buono A, Testa V, et al. Safety and outcome of surgical debridement of insertional Achilles tendinopathy using a transverse (Cincinnati) incision. J Bone Joint Surg Br 2011;93:1503–7.
58. Miao XD, Jiang H, Wu YP, et al. Treatment of calcified insertional achilles tendinopathy by the posterior midline approach. J Foot Ankle Surg 2016;55(3):529–34.
59. Jerosch J, Sokkar S, Dücker M, et al. Endoscopic calcaneoplasty (ECP) in Haglund's syndrome. Indication, surgical technique, surgical findings and results. Z Orthop Unfall 2012;150:250–6.
60. Kaynak G, Öğüt T, Yontar NS, et al. Endoscopic calcaneoplasty: five-year results. Acta Orthop Traumatol Turc 2013;47:261–5.
61. Appala Raju S, Rajasekhara Rao G, Vijayabhushanam M, et al. Comparison of open versus endoscopic calcaneoplasty for haglunds deformity: a short term analysis. J Evolut Med Dental Sci 2015;4:1930–4.
62. Wiegerinck JI, Kok AC, van Dijk CN. Surgical treatment of chronic retrocalcaneal bursitis. Arthroscopy 2012;28:283–93.
63. Javali V, Reddy VN. Haglund's disease: surgical outcome of calcaneal osteotomy. Int J Res Orthop 2017;3:278–81.
64. Van Dijk CN, van Dyk GE, Scholten PE, et al. Endoscopic calcaneoplasty. Am J Sports Med 2001;29:185–9.
65. Leitze Z, Sella EJ, Aversa JM. Endoscopic decompression of the retrocalcaneal space. J Bone Joint Surg Am 2003;85A:1488–96.
66. Jerosch J, Nasef NM. Endoscopic calcaneoplasty—rationale, surgical technique, and early results: a preliminary report. Knee Surg Sports Traumatol Arthrosc 2003;11:190–5.
67. Wu Z, Hua Y, Li Y, et al. Endoscopic treatment of Haglund's syndrome with a three portal technique. Int Orthop 2012;36:1623–7.
68. Bulstra GH, van Rheenen TA, Scholtes VA, et al. Can we measure the heel bump? Radiographic evaluation of Haglund's deformity. J Foot Ankle Surg 2015;54: 338–40.
69. Pavlov H, Heneghan MA, Hersh A, et al. The Haglund syndrome: initial and differential disgnosis. Radiology 1981;143:83–8.
70. Pfeffer G, Gonzalez T, Zapf M, et al. Achilles pullout strength after open calcaneoplasty for Haglund's syndrome. Foot Ankle Int 2018;39(8):966–9.

71. Roth KE, Mueller R, Schwand E, et al. Open versus endoscopic bone resection of the dorsolateral calcaneal edge: a cadaveric analysis comparing three dimensional CT scans. J Foot Ankle Res 2014;7(1):56.
72. Lohrer H, Nauck T, Dorn NV, et al. Comparison of endoscopic and open resection for Haglund tuberosity in a cadaver study. Foot Ankle Int 2006;27(6):445–50.
73. Ortmann FW, McBryde AM. Endoscopic bony and soft tissue decompression of the retrocalcaneal space for the treatment of Haglund deformity and retrocalcaneal bursitis. Foot Ankle Int 2007;28(2):149–53.
74. Lui TH. Endoscopic calcaneoplasty and Achilles tendoscopy with the patient in supine position. Arthrosc Tech 2016;5:e1475–9.
75. Jerosch J. Endoscopic calcaneoplasty. Foot Ankle Clin N Am 2015;20:149–65.
76. Georgiannos D, Lampridis V, Vasiliadis A, et al. Treatment of insertional Achilles pathology with dorsal wedge calcaneal osteotomy in athletes. Foot Ankle Int 2017;38(4):381–7.
77. Lui TH. Percutaneous posterior calcaneal osteotomy. J Foot Ankle Surg 2015;54:1188–92.
78. Talusan PG, Cata E, Tan EW, et al. Safe zone for neural structures in medial displacement calcaneal osteotomy: a cadaveric and radiographic investigation. Foot Ankle Int 2015;36:1493–8.
79. Kolodziej P, Glisson RR, Nunley JA. Risk of avulsion of the Achilles tendon after partial excision for treatment of insertional tendonitis and Haglund's deformity: a biomechanical study. Foot Ankle Int 1999;20(7):433–7.
80. DeOrio MJ, Easley ME. Surgical strategies: insertional achilles tendinopathy. Foot Ankle Int 2008;29:542–50.
81. Hegewald KW, Doyle MD, Todd NW, et al. Minimally invasive approach to achilles tendon pathology. J Foot Ankle Surg 2016;55:166–8.
82. Lui TH. Reattachment of Achilles tendon after endoscopic calcaneoplasty. Foot Ankle Int 2007;28:742–5.
83. Jiang Y, Li Y, Tao T, et al. The double-row suture technique: a better option for the treatment of Haglund syndrome. Biomed Res Int 2016;2016:1895948.
84. McBeth ZL, Galvin JW, Robbins J. Proximal to distal exostectomy for the treatment of insertional achilles tendinopathy. Foot Ankle Spec 2018;11(4):362–4.
85. Boden SA, Boden AL, Mignemi D, et al. Liquifying PLDLLA anchor fixation in Achilles reconstruction for insertional tendinopathy. Foot Ankle Spec 2018;11(2):162–7.
86. Michels F, Guillo S, King A, et al. Endoscopic calcaneoplasty combined with Achilles tendon repair. Knee Surg Sports Traumatol Arthrosc 2008;16(11):1043–6.
87. Tallerico VK, Greenhagen RM, Lowery C. Isolated gastrocnemius recession for treatment of insertional Achilles tendinopathy: a pilot study. Foot Ankle Spec 2015;8(4):260–5.
88. Villanueva M, Iborra A, Rodríguez G, et al. Ultrasound-guided gastrocnemius recession: a new ultra–minimally invasive surgical technique. BMC Musculoskelet Disord 2016;17:409.
89. Lui TH. Endoscopic gastrocnemius intramuscular aponeurotic recession. Arthrosc Tech 2015;4(5):e615–8.
90. Lui TH. Modified endoscopic release of gastrocnemius aponeurosis. J Foot Ankle Surg 2015;54:140–2.
91. Hunt KJ, Cohen BE, Davis WH, et al. Surgical treatment of insertional Achilles tendinopathy with or without flexor hallucis longus tendon transfer: a prospective, randomized study. Foot Ankle Int 2015;36(9):998–1005.

92. Staggers JR, Smith K, de C Netto C, et al. Reconstruction for chronic Achilles tendinopathy: comparison of flexor hallucis longus (FHL) transfer versus V-Y advancement. Int Orthop 2018;42(4):829–34.
93. Lui TH. Endoscopic-assisted flexor hallucis longus transfer: harvest of the tendon at zone 2 or zone 3. Arthrosc Tech 2015;4:e811–4.
94. Lui TH. Flexor hallucis longus tendoscopy: a technical note. Knee Surg Sports Traumatol Arthrosc 2009;17:107–10.
95. Lui TH. Whole length flexor hallucis longus transfer with a minimally invasive approach: technique tip. Foot Ankle Int 2011;32:730–4.
96. Lui TH. Arthroscopic ganglionectomy of the foot and ankle. Knee Surg Sports Traumatol Arthrosc 2014;22:1693–700.
97. Schon LC, Shores JL, Faro FD, et al. Flexor hallucis longus tendon transfer in treatment of Achilles tendinosis. J Bone Joint Surg Am 2013;95:54–60.
98. Bohu Y, Lefèvre N, Bauer T, et al. Surgical treatment of Achilles tendinopathies in athletes. Multicenter retrospective series of open surgery and endoscopic techniques. Orthop Traumatol Surg Res 2009;95(8):72–7.

Surgical Strategies for the Treatment of Insertional Achilles Tendinopathy

Alexej Barg, MD*, Todd Ludwig, MD

KEYWORDS

- Insertional Achilles tendinopathy • Insertional Achilles calcifications
- Haglund deformity • Knotless double-row footprint reconstruction

KEY POINTS

- Insertional Achilles tendinopathy is a common Achilles tendon disorder that often is associated with increasing age, repetitive microtrauma from constant overuse of the Achilles tendon, and/or increased vascularity.
- Most available studies suggest that patients with insertional Achilles tendinopathy should first be presented with nonsurgical treatment options, including eccentric calf-muscle training, high-energy extracorporeal shock wave therapy, and dry needling.
- Patients who have failed exhaustive conservative treatment for a period of 3 months to 6 months should be counseled about surgical treatment options unless contraindicated by general or procedure-specific complications.
- Surgical treatment includes débridement of insertional calcifications with a partial detachment of the distal Achilles tendon, débridement of intratendinous degenerative tissue, resection of any Haglund deformity, and reattachment of the distal Achilles tendon.
- Postoperative complications are not rare, and wound healing issues are the most common complication.
- Surgical treatment of insertional Achilles tendinopathy frequently results in substantial pain relief and functional improvement; however, complete rehabilitation, including return to sports activities, often is delayed up to 1 year postoperatively.

INTRODUCTION

Heel pain is a common disorder, but it is often poorly understood and managed (**Table 1**).[1] Clain and Baxter[2] classified Achilles tendon pain as arising either from the insertional portion of the tendon (insertional Achilles tendinopathy)[1,3–5] or from the noninsertional region of the tendon (noninsertional Achilles tendinopathy).[6–8]

Department of Orthopaedics, University of Utah, 590 Wakara Way, Salt Lake City, UT 84108, USA
* Corresponding author.
E-mail address: alexej.barg@hsc.utah.edu

Foot Ankle Clin N Am 24 (2019) 533–559
https://doi.org/10.1016/j.fcl.2019.04.005
1083-7515/19/

Table 1 Differential diagnosis of heel pain	
Posterior heel pain	Insertional Achilles tendinopathy Noninsertional Achilles tendinopathy Acute/chronic paratendinopathy Acute/chronic complete/partial Achilles tendon rupture Retrocalcaneal bursitis Superficial calcaneal bursitis Tight gastrocsoleus complex Flexor hallucis longus tendinopathy Gout Seronegative arthropathy
Plantar heel pain	Plantar fasciitis Calcaneus stress fracture Tarsal tunnel syndrome Rheumatoid arthritis Infection (especially in patients with diabetes)

Adapted from Solan M, Davies M. Management of insertional tendinopathy of the Achilles tendon. Foot Ankle Clin 2007;12(4):597–615; with permission.

Van Dijk and colleagues[9] systematically worked through the terminology of Achilles tendon pathology, which has become inconsistent and confusing with an increasing quantity of published literature. They proposed 6 different pathologies: (1) midportion Achilles tendinopathy, (2) acute paratendinopathy, (3) chronic paratendinopathy, (4) insertional Achilles tendinopathy, (5) retrocalcaneal bursitis, and (6) superficial calcaneal bursitis.[9]

In the current literature, insertional Achilles tendinopathy often is related to the Haglund deformity, which was described by Swedish orthopedic surgeon Patrick Haglund in 1928.[10] Albert,[11] however, was the first to describe heel pain as "Achillodynia" in 1893. Two years later, Rössler[12] analyzed patients with heel pain and suggested that achillodynia may be related to bursal inflammation between the insertion of the Achilles tendon and the calcaneus tuberosity. In 1898, Painter[13] performed a histologic analysis of the calcaneal exostosis in patients with retrocalcaneal bursitis. He concluded that exostoses are most likely "manifestations of an osteo-arthritic process."[13] Haglund[10] finally described 2 separate bursae around the insertion of the Achilles tendon: 1 located between the calcaneus and the skin ("bursa Achillea infero-posterior") and the other between the Achilles tendon and the calcaneus ("bursa Achillea supero-anterior"). In 1954, Dickinson and colleagues[14] introduced the term "pump bump" to characterize a visible and palpable enlargement of the posterolateral aspect of the heel at the site of the Achilles tendon insertion.

Most studies suggest that patients with insertional Achilles tendinopathy should first be presented with a nonsurgical treatment.[1,3–5] Surgical management should be considered, however, should conservative treatment fail. Different surgical techniques have been discussed in the current literature, including minimally invasive percutaneous approaches[15–19] and open approaches.[1,3–5,20–22] This article highlights the surgical treatment of insertional Achilles tendinopathy using open transtendinous approach, débridement of insertional calcifications, resection of Haglund exostosis, reattachment of the distal Achilles tendon, and, if needed, repair of the distal Achilles tendon.

INDICATIONS AND CONTRAINDICATIONS

The indications for surgical treatment of insertional Achilles tendinopathy are persisting pain and limitations in daily and/or sports activities. Patients should have failed exhaustive conservative treatment for a period of 3 to 6 months.

Contraindications for surgical treatment may be general or procedure-specific. General contraindications include acute or chronic infection with or without osteomyelitis, severe vascular or neurologic deficiency, compromised soft tissue and skin conditions (eg, patients with several prior surgeries), poorly controlled diabetes, and tobacco use. One procedure-specific contraindication is severe damage/degeneration of the Achilles tendon (in this case, other treatment options, including potential use of an allograft, should be discussed). Another specific contraindication is patient noncompliance; rehabilitation takes several months and requires that patients remain non-weightbearing for at least 6 weeks postoperatively. Furthermore, based on the authors' experience, significant pain relief may take a substantial amount of time (up to 12 months or longer), and patients should be aware of this. Finally, there are remarkably high rates of intraoperative, perioperative, and postoperative complications, and these facts should be clearly presented to patients.[1,3–5]

PHYSICAL EXAMINATION

Routine physical examination starts with a careful inspection of the foot and ankle while walking and standing. The hindfoot alignment (varus vs valgus vs neutral) is clinically assessed from behind the patient while the patient is standing. Patients often present with painful thickening of the soft tissues, a prominence at the Achilles tendon insertion (the so-called pump bump), and prominent heel-swelling (typically more on the lateral aspect of the heel) (**Fig. 1**). Local skin and soft tissue conditions should be noted, especially in patients with previous surgeries. The Achilles tendon should

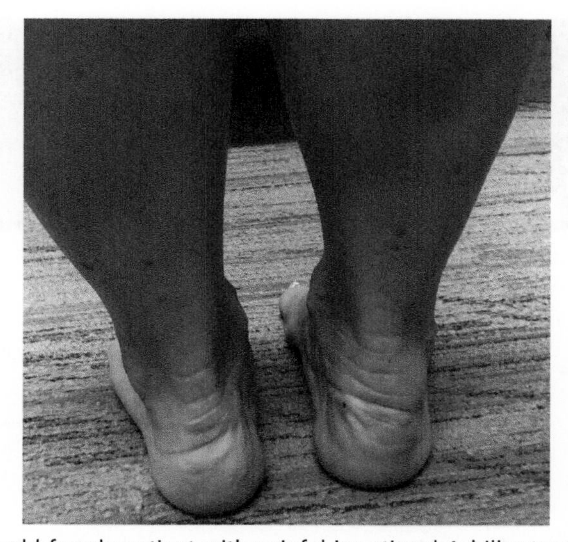

Fig. 1. A 53-year old female patient with painful insertional Achilles tendinopathy on the right side. Note painful thickening of the soft tissues, prominence at the Achilles tendon insertion—the so-called pump bump—and prominent swelling of the heel, typically more on the lateral aspect.

be carefully inspected and palpated with attention to the following: contour of the tendon, musculotendinous conjunction, muscle belly, areas of swelling and crepitation, skin color and temperature, palpable tendon defects, and/or nodules. The assessment of functional status includes activation of the gastrocsoleus complex by tiptoeing (bilateral and 1-leg stand). For patients with Achilles tendinopathy, ankle stability (medial, lateral, and rotational) should be assessed clinically.

IMAGING

Preoperative radiographic assessment routinely starts with conventional weightbearing radiographs, including mortise and lateral views of the ankle and a hindfoot alignment view (**Fig. 2**).[23] The lateral ankle view, in particular, is crucial for identifying intratendinous and/or insertional calcifications and prominent Haglund deformities (**Fig. 3**). In the current literature, 2 different methods for quantitative assessment of a Haglund deformity exist. Fowler and Philip[24] described an angle between the plantar surface of the calcaneal tuberosity and the tangent to the most prominent aspect of the posterior contour of the tuberosity (**Fig. 4**). Values greater than 75° should be interpreted as pathologic.[24] Another measurement was described by Pavlov and colleagues.[25] It is based on 2 parallel pitch lines: 1 along the most prominent aspects of the plantar surface of the calcaneal tuberosity and the other starting at the most posterior point of the posterior facet of the subtalar joint (**Fig. 5**). A pathologic Haglund deformity crosses the superior line and was found to significantly correlate with clinical symptoms.[25]

Advanced imaging modalities include sonography and MRI. Sonography usually is inexpensive and has a distinct advantage of facilitating dynamic assessment. Sonography also can assess the paratenon, and increased paratenon thickness often is associated with Achilles tendinopathy.[26] Sonography also can assess the insertion

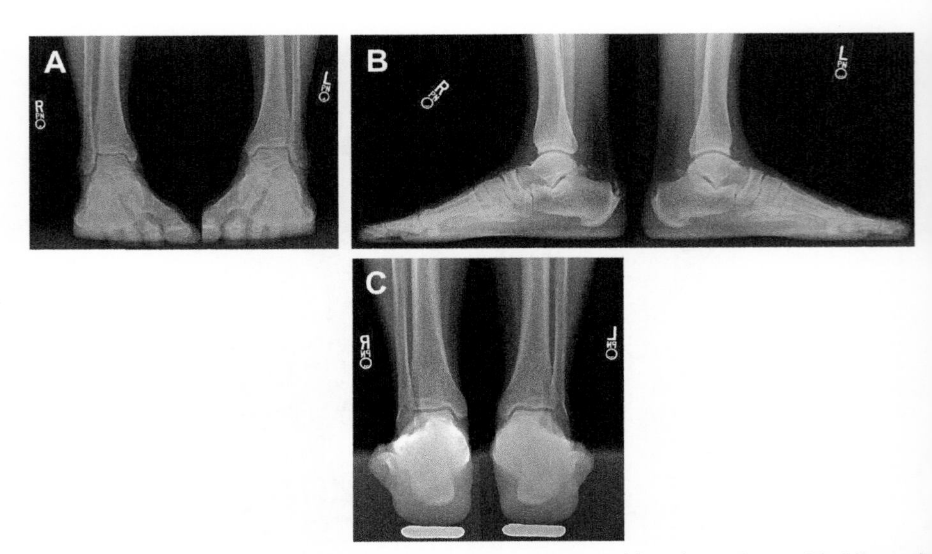

Fig. 2. Preoperative radiographic assessment in a 40-year old male patient with bilateral insertional Achilles tendinopathy. (*A*) Weightbearing mortise view of both ankles. (*B*) Weightbearing lateral view of both feet. (*C*) Weightbearing bilateral hindfoot alignment view.

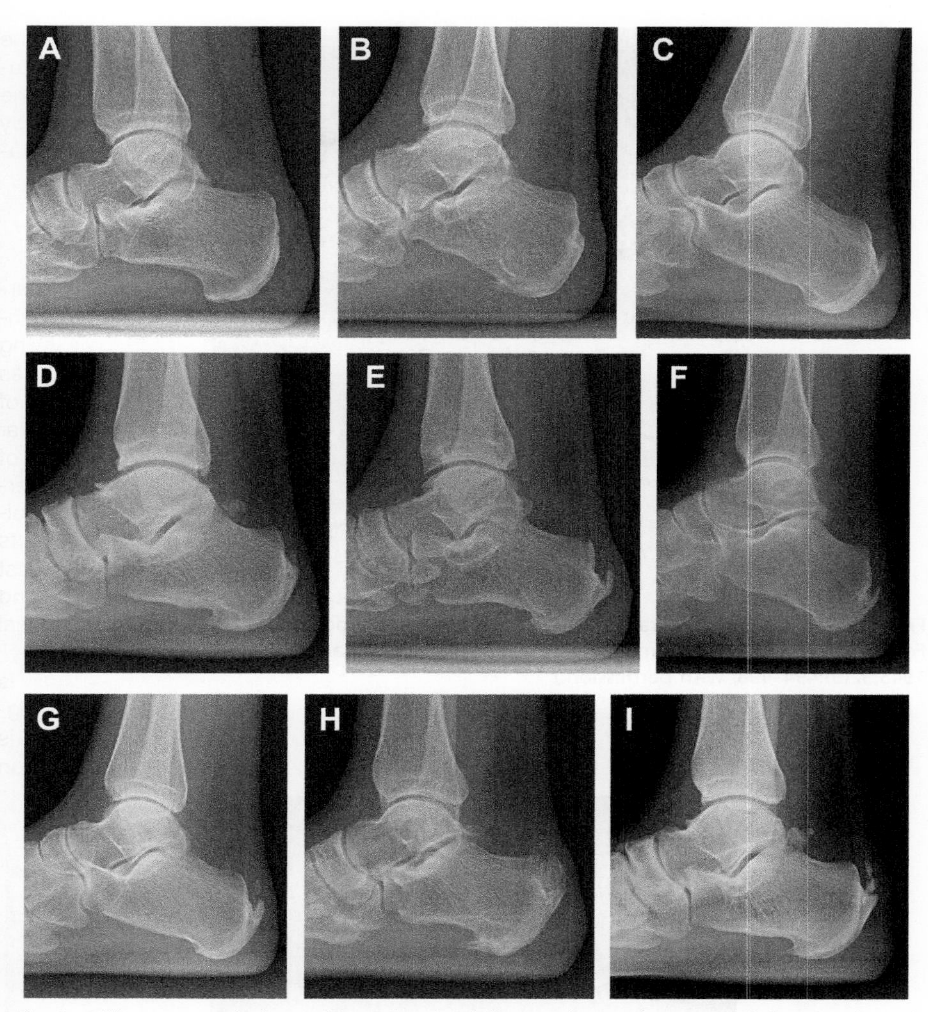

Fig. 3. Different morphology of insertional Achilles tendinopathy on weightbearing lateral radiographs. (*A*) Without ossifications at the insertion of the Achilles tendon. (*B*) Very mild ossifications at the insertion of the Achilles tendon. (*C*) Mild ossifications at the insertion of the Achilles tendon. (*D*) Mild ossifications at the insertion of the Achilles tendon with some intratendinous ossifications. (*E*) Moderate ossifications at the insertion of the Achilles tendon. (*F*) Moderate filiform ossifications at the insertion of the Achilles tendon. (*G*) Moderate ossifications at the insertion of the Achilles tendon with intratendinous ossifications. (*H*) Severe ossifications at the insertion of the Achilles tendon. (*I*) Severe ossifications at the insertion of the Achilles tendon with intratendinous ossifications.

of the Achilles tendon in great detail, illuminating potential calcaneal cysts in the tuber calcanei (**Fig. 6**). Exact sonographic assessment of the Achilles tendon, however, often requires substantial experience to correctly capture and interpret images. In the past 2 decades, axial-strain sonoelastography has been used increasingly to assess Achilles tendinopathy. Providing biomechanical information that conventional sonography fails to capture,[27–30] sonoelastography has demonstrated that patients

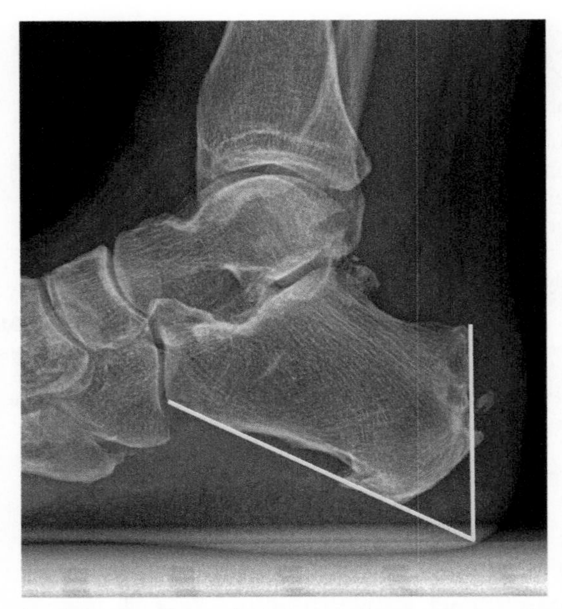

Fig. 4. Weightbearing lateral radiograph demonstrating posterior calcaneal angle. (*From* Fowler A, Philip JF. Abnormality of the calcaneus as a cause of painful heel. Br J Surg 1945;32(5):494–498; with permission.)

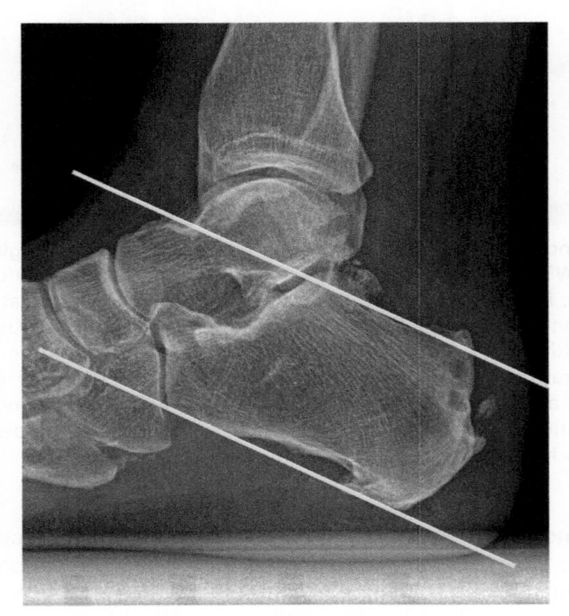

Fig. 5. Weightbearing lateral radiograph demonstrating parallel pitch lines. (*Data from* Pavlov H, Heneghan MA, Hersh A, Goldman AB, Vigorita V. The Haglund syndrome: initial and differential diagnosis. Radiology 1982;144(1):83–88.)

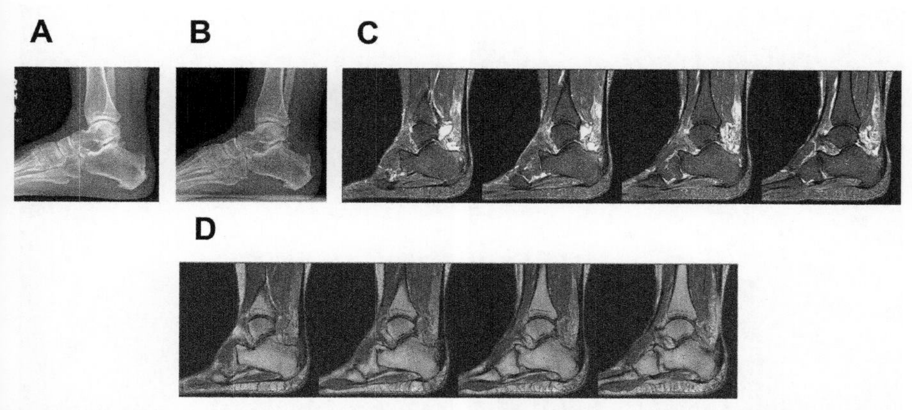

Fig. 6. (*A*) A 53-year old female patient with painful insertional Achilles tendinopathy on the right side (the same patient as in **Fig. 1**). (*B*) Two years later, worsening of symptoms with increasing insertional calcifications. (*C*) (from medial to lateral) Short tau inversion recovery and (*D*) (from medial to lateral) Proton density–weighted sagittal sequences demonstrate prominent insertional Achilles tendinopathy with partial thickness, interstitial split tearing, adjacent reactive posterior superior calcaneal marrow edema with cystic changes, and a prominent Haglund deformity with a small volume retrocalcaneal bursitis.

with insertional Achilles tendinopathy have an increased hardness of the tendon relative to asymptomatic controls.[31]

MRI is relatively expensive, especially compared with sonography, and cannot be performed under dynamic conditions. It provides detailed anatomic and 3-D information regarding the amount of degeneration/damage present in the distal Achilles tendon.[32–34] In general, sonography and MRI may provide similar information for patients with chronic Achilles tendinopathy.[35] Nicholson and colleagues[36] evaluated the MRIs of 157 patients (176 feet) who were treated for insertional posterior heel pain. The investigators have suggested their own classification of distal Achilles tendinopathy (**Fig. 7**, **Table 2**). They demonstrated that patients with substantial intramural degeneration respond less successfully to conservative treatment. Early identification of these patients and appropriate discussion of possible surgical treatments may result in earlier functional improvement.[36]

SURGICAL TECHNIQUE

Either general or regional anesthesia can be used for surgery. The patient is placed prone on a well-padded chest roll with feet overhanging the edge of the table. The operative lower leg is positioned on a stable radiolucent cushion with the knee in slight flexion. Esmarch exsanguination and a thigh tourniquet can be applied unless contraindicated.

Skin landmarks include the calcaneal tuberosity, the contour of the distal Achilles tendon, and the planned midline incision (**Fig. 8**). A 6-cm to 8-cm longitudinal midline incision is made over the posterior aspect of the Achilles tendon, starting at the distal part of tuber calcanei, extending down the Haglund exostosis, and ending over the distal part of the Achilles tendon (**Fig. 9**). Alternatively, a medial or lateral approach can be chosen to avoid the midline watershed region and reduce the risk of scar sensitivity with shoe wear.[5] An alternative approach, however, may not provide optimal access to the tendon for repair and débridement and may increase the risk of injury to neurovascular structures. Incision length

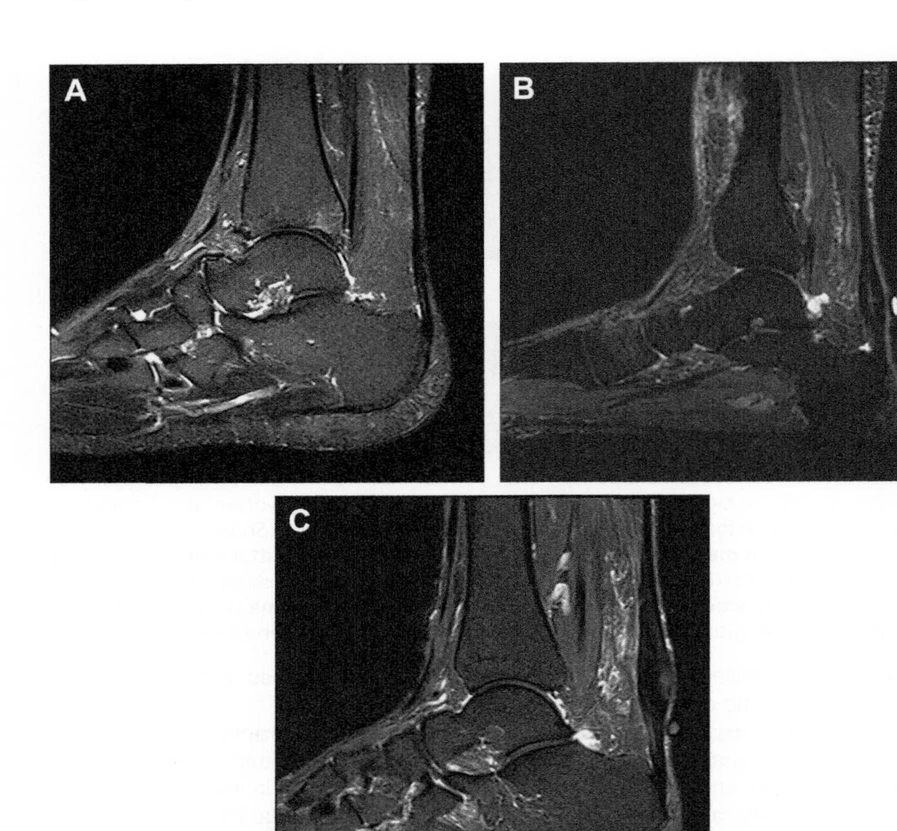

Fig. 7. MRI-based classification of degenerative changes in patients with insertional Achilles tendinopathy (for detailed description, see **Table 2**).[36] (*A*) Type I. (*B*) Type II. (*C*) Type III.

varies depending on the extent of the lesion and/or degeneration of the Achilles tendon. After the skin incision is complete, blunt dissection of the subcutaneous tissues is performed with special attention paid to not injure neurovascular structures. The incision and preparation are made full-thickness down to the Achilles

Table 2
MRI-based classification of degenerative changes in patients with insertional Achilles tendinopathy

Type I	• Tendon thickening (6–8 mm) • Nonuniform intramural splits or foci of punctuate degeneration
Type II	• Tendon thickening (more than 8 mm) • Uniform intramural degeneration = <50% of the width of the tendon
Type III	• Tendon thickening (more than 8 mm) • Uniform intramural degeneration = more than 50% of the width of the tendon

From Nicholson CW, Berlet GC, Lee TH. Prediction of the success of nonoperative treatment of insertional Achilles tendinosis based on MRI. Foot Ankle Int 2007;28(4):472–477; with permission.

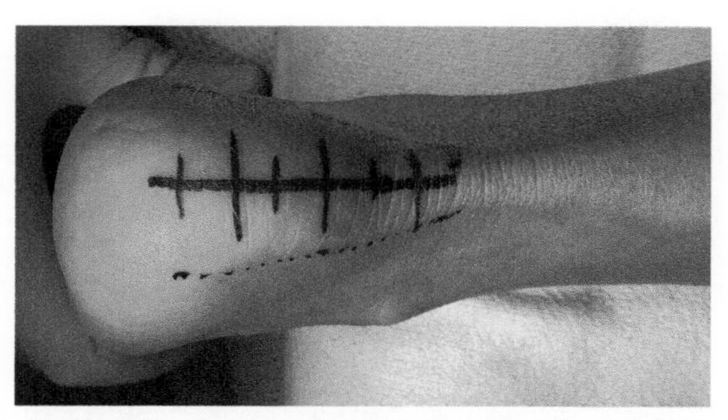

Fig. 8. Skin landmarks, including calcaneal tuberosity, contour of the distal Achilles tendon, and the planned midline incision.

paratenon, which may help ensure postoperative wound healing. A longitudinal incision of the paratenon is then performed, followed by careful dissection of the paratenon from the tendon (**Fig. 10**). The Achilles tendon itself has no synovial sheath; however, it is surrounded by the paratenon—a double-layered sheath composed of an inner, visceral layer and an outer, parietal layer. The paratenon has an abundance of nerves and blood vessels and provides the main blood supply to the Achilles tendon.[37,38] After the paratenon is incised and mobilized, the Achilles tendon is carefully exposed, inspected, and palpated. Special attention is paid to the thickness of the Achilles tendon as well as any defects or intratendinous ossifications. The tendon is then split longitudinally via a midline incision. The split tendon is evaluated for degenerative/necrotic changes and intratendinous ossifications. All tendinotic tissue, as well as ossifications, should be completely débrided and resected. Incomplete débridement is associated with the risk of persisting pain and postoperative symptoms.[3] Intratendinous débridement is followed by further preparation to the distal insertion of the Achilles tendon at the tuber calcanei. Usually, a 70% to 80% detachment of the distal Achilles tendon is needed to expose the tuber calcanei and the Haglund exostosis (**Fig. 11**). The Haglund exostosis is removed using an osteotome or an oscillating saw. Complete exostosis removal is confirmed by a clinical (inspection and palpation) and fluoroscopic check. Any insertional spurs are then removed using an osteotome. A majority of insertional spurs are located centrally and are well exposed for removal (**Fig. 12**). Medical and lateral spurs also should be identified and, if present, completely resected. Therefore, a fluoroscopic check of tuber calcanei should be performed in different planes: neutral position (central spurs), internally rotated (lateral spurs), and externally rotated (medial spurs) (**Fig. 13**). Incomplete spur removal may result in persisting

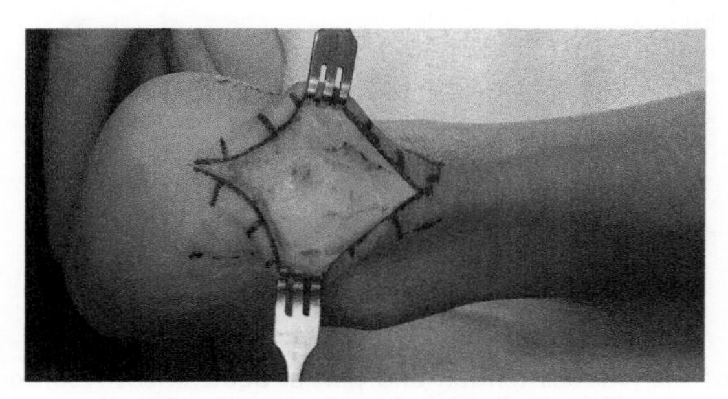

Fig. 9. Posterior approach with a 6-cm to 8-cm longitudinal midline incision.

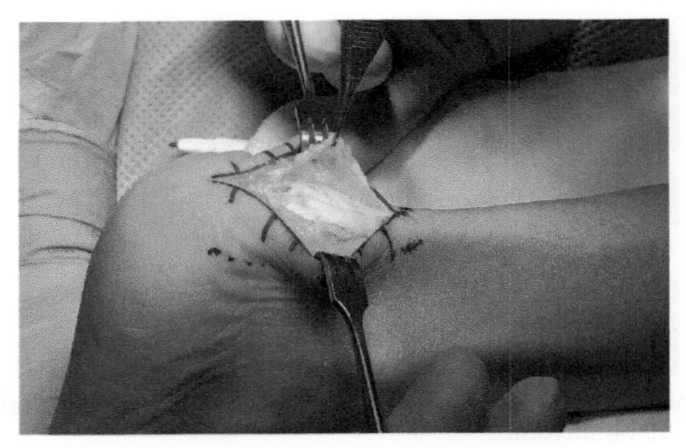

Fig. 10. Careful dissection of paratenon from the Achilles tendon.

pain and tenderness. The distal insertional débridement is followed by reattachment of the Achilles tendon. In patients with severe Achilles tendinosis, flexor hallucis longus tendon transfer should be performed.[39–43] Different surgical techniques have been described in the current literature for Achilles tendon reattachment (**Table 3**). The authors' preferred surgical technique includes using a knotless double-row footprint reconstruction. First, 2 proximal holes are drilled and tapped, followed by placement of 2 4.75-mm absorbable anchors with 2-mm width nonresorbable tapes. Both tapes are passed through the proximal Achilles tendon on the medial and lateral sides (**Fig. 14**). Two distal holes are drilled and tapped using the same technique as the proximal fixation row. The split Achilles tendon is closed using resorbable sutures. The distal anchors are preloaded with 1 suture tail from the ipsilateral proximal anchor and 1 suture tail from the contralateral proximal anchor (**Fig. 15**). The foot is held in a plantar flexed position, and the tape tension is adjusted within the eyelet of the distal anchor. Both distal anchors are placed under tension. Special attention is paid to ensure that both anchors are flush to the bone surface. The tape tails are cut flush to the anchor, resulting in the final knotless repair. The wound is copiously irrigated. The paratenon is carefully closed using 2-0 absorbable sutures (**Fig. 16**) and followed by wound closure in layers. A sterile dressing is applied with plenty of cast padding to avoid any pressure around the wound. The hindfoot is placed in a splint or a 3-D tall boot with 3 heel wedges, positioning the foot in 15° to 20° of plantarflexion.

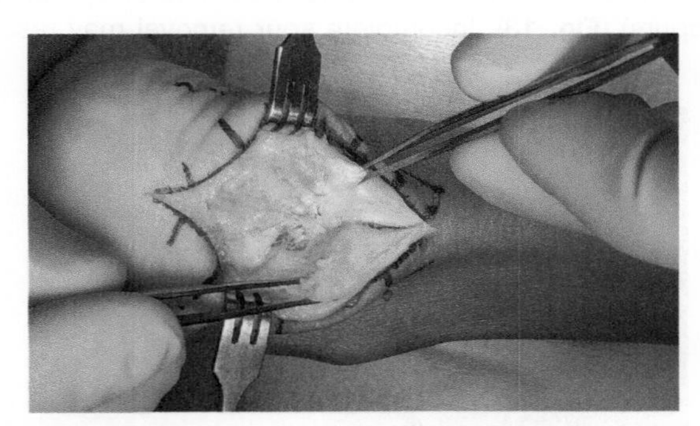

Fig. 11. Splitting of the Achilles tendon and partial detachment resulting in exposure of insertion of the Achilles tendon.

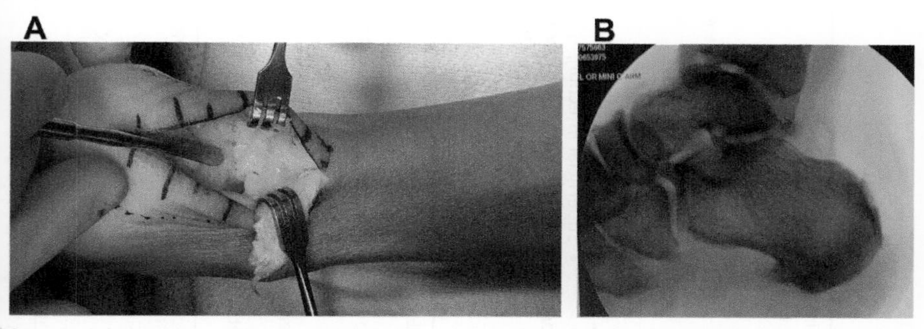

Fig. 12. (*A*) Resection of Haglund exostosis and débridement of central part of insertional calcifications. (*B*) Fluoroscopy demonstrates appropriate débridement with the foot held in neutral rotation.

In general, postoperative rehabilitation is similar to that of patients treated for acute Achilles tendon rupture.[44,45] The authors recommend 6 weeks at 10 kg partial weightbearing and protected in a 3-D tall boot. Every 2 weeks, 1 of 3 heel wedges is removed, resulting in a plantar flexion reduction of 5° to 10°. At the 6-week

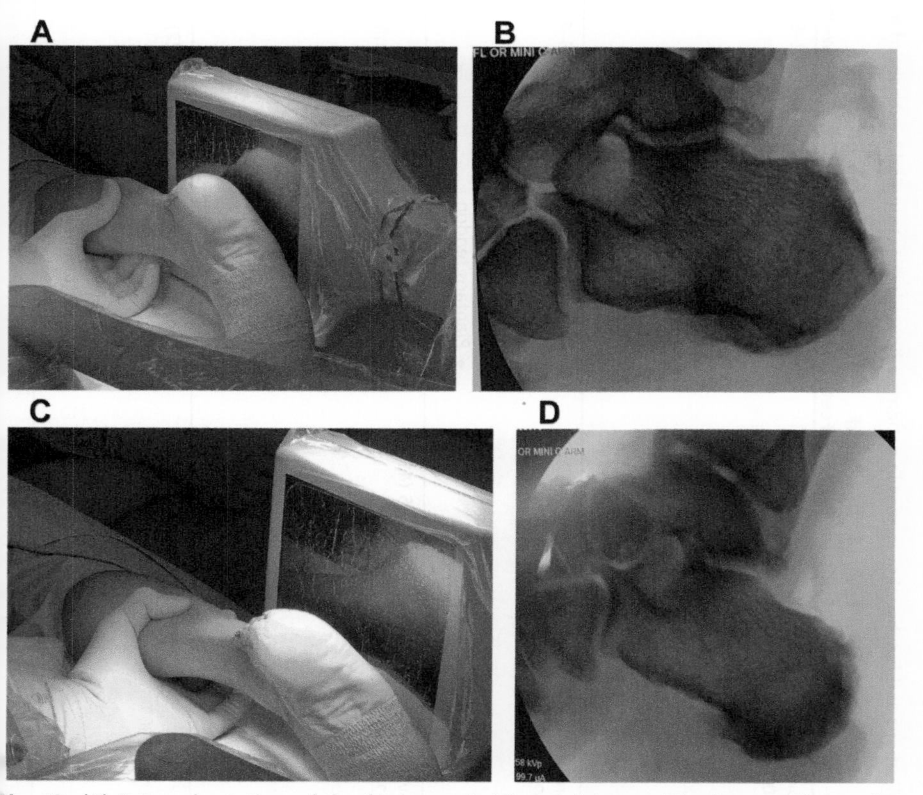

Fig. 13. (*A*) External rotation of the foot reveals (*B*) remaining ossifications on the medial aspect of the tuber calcanei. (*C*) Internal rotation of the foot reveals (*D*) remaining ossifications on the lateral aspect of the tuber calcanei.

Table 3
Complications and functional outcomes in patients who underwent surgical treatment of insertional Achilles tendinopathy

Study	Study Type	Level of Evidence	Number of Patients (Feet)	Surgical Technique (no. of patients)	Follow-up (mo)	Outcome (range)	Complications (no. of patients)
Watson et al,[83] 2000	RS, SC	IV	16 (19)	• Prone position • Posterolateral approach • Haglund resection using osteotome or oscillating saw • AT reattachment using periosteum sutures	47 (22–81)	• Average time to maximum symptomatic improvement 10.6 mo (3–18 mo) • AOFAS pain subscore (0–40): 34.2	• No wound healing complications • AT avulsion (1) at fall • Insertional Achilles tendinopathy recurrence requiring revision surgery (1) • Sural nerve neuritis, completely resolved (3)
McGarvey et al,[84] 2002	RS, SC	IV	21 (22)	• Prone position • Midline incision • AT reattachment using bone-anchored sutures • Plantaris tendon augmentation (1)	33 (26–40)	• 13 patients pain-free without any restrictions in their activity • 18 patients satisfied	• Superficial infection, resolved with oral ABX (1) • Scar hypersensitivity (2), scar numbness (4)
Yodlowski et al,[80] 2002	RS, SC	IV	35 (41)	• Prone position • Posterolateral approach • Haglund resection using osteotome • AT débridement without detachment • AT reattachment in only 1 case	39 (minimum 20)	• Pain score (0–6): $4.7 \pm 1.1 \rightarrow 1.5 \pm 1.3$ • 14 patients: complete symptoms relief; 17 patients: significant improvement; 4 patients: improvement • All 26 athletes were able to return to sports	• No wound-healing complications • Scar hypersensitivity (14) • DVT (1)
Calder and Saxby,[85] 2003	RS, SC	IV	45 (52)	• Prone position • Midline incision • Haglund resection using osteotome • AT reattachment in 3 patients	8 (6–22)	NR	• AT avulsion (2), no revision surgery • Superficial infection, resolved with oral ABX (3)

Den Hartog,[86] 2003	RS, SC	IV	26 (29)	• Prone position • L-shaped incision • Haglund resection using osteotome • AT reattachment using 2 bone anchors • FHL tendon transfer augmentation	35 (12–58)	• AOFAS hindfoot score (0–100): 41.7 (23–63) → 90.1 (49–100) • AOFAS pain subscore (0–40): 7.4 (0–20) → 35.7 (20–40)	• Medial calcaneal nerve dysesthesia (2)
Maffulli et al,[87] 2004	PS, SC	IV	21 (21)	• Prone position • Midline incision (19), hockey stick incision laterally (2) • AT reattachment using 2 bone anchors	48 (24–84)	• 11 Excellent results, 5 good results • 5 patients could not return to normal activity level	• Superficial infection, resolved with oral ABX (2) • Scar hypersensitivity (3)
Johnson et al,[88] 2006	RS, SC	IV	25 (25)	• Prone position • Midline incision • AT reattachment using 2 bone anchors	34 (11–64)	• Total ankle-hindfoot scale (0–100): 53 → 89 • Pain score (0–40): 7 → 33 • Function score (0–50): 36 → 46	• DVT (1)
Wagner et al,[22] 2006	RS, SC	IV	39 (39)	• Prone position • Posteromedial J-shaped incision • AT reattachment using 2 bone anchors	33	• 92% satisfaction rate	• Superficial infection, resolved with oral ABX (6) • Sural nerve pain (2)
Carmont and Maffulli,[76] 2007	RS, SC	IV	40 (40)	• Prone position • Transverse skin incision (Cincinnati incision) • Haglund resection using osteotome • AT reattachment using transosseous sutures or anchors	NR	• Average time to return to previous activities 9 mo (6–15 mo)	• Delayed wound healing (1) • Wound infection, resolved with oral ABX (3) and I&D (1)

(*continued on next page*)

Table 3
(continued)

Study	Study Type	Level of Evidence	Number of Patients (Feet)	Surgical Technique (no. of patients)	Follow-up (mo)	Outcome (range)	Complications (no. of patients)
Elias et al,[89] 2009	RS, SC	IV	40 (40)	• Prone position • Midline incision • Haglund resection using osteotome • FHL tendon transfer augmentation • AT reattachment using 2 bone anchors	27 (18–68)	• AOFAS hindfoot score (0–100): 56 (29–82) → 96 (69–100) • VAS (0–10): 7.5 → 0.3 • 95% satisfaction rate	• AT longitudinal split tear (1)
Philippot et al,[90] 2010	RS, SC	IV	24 (25)	• Lateral decubitus position • Posterolateral incision • Haglund resection using osteotome • Augmentation with bone-quadriceps tendon graft	52 (12–156)	• Average time to return to work 3.7 mo (2–8 mo) • Average time to return to sport activities 6.7 mo (3–12 mo) • Tegner scale (0–10): 4.5 → 5.2 • AOFAS hindfoot score (0–100): 98 (87–100)	• Superficial infection, resolved with local care (1) • DVT (1) • Complex regional pain syndrome, resolved completely (2) • Knee pain (2)
Maffulli et al,[91] 2011	PS, SC	IV	30 (30)	• Prone position • Transverse skin incision (Cincinnati incision) • Haglund resection using osteotome	39 (37–73)	• VISA-A score (0–100): 62 (49–75) → 88 (77–96)	• Superficial infection, resolved with oral ABX (6)
Nunley et al,[81] 2011	RS, SC	IV	27 (29)	• Prone position • Midline incision • Haglund resection using oscillating saw • AT reattachment using 2 bone anchors	48 (35–97)	• Average time to pain relief 5.7 mo (2–16 mo) • AOFAS hindfoot score (0–100): 96 • 22 patients completely pain free	• Superficial infection, resolved with oral ABX (1) • Recurrent calcifications: small (7), moderate (1), large (3)
Lim et al,[92] 2012	PS, SC	IV	8 (8)	• Prone position • Midline incision • Haglund resection using osteotome • AT reattachment using 2	12 (3–24)	• All patients were pain free • AOFAS hindfoot score (0–100): 58 → 100	• Wound infection (1) • Painful scar (1)

Miyamoto et al,[82] 2012	RS, SC	IV	49 (49)	• Posterolateral incision • Haglund resection using osteotome • Augmentation with bone–patellar tendon graft	32 (25–48)	• AT rupture score (0–100): 92.5 (85–100) • VAS (0–10): 90 (85–100) → 5 (0–10) • Average time to full sports activity 13.5 mo (12–14 mo)	NR
Oshri et al,[93] 2012	RS, SC	IV	20 (21)	• Prone position • Posterolateral incision	NR	• VAS (0–10): 7.9 ± 1.8 → 3.7 ± 3.8 • AOFAS hindfoot score (0–100): 52.0 ± 22.9 → 83.1 ± 21.3	None
Witt and Hyer,[94] 2012	RS, SC	IV	4 (4)	• Prone position • Midline incision • Haglund resection using oscillating saw • AT reattachment using knotless footprint reconstruction	24 (18–27)	• VAS (0–10): 1 (0–4) • Foot function index: 3.4 (0–10.7)	None
Greenhagen et al,[95] 2013	RS, SC	IV	30 (30)	• Prone position • Midline incision • Haglund resection using oscillating saw or osteotome • AT reattachment using knotless footprint reconstruction	29 (7–65)	• AOFAS hindfoot score (0–100): 57 ± 14 → 92 ± 10	• Persisting pain (1)
Rigby et al,[79] 2013	RS, SC	IV	43 (43)	• Prone position • Slightly medial incision • Haglund resection using oscillating saw • AT reattachment using knotless footprint reconstruction	24 (10–49)	• AOFAS hindfoot score (0–100): 90 (65–100) • VAS (0–10): 6.8 (2–10) → 1.3 (0–6)	• Wound healing problems, resolved with I&D (2) • Superficial infection (1)

(continued on next page)

Table 3 (*continued*)

Study	Study Type	Level of Evidence	Number of Patients (Feet)	Surgical Technique (no. of patients)	Follow-up (mo)	Outcome (range)	Complications (no. of patients)
Schon et al,[96] 2013	RS, SC	IV	46 (48)	• Prone position • Slightly medial incision • Haglund resection • FHL tendon transfer augmentation	24	• VAS (0–10): 6.7 ± 2.3 → 0.8 ± 2.0 • SF-36 (0–100): 34.3 ± 8.0 → 49.0 ± 9.3 • AOS pain (0–100): 54.4 ± 19.2 → 1.9 ± 2.7 • AOS function (0–100): 62.6 ± 21.4 → 11.0 ± 24.2	• Superficial infection/ delayed wound healing (6)
Lin et al,[97] 2014	RS, SC	IV	44 (44)	• Prone position • Posterolateral incision • Haglund resection using oscillating saw • AT reattachment using 2 bone anchors	12	• AOFAS hindfoot score (0–100): 43.5 → 86.5	• Superficial infection, resolved with local care (3)
El-Tantawy and Azzam,[39] 2015	PS, SC	IV	13 (13)	• Prone position • J-shaped paramedian incision • Haglund resection using osteotome • FHL tendon transfer augmentation	24.5 (18–38)	• 10 patients completely pain free, 3 patients with mild occasional pain • AOFAS hindfoot score (0–100): 58 (48–62) → 98 (78–100)	• Superficial infection, resolved with local care (2)
McAlister and Hyer,[78] 2015	RS, SC	IV	98 (100)	• Prone position • Midline incision • Haglund resection using osteotome • AT reattachment using 2 bone anchors	6 (4–38)	NR	• Wound complications (9), resolved with I&D (7) • DVT (3) • Failure of bone-tendon repair requiring revision (2) • Recurrent pain and tendinitis requiring revision (2)

Hunt et al,[75] 2015	PS, SC	I	39 (39)	• Prone position • Midline, posterolateral, or posteromedial incision • FHL tendon transfer augmentation (21) • AT reattachment using 2 bone anchors	12	• VAS (0–10): 68 ± 20 → 15 ± 19 (control); 64 ± 21 → 10 ± 18 (FHL transfer) • AOFAS hindfoot score (0–100): 57 ± 13 → 91.5 ± 13 (control); 61 ± 10 → 92 ± 15 (FHL transfer) • 87% satisfaction rate	• Wound complications, including superficial wound dehiscence (6), skin blistering or cellulitis (2), delayed wound healing (2), periincisional maceration (2)
Ettinger et al,[20] 2016	RS, SC	IV	40 (40)	• Prone position • Midline incision • Haglund resection using osteotome • AT reattachment using single anchor, 2 anchors, or double-row anchors	16 (12–27)	• AOFAS hindfoot score (0–100): 59 (30–99) → 86.5 (60–100) • Pain (rest) (0–10): 3.9 → 0.8 • Pain walking (0–10): 7.2 → 1.7 • Pain exercise (0–10): 8.5 → 2.6	• Hematoma requiring revision (1) • Superficial infection, resolved with local care (3) • DVT (2) • Painful scar (1)
Gillis and Lin,[77] 2016	RS, SC	IV	14 (16)	• Prone position • Midline incision • Haglund resection using osteotome • AT reattachment using knotless footprint reconstruction	18 (11–25)	• AOFAS hindfoot score (0–100): 87 • SF-36 physical function (0–100): 78 • VAS (0–10): 7.3 → 1.8	• Wound infection, resolved with I&D (1)
Miao et al,[98] 2016	RS, SC	IV	34 (34)	• Prone position • Midline incision • Haglund resection using osteotome • AT reattachment using 2 bone anchors	45 (24–84)	• VAS (0–10): 6.5 → 2.1 • Tegner score (0–10): 2.4 → 4.8 • VISA-A score (0–100): 49 → 88	• Chronic persistent allergic reaction to sutures (1)

Abbreviations: ABX, antibiotics; AOFAS, American Orthopaedic Foot and Ankle Society; AOS, ankle osteoarthritis scale; AT, Achilles tendon; DVT, deep vein thrombosis; FHL, flexor hallucis longus; I&D, irrigation and débridement; NR, not reported; PS, prospective; RS, retrospective; SC, single-center; SF-36, 36-item Short-Form Health Survey; VAS, visual analog scale; VISA-A, Victorian Institute of Sport tendon study group.

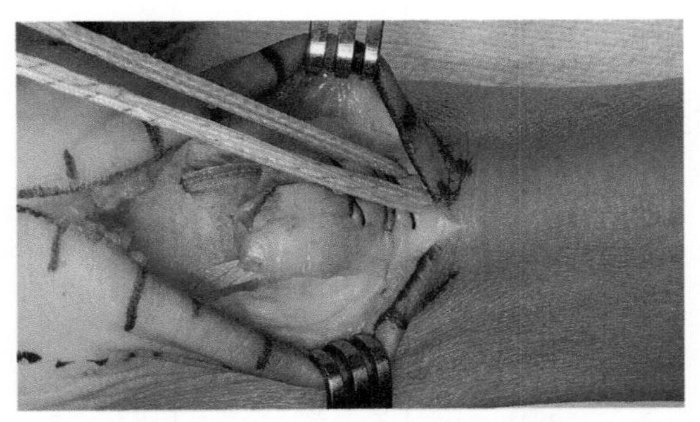

Fig. 14. Fixation tape is passed through the proximal Achilles tendon on the medial and lateral sides.

follow-up, the authors proceed with a gradual increase in weightbearing, starting with 25% and further increasing by 25% every 2 to 3 days, followed by a transition to normal shoes after full weightbearing is achieved. Full return to sports activities is variable, with a recovery time of 4 to 6 months, and it often depends on progress in physical therapy.

DISCUSSION

The anatomy of the distal Achilles tendon and its insertion on the calcaneal tuberosity is complex and demonstrates different patterns.[46–49] The pathogenesis of the insertional Achilles tendinopathy is not fully understood. Although Achilles tendinopathy is a common problem, there are a limited number of reliable epidemiologic studies. Up to 6% of the entire population reports at least 1 episode of Achilles tendon pain during their lifetime and approximately one-third complain of insertional Achilles tendinopathy.[50] A majority of symptomatic patients with insertional Achilles tendinopathy seem to have a degenerative etiology, which may be associated with increasing age, repetitive microtrauma due to constant overuse of the Achilles tendon, and increased vascularity.[5,50,51]

There is strong consensus across the available literature that patients with insertional Achilles tendinopathy should first be treated conservatively.[1,3–5,50–53] Patients

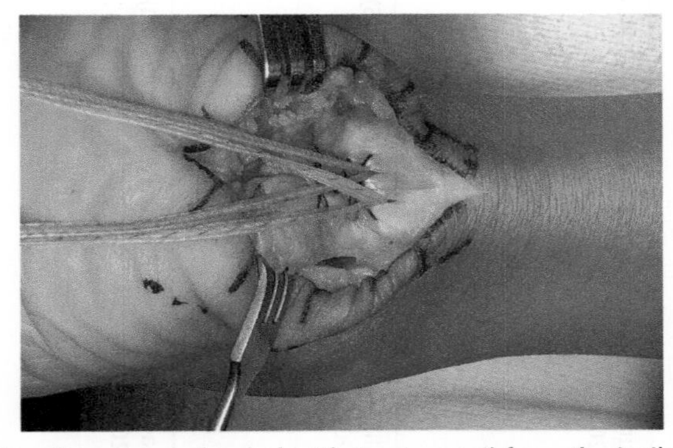

Fig. 15. The distal anchors are preloaded with 1 suture tail from the ipsilateral proximal anchor and 1 suture tail from the contralateral proximal anchor.

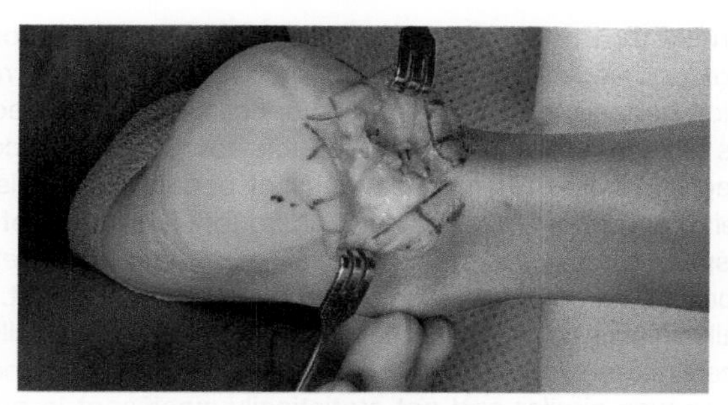

Fig. 16. Paratenon closure using 2-0 absorbable sutures.

with Achilles tendon disorders often present with concomitant hindfoot malalignment.[54] Therefore, nonoperative treatment often starts with a custom-made orthotics to address hindfoot malalignment.

Eccentric calf-muscle training often is part of conservative treatment plans for patients with Achilles tendinopathy.[55–59] Eccentric training results in decreased paratendon capillary blood flow and preserved paratendon oxygen saturation.[60] Although eccentric calf-muscle exercises may substantially improve symptoms for patients with chronic painful midportion Achilles tendinopathy, there is no demonstrated improvement for patients with insertional tendinopathy.[55]

High-energy extracorporeal shock wave therapy is another conservative treatment modality for insertional Achilles tendinopathy.[59,61–64] A randomized, controlled trial demonstrated that shock wave therapy has superior results, including pain relief, functional improvement, and return to activities, compared with eccentric calf-muscle training.[59] A combination of both treatment modalities (shock wave therapy and eccentric training), however, may increase the success rate of nonoperative treatment.[61]

Dry needling is another nonoperative treatment option for patients with tendinopathy.[65] Especially in combination with percutaneous paratenon decompression, dry needling is a well-tolerated procedure that often results in pain relief and improved functional outcome.[66]

For patients who have failed exhaustive conservative treatment for a period of 3 months to 6 months, surgical treatment should be discussed, unless contraindicated by general or procedure-specific complications. Most surgical techniques described in the current literature are open procedures (see **Table 3**). A posterior approach to the heel with a midline incision is the most common surgical approach for open procedures. These may consist of débridement of the insertional calcifications and/or resection of Haglund deformity (not all studies), with subsequent reattachment of the distal Achilles tendon (see **Table 3**). In the authors' opinion, the following must be performed: (1) débridement of the distal Achilles tendon (including resection of insertional calcifications), débridement of intratendinous degeneration, and bursectomy, and (2) resection of the Haglund deformity. An immunohistochemical study of 10 biopsies from patients with insertional Achilles tendinopathy demonstrated a high degree of innervation of both bursae (subcutaneous and retrocalcaneal), the Haglund deformity, and the distal Achilles tendon.[67] Therefore, incomplete resection of the Haglund deformity and/or débridement of the distal Achilles tendon may result in persisting postoperative pain and symptoms.

Bone-anchor suture repair is the most common method in the available literature for distally reattaching the Achilles tendon (see **Table 3**). Recently, knotless double-row footprint reconstruction has been described for distal Achilles tendon reattachment. The superiority of double-row repair has been demonstrated in rotator cuff surgery.[68–72] Two biomechanical cadaver studies specifically addressed the stability of the distal Achilles tendon after the knotless double-row footprint reconstruction.[73,74] Pilson and colleagues[74] used 9 matched pairs of cadaveric Achilles tendons with attached calcanei to compare single-row versus double-row repair of the distal Achilles tendon. All specimens were loaded to failure, which was defined as suture breakage or pullout, midsubstance tendon rupture, or anchor pullout. The most common mode of failure was suture failure, including suture knot pulling through the tendon substance (10 specimens) and suture breakage (2 specimens). The mean peak load to failure was similar and not statistically significant in both groups, with 432.9 N (range 150.3–940.5 N) and 422.0 N (range 181.4–672.7 N) in single-row and double-row specimen groups, respectively ($P = .46$). Also, the mean energy expenditure to failure was similar at 5.7 J and 8.17 J in the single-row and double-row specimen groups, respectively ($P = .069$). Beitzel and colleagues[73] used 9 matched pairs of human cadaveric Achilles tendons with attached calcanei to compare single-row versus double-row repair of the distal Achilles tendon. Testing included footprint area measurements over time, displacement after cyclic loading (2000 cycles), and final load at failure. The double-row fixation resulted in a statistically higher footprint area measurement initially and 5 minutes after reconstruction ($P = .009$ and $P = .01$, respectively), but not after 24 hours ($P = .713$). Displacement after cyclic loading was comparable in both groups: 1.9 mm $\pm$ 0.9 mm and 2.4 mm $\pm$ 0.8 mm on the medial aspect and 1.7 mm $\pm$ 1.0 mm and 2.3 mm $\pm$ 0.8 mm on the lateral aspect in the single-row and double-row specimen groups ($P = .45$ and $P = .24$), respectively. Suture tearing through the ligament was the mode of failure for all but 1 specimen (failure due to anchor pullout). The double-row reconstruction specimen group demonstrated statistically significant higher values for peak load (433.9 N $\pm$ 84.3 N vs 212.0 N $\pm$ 49.7 N, $P = .042$), load at yield (354.7 N $\pm$ 106.2 N vs 198.7 N $\pm$ 39.5 N, $P = .01$), and slope (51.8 N/mm $\pm$ 9.9 N/mm vs 66.7 N/mm $\pm$ 16.2 N/mm, $P = .021$).[73]

As with every foot and ankle procedure, surgical treatment of insertional Achilles tendinopathy is associated with a remarkably high rate of postoperative complications (see **Table 3**). Wound healing problems are the most common complications, with an incidence of up to 30.8%.[75] Most cases can be managed conservatively with local wound care and oral antibiotics; however, cases of persisting infection or deep infection often require surgical débridement and irrigation.[76–79] The authors recommend wound closure using a no-touch technique and dressings that reduce the pressure around the incision (**Fig. 17**) to avoid wound healing issues. Deep vein thrombosis is another perioperative complication in patients with insertional Achilles tendinopathy (see **Table 3**). There is no consensus with regard to postoperative thrombosis prophylaxis. Based on the current literature, the rate of scar hypertrophy and hypersensitivity can range up to 34.1% (see **Table 3**).[80] The recurrence rate of insertional calcifications is not clear (**Fig. 18**); only 1 study so far has addressed this problem specifically. Nunley and colleagues[81] performed a retrospective review of 29 surgical procedures in 27 patients. The mean follow-up in this study was 4 years, with a range between 2.9 and 8.1 years. At the latest follow-up, lateral radiographs demonstrated recurrent calcifications in 11 feet (37.9%): small calcifications (less than 0.5 cm) in 7 feet, moderate (0.5–1 cm) in 1 foot, and large (more than 1 cm) in 3 feet. All patients were pain-free despite the recurrent calcifications.[81]

A majority of patients who undergo surgical treatment for insertional Achilles tendinopathy report good pain relief and functional improvement postoperatively (see

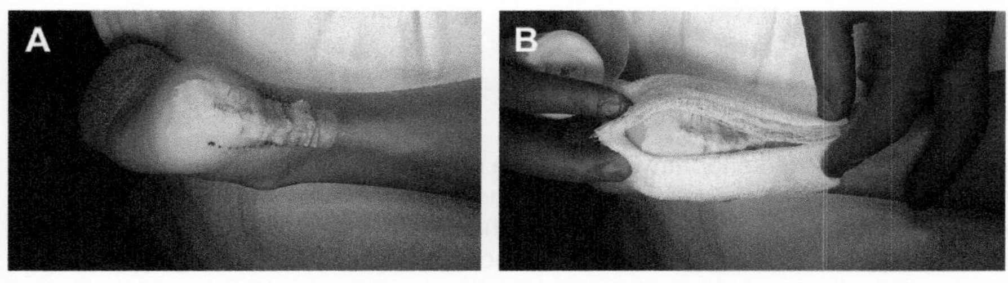

Fig. 17. Postoperative dressing using (*A*) nonadhering protective gauze and (*B*) rolled gazes to reduce the pressure over the incision.

Table 3); however, the rate of patients who are completely pain-free is not 100%. Therefore, patients should be preoperatively informed that pain may be substantially reduced by surgery, but they should not expect complete pain relief. Furthermore, the postoperative rehabilitation time until return to sports activities and substantial pain relief can be long (sometimes more than 1 year).[76,81–83]

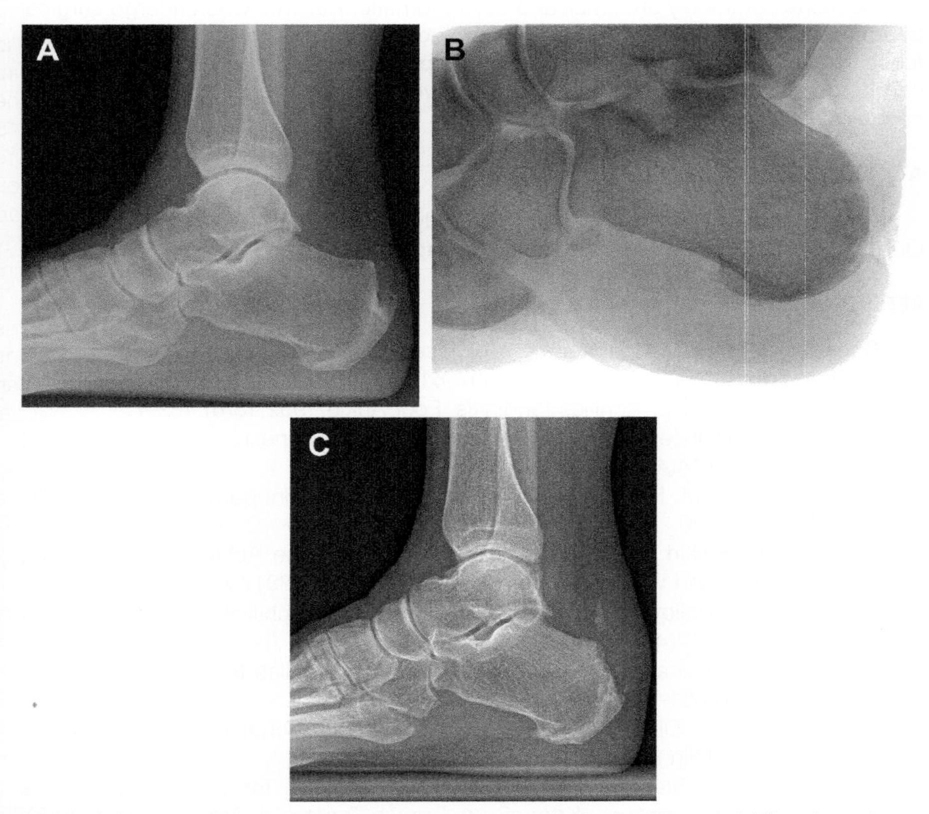

Fig. 18. (*A*) Preoperative weightbearing lateral radiograph of a 61-year old female patient. (*B*) Intraoperative fluoroscopy after the débridement. (*C*) Postoperative weightbearing lateral radiograph demonstrates partial recurrence of insertional calcifications 2 years after the surgery.

Thus, a prolonged recovery time should be another part of the preoperative consent.

SUMMARY

Insertional Achilles tendinopathy is one of the most common Achilles tendon disorders and often results in substantial heel pain and functional disability. There is a strong consensus across the published literature that treatment of patients with insertional Achilles tendinopathy should start with nonoperative modalities. Surgery should be planned for patients who have failed exhaustive conservative treatment for a period of 3 to 6 months and includes careful débridement of insertional calcifications, which often requires a substantial detachment of the distal Achilles tendon. Débridement of insertional calcification is followed by débridement of intratendinous degenerative tissue and resection of the Haglund deformity. Different surgical techniques have been described for reattachment of the distal Achilles tendon. The authors' preferred surgical technique includes the knotless double-row footprint reconstruction. Postoperative complications are not rare. Wound healing problems are the most common complication, although they can often be managed without further operative intervention. The rate of recurrent calcifications remains unclear, although recurrent insertional calcifications commonly are small and asymptomatic. Patients who undergo surgical treatment of insertional Achilles tendinopathy often report substantial pain relief and functional improvement, including a return to sports activities. Complete rehabilitation can be delayed up to 12 months postoperatively, however, and patients should be carefully informed about this possibility.

ACKNOWLEDGMENTS

The authors thank Maxwell Weinberg, a study coordinator at the University of Utah Orthopaedic Center, who provided editorial support.

REFERENCES

1. Solan M, Davies M. Management of insertional tendinopathy of the Achilles tendon. Foot Ankle Clin 2007;12(4):597–615.
2. Clain MR, Baxter DE. Achilles tendinitis. Foot Ankle 1992;13(8):482–7.
3. Den Hartog BD. Insertional Achilles tendinosis: pathogenesis and treatment. Foot Ankle Clin 2009;14(4):639–50.
4. Krishna Sayana M, Maffulli N. Insertional Achilles tendinopathy. Foot Ankle Clin 2005;10(2):309–20.
5. Shakked RJ, Raikin SM. Insertional tendinopathy of the Achilles: debridement, primary repair, and when to augment. Foot Ankle Clin 2017;22(4):761–80.
6. Hennessy MS, Molloy AP, Sturdee SW. Noninsertional Achilles tendinopathy. Foot Ankle Clin 2007;12(4):617–41.
7. Murphy GA. Surgical treatment of non-insertional Achilles tendinitis. Foot Ankle Clin 2009;14(4):651–61.
8. Singh A, Calafi A, Diefenbach C, et al. Noninsertional Tendinopathy of the Achilles. Foot Ankle Clin 2017;22(4):745–60.
9. Van Dijk CN, Van Sterkenburg MN, Wiegerinck JI, et al. Terminology for Achilles tendon related disorders. Knee Surg Sports Traumatol Arthrosc 2011;19(5):835–41.
10. Haglund P. Beitrag zur Klinik der Achillessehne. Zeitschr Orthop Chir 1928;49(1):49–58.

11. Albert E. Achillodynie, 34. Wien: Wien Med Press; 1893. p. 41–3 (1).
12. Rössler A. Zur Kenntniss der Achillodynie. Deutsch Ztschr Chir 1895;52(1): 274–91.
13. Painter CF. Inflammation fo the post-calcaneal bursa associated with exostosis. J Bone Joint Surg 1898;s1-11(1):169–80.
14. Dickinson PH, Coutts MB, Woodward EP, et al. Tendo Achillis bursitis. Report of twenty-one cases. J Bone Joint Surg Am 1966;48(1):77–81.
15. Carreira D, Ballard A. Achilles tendoscopy. Foot Ankle Clin 2015;20(1):27–40.
16. Cerrato R, Switaj P. Using arthroscopic techniques for Achilles pathology. Foot Ankle Clin 2017;22(4):781–99.
17. Jerosch J. Endoscopic calcaneoplasty. Foot Ankle Clin 2015;20(1):149–65.
18. Syed TA, Perera A. A proposed staging classification for minimally invasive management of Haglund's syndrome with percutaneous and endoscopic surgery. Foot Ankle Clin 2016;21(3):641–64.
19. Van Dijk CN. Hindfoot endoscopy. Foot Ankle Clin 2006;11(2):391–414, vii.
20. Ettinger S, Razzaq R, Waizy H, et al. Operative treatment of the insertional achilles tendinopathy through a transtendinous approach. Foot Ankle Int 2016;37(3):288–93.
21. Kang S, Thordarson DB, Charlton TP. Insertional Achilles tendinitis and Haglund's deformity. Foot Ankle Int 2012;33(6):487–91.
22. Wagner E, Gould JS, Kneidel M, et al. Technique and results of Achilles tendon detachment and reconstruction for insertional Achilles tendinosis. Foot Ankle Int 2006;27(9):677–84.
23. Saltzman CL, El-Khoury GY. The hindfoot alignment view. Foot Ankle Int 1995; 16(9):572–6.
24. Fowler A, Philip JF. Abnormality of the calcaneus as a cause of painful heel. Br J Surg 1945;32(5):494–8.
25. Pavlov H, Heneghan MA, Hersh A, et al. The Haglund syndrome: initial and differential diagnosis. Radiology 1982;144(1):83–8.
26. Stecco A, Busoni F, Stecco C, et al. Comparative ultrasonographic evaluation of the Achilles paratenon in symptomatic and asymptomatic subjects: an imaging study. Surg Radiol Anat 2015;37(3):281–5.
27. De Zordo T, Chhem R, Smekal V, et al. Real-time sonoelastography: findings in patients with symptomatic achilles tendons and comparison to healthy volunteers. Ultraschall Med 2010;31(4):394–400.
28. De Zordo T, Fink C, Feuchtner GM, et al. Real-time sonoelastography findings in healthy Achilles tendons. AJR Am J Roentgenol 2009;193(2):W134–8.
29. Klauser AS, Miyamoto H, Tamegger M, et al. Achilles tendon assessed with sonoelastography: histologic agreement. Radiology 2013;267(3):837–42.
30. Tan S, Kudas S, Ozcan AS, et al. Real-time sonoelastography of the Achilles tendon: pattern description in healthy subjects and patients with surgically repaired complete ruptures. Skeletal Radiol 2012;41(9):1067–72.
31. Zhang Q, Cai Y, Hua Y, et al. Sonoelastography shows that Achilles tendons with insertional tendinopathy are harder than asymptomatic tendons. Knee Surg Sports Traumatol Arthrosc 2017;25(6):1839–48.
32. Bleakney RR, White LM. Imaging of the Achilles tendon. Foot Ankle Clin 2005; 10(2):239–54.
33. Haygood TM. Magnetic resonance imaging of the musculoskeletal system: part 7. The ankle. Clin Orthop Relat Res 1997;336(1):318–36.
34. Shalabi A. Magnetic resonance imaging in chronic Achilles tendinopathy. Acta Radiol Suppl (Stockholm) 2004;432(1):1–45.

35. Astrom M, Gentz CF, Nilsson P, et al. Imaging in chronic achilles tendinopathy: a comparison of ultrasonography, magnetic resonance imaging and surgical findings in 27 histologically verified cases. Skeletal Radiol 1996;25(7):615–20.
36. Nicholson CW, Berlet GC, Lee TH. Prediction of the success of nonoperative treatment of insertional Achilles tendinosis based on MRI. Foot Ankle Int 2007; 28(4):472–7.
37. Carr AJ, Norris SH. The blood supply of the calcaneal tendon. J Bone Joint Surg Br 1989;71(1):100–1.
38. Cohen JC. Anatomy and biomechanical aspects of the gastrocsoleus complex. Foot Ankle Clin 2009;14(4):617–26.
39. El-Tantawy A, Azzam W. Flexor hallucis longus tendon transfer in the reconstruction of extensive insertional Achilles tendinopathy in elderly: an improved technique. Eur J Orthop Surg Traumatol 2015;25(3):583–90.
40. Lin JL. Tendon transfers for Achilles reconstruction. Foot Ankle Clin 2009;14(4): 729–44.
41. Maffulli N, Ajis A, Longo UG, et al. Chronic rupture of tendo Achillis. Foot Ankle Clin 2007;12(4):583–96.
42. Neufeld SK, Farber DC. Tendon transfers in the treatment of Achilles' tendon disorders. Foot Ankle Clin 2014;19(1):73–86.
43. Padanilam TG. Chronic Achilles tendon ruptures. Foot Ankle Clin 2009;14(4): 711–28.
44. Saltzman CL, Tearse DS. Achilles tendon injuries. J Am Acad Orthop Surg 1998; 6(5):316–25.
45. Strom AC, Casillas MM. Achilles tendon rehabilitation. Foot Ankle Clin 2009;14(4): 773–82.
46. Ballal MS, Walker CR, Molloy AP. The anatomical footprint of the Achilles tendon: a cadaveric study. Bone Joint J 2014;96-b(10):1344–8.
47. Hall RL, Shereff MJ. Anatomy of the calcaneus. Clin Orthop Relat Res 1993; 290(1):27–35.
48. Kelikian AS, Sarrafian SK. Sarrafian's anatomy of the foot and ankle: descriptive, topographic, functional. Philadelphia: Lippincott Williams & Wilkins; 2011.
49. Edama M, Kubo M, Onishi H, et al. Structure of the Achilles tendon at the insertion on the calcaneal tuberosity. J Anat 2016;229(5):610–4.
50. Chimenti RL, Cychosz CC, Hall MM, et al. Current concepts review update: insertional Achilles tendinopathy. Foot Ankle Int 2017;38(10):1160–9.
51. Irwin TA. Current concepts review: insertional achilles tendinopathy. Foot Ankle Int 2010;31(10):933–9.
52. Kearney R, Costa ML. Insertional achilles tendinopathy management: a systematic review. Foot Ankle Int 2010;31(8):689–94.
53. Roche AJ, Calder JD. Achilles tendinopathy: a review of the current concepts of treatment. Bone Joint J 2013;95-b(10):1299–307.
54. Waldecker U, Hofmann G, Drewitz S. Epidemiologic investigation of 1394 feet: coincidence of hindfoot malalignment and Achilles tendon disorders. Foot Ankle Surg 2012;18(2):119–23.
55. Fahlstrom M, Jonsson P, Lorentzon R, et al. Chronic Achilles tendon pain treated with eccentric calf-muscle training. Knee Surg Sports Traumatol Arthrosc 2003; 11(5):327–33.
56. Jonsson P, Alfredson H, Sunding K, et al. New regimen for eccentric calf-muscle training in patients with chronic insertional Achilles tendinopathy: results of a pilot study. Br J Sports Med 2008;42(9):746–9.

57. Kedia M, Williams M, Jain L, et al. The effects of conventional physical therapy and eccentric strengthening for insertional achilles tendinopathy. Int J Sports Phys Ther 2014;9(4):488–97.
58. Mccormack JR, Underwood FB, Slaven EJ, et al. Eccentric exercise versus eccentric exercise and soft tissue treatment (Astym) in the management of insertional Achilles tendinopathy. Sports Health 2016;8(3):230–7.
59. Rompe JD, Furia J, Maffulli N. Eccentric loading compared with shock wave treatment for chronic insertional achilles tendinopathy. A randomized, controlled trial. J Bone Joint Surg Am 2008;90(1):52–61.
60. Knobloch K, Kraemer R, Jagodzinski M, et al. Eccentric training decreases paratendon capillary blood flow and preserves paratendon oxygen saturation in chronic achilles tendinopathy. J Orthop Sports Phys Ther 2007;37(5):269–76.
61. Al-Abbad H, Simon JV. The effectiveness of extracorporeal shock wave therapy on chronic achilles tendinopathy: a systematic review. Foot Ankle Int 2013;34(1):33–41.
62. Furia JP. High-energy extracorporeal shock wave therapy as a treatment for insertional Achilles tendinopathy. Am J Sports Med 2006;34(5):733–40.
63. Lee JY, Yoon K, Yi Y, et al. Long-term outcome and factors affecting prognosis of extracorporeal shockwave therapy for chronic refractory Achilles tendinopathy. Ann Rehabil Med 2017;41(1):42–50.
64. Taylor J, Dunkerley S, Silver D, et al. Extracorporeal shockwave therapy (ESWT) for refractory Achilles tendinopathy: a prospective audit with 2-year follow up. Foot (Edinb) 2016;26(1):23–9.
65. Krey D, Borchers J, Mccamey K. Tendon needling for treatment of tendinopathy: a systematic review. Phys Sportsmed 2015;43(1):80–6.
66. Yeo A, Kendall N, Jayaraman S. Ultrasound-guided dry needling with percutaneous paratenon decompression for chronic Achilles tendinopathy. Knee Surg Sports Traumatol Arthrosc 2016;24(7):2112–8.
67. Andersson G, Backman LJ, Christensen J, et al. Nerve distributions in insertional Achilles tendinopathy - a comparison of bone, bursae and tendon. Histol Histopathol 2017;32(3):263–70.
68. Brady PC, Arrigoni P, Burkhart SS. Evaluation of residual rotator cuff defects after in vivo single- versus double-row rotator cuff repairs. Arthroscopy 2006;22(10):1070–5.
69. Kim DH, Elattrache NS, Tibone JE, et al. Biomechanical comparison of a single-row versus double-row suture anchor technique for rotator cuff repair. Am J Sports Med 2006;34(3):407–14.
70. Ma CB, Comerford L, Wilson J, et al. Biomechanical evaluation of arthroscopic rotator cuff repairs: double-row compared with single-row fixation. J Bone Joint Surg Am 2006;88(2):403–10.
71. Mazzocca AD, Bollier MJ, Ciminiello AM, et al. Biomechanical evaluation of arthroscopic rotator cuff repairs over time. Arthroscopy 2010;26(5):592–9.
72. Tuoheti Y, Itoi E, Yamamoto N, et al. Contact area, contact pressure, and pressure patterns of the tendon-bone interface after rotator cuff repair. Am J Sports Med 2005;33(12):1869–74.
73. Beitzel K, Mazzocca AD, Obopilwe E, et al. Biomechanical properties of double- and single-row suture anchor repair for surgical treatment of insertional Achilles tendinopathy. Am J Sports Med 2013;41(7):1642–8.
74. Pilson H, Brown P, Stitzel J, et al. Single-row versus double-row repair of the distal Achilles tendon: a biomechanical comparison. J Foot Ankle Surg 2012;51(6):762–6.

75. Hunt KJ, Cohen BE, Davis WH, et al. Surgical treatment of insertional Achilles tendinopathy with or without flexor hallucis longus tendon transfer: a prospective, randomized study. Foot Ankle Int 2015;36(9):998–1005.
76. Carmont MR, Maffulli N. Management of insertional Achilles tendinopathy through a Cincinnati incision. BMC Musculoskelet Disord 2007;8(1):82.
77. Gillis CT, Lin JS. Use of a central splitting approach and near complete detachment for insertional calcific Achilles tendinopathy repaired with an Achilles bridging suture. J Foot Ankle Surg 2016;55(2):235–9.
78. Mcalister JE, Hyer CF. Safety of achilles detachment and reattachment using a standard midline approach to insertional enthesophytes. J Foot Ankle Surg 2015;54(2):214–9.
79. Rigby RB, Cottom JM, Vora A. Early weightbearing using Achilles suture bridge technique for insertional Achilles tendinosis: a review of 43 patients. J Foot Ankle Surg 2013;52(5):575–9.
80. Yodlowski ML, Scheller AD Jr, Minos L. Surgical treatment of Achilles tendinitis by decompression of the retrocalcaneal bursa and the superior calcaneal tuberosity. Am J Sports Med 2002;30(3):318–21.
81. Nunley JA, Ruskin G, Horst F. Long-term clinical outcomes following the central incision technique for insertional Achilles tendinopathy. Foot Ankle Int 2011;32(9):850–5.
82. Miyamoto W, Takao M, Matsushita T. Reconstructive surgery using autologous bone-patellar tendon graft for insertional Achilles tendinopathy. Knee Surg Sports Traumatol Arthrosc 2012;20(9):1863–7.
83. Watson AD, Anderson RB, Davis WH. Comparison of results of retrocalcaneal decompression for retrocalcaneal bursitis and insertional achilles tendinosis with calcific spur. Foot Ankle Int 2000;21(8):638–42.
84. Mcgarvey WC, Palumbo RC, Baxter DE, et al. Insertional Achilles tendinosis: surgical treatment through a central tendon splitting approach. Foot Ankle Int 2002;23(1):19–25.
85. Calder JD, Saxby TS. Surgical treatment of insertional Achilles tendinosis. Foot Ankle Int 2003;24(2):119–21.
86. Den Hartog BD. Flexor hallucis longus transfer for chronic Achilles tendonosis. Foot Ankle Int 2003;24(3):233–7.
87. Maffulli N, Testa V, Capasso G, et al. Calcific insertional Achilles tendinopathy: reattachment with bone anchors. Am J Sports Med 2004;32(1):174–82.
88. Johnson KW, Zalavras C, Thordarson DB. Surgical management of insertional calcific achilles tendinosis with a central tendon splitting approach. Foot Ankle Int 2006;27(4):245–50.
89. Elias I, Raikin SM, Besser MP, et al. Outcomes of chronic insertional Achilles tendinosis using FHL autograft through single incision. Foot Ankle Int 2009;30(3):197–204.
90. Philippot R, Wegrzyn J, Grosclaude S, et al. Repair of insertional achilles tendinosis with a bone-quadriceps tendon graft. Foot Ankle Int 2010;31(9):802–6.
91. Maffulli N, Del Buono A, Testa V, et al. Safety and outcome of surgical debridement of insertional Achilles tendinopathy using a transverse (Cincinnati) incision. J Bone Joint Surg Br 2011;93(11):1503–7.
92. Lim S, Yeap E, Lim Y, et al. Outcome of calcaneoplasty in insertional achilles tendinopathy. Malays Orthop J 2012;6(SupplA):28–34.
93. Oshri Y, Palmanovich E, Brin YS, et al. Chronic insertional Achilles tendinopathy: surgical outcomes. Muscles Ligaments Tendons J 2012;2(2):91–5.

94. Witt BL, Hyer CF. Achilles tendon reattachment after surgical treatment of insertional tendinosis using the suture bridge technique: a case series. J Foot Ankle Surg 2012;51(4):487–93.
95. Greenhagen RM, Shinabarger AB, Pearson KT, et al. Intermediate and long-term outcomes of the suture bridge technique for the management of insertional achilles tendinopathy. Foot Ankle Spec 2013;6(3):185–90.
96. Schon LC, Shores JL, Faro FD, et al. Flexor hallucis longus tendon transfer in treatment of Achilles tendinosis. J Bone Joint Surg Am 2013;95(1):54–60.
97. Lin HA, Chong HA, Yeo W. Calcaneoplasty and reattachment of the Achilles tendon for insertional tendinopathy. J Orthop Surg (Hong Kong) 2014;22(1):56–9.
98. Miao XD, Jiang H, Wu YP, et al. Treatment of calcified insertional Achilles tendinopathy by the posterior midline approach. J Foot Ankle Surg 2016;55(3):529–34.

Moving?

Make sure your subscription moves with you!

To notify us of your new address, find your **Clinics Account Number** (located on your mailing label above your name), and contact customer service at:

Email: journalscustomerservice-usa@elsevier.com

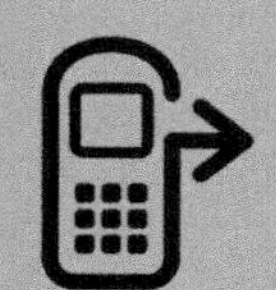

800-654-2452 **(subscribers in the U.S. & Canada)**
314-447-8871 **(subscribers outside of the U.S. & Canada)**

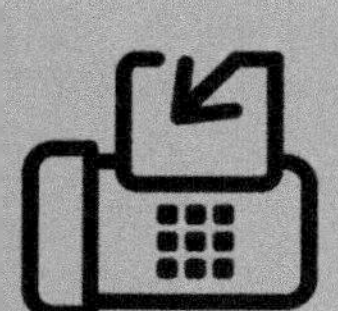

Fax number: 314-447-8029

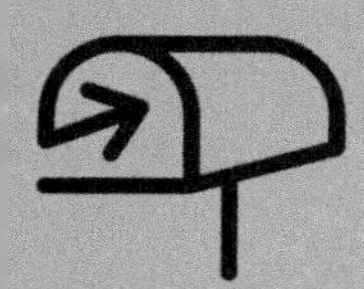

Elsevier Health Sciences Division
Subscription Customer Service
3251 Riverport Lane
Maryland Heights, MO 63043

*To ensure uninterrupted delivery of your subscription, please notify us at least 4 weeks in advance of move.

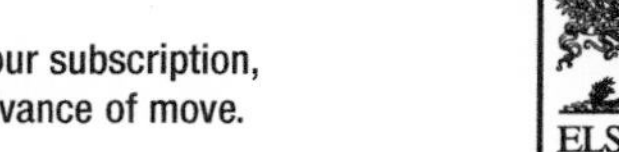

Printed and bound by CPI Group (UK) Ltd, Croydon, CR0 4YY

Printed and bound by CPI Group (UK) Ltd, Croydon, CR0 4YY

08/05/2025

01864745-0010